FDA: Failure, Deception, Abuse

FDA: Failure, Deception, Abuse

*The Story of an Out-of-Control
Government Agency and What it
Means for Your Health*

from Life Extension Foundation

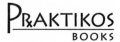

PRAKTIKOS
BOOKS

DISCLAIMER

Ideas and information in this book are based upon the experience and training of the author and the scientific information currently available. The suggestions in this book are definitely not meant to be a substitute for careful medical evaluation and treatment by a qualified, licensed health professional. The author and publisher do not recommend changing or adding medication or supplements without consulting your personal physician. They specifically disclaim any liability arising directly or indirectly from the use of this book.

Praktikos Books
P.O. Box 118
Mount Jackson, VA 22842
888.542.9467   info@praktikosbooks.com

FDA: Failure, Deception, Abuse: The Story of an Out-of-Control Government Agency and What it Means for Your Health © 2010 by Praktikos Books. All rights reserved. Printed in the United States of America. No part of this book may be used or reproduced in any manner whatsoever without written permission except in the case of brief quotations used in critical articles and reviews.

Praktikos Books are produced in alliance with Axios Press.

Library of Congress Cataloging-in-Publication Data

FDA—failure, deception, abuse : the story of an out-of-control government agency and what it means for your health / from Life Extension Foundation.
    p. cm.
    Includes bibliographical references and index.
    ISBN 978-1-60766-001-9 (hardcover)

    1. United States. Food and Drug Administration. I. Life Extension Foundation.

RA401.A3.F43 2010

362.1—dc22

2009038263

Contents

Preface. ix

Introduction

Victory Over the FDA 3

2009

The Unscientific Bioidentical Hormone Debate 29
Why American Healthcare is Headed for Collapse 39
The Generic Drug Rip-off 51
Ending the Atrocities 65
Millions of Needless Deaths 79

2008

Would You Tolerate This Abuse? 93
The FDA Indicts Itself 103
The FDA's Cruel Hoax 111

2007

The Little-Known Dangers of Acetaminophen 117
The Abigail Alliance: Motivated by Tragic Circumstances,
   Families Battle an Uncaring Bureaucracy 125

Life-Saving Cancer Drugs Not Approved by the FDA. 137
FDA Drops the Ball on Avandia® Warning. 143
The Untapped Healing Potential of DMSO 145
Does Green Tea Prevent Cardiovascular Disease? 151

2006

Lifesaving Benefits of Storing Your Own Blood 163
Fish Oil Now Available by Prescription!. 171
Popular Misconceptions About Skin Cancer Prevention. .181
FDA Threatens to Raid Cherry Orchards 185

2005

Inside the FDA's Brain 199
Drug Makers Abuse FDA Approval Process. 205
FDA Fails to Protect Domestic Drug Supply 207
Inside the Vioxx® Debacle 215

2004

Pharmacies Sue FDA Over Compounding Limits. 229
FDA Permits New Fish Oil Health Claim. 231
FDA Approves Deadly Drugs, Delays Lifesaving
   Therapies. 237
Dangerous Medicine. 249
Dr. Julian Whitaker Files a Petition Against the FDA. . . .253

2003

Patient Advocates Sue FDA Over Drug Access 261
FDA's Lethal Impediment 263
The FDA's Safety Charade. 273
Supplement Benefit Claims Finally Allowed by the FDA. .275
A New Day at FDA?. 279
Medications Side Effects 289

2002

The FDA Versus the American Consumer 323
Supreme Court Roundup 337

2001

Dying from Deficiency 343
Are Offshore Drugs Dangerous? 349
Drugs the FDA Says You Can't Have. 355
What's Wrong with the FDA 367
FDA Suffers Second Massive Legal Defeat in
    "Pearson vs. Shalala II" 369
FDA Loses Case against Compounding Pharmacies on
    First Amendment Grounds. 377
Need to Reform the FDA 379

2000

Life Extension Wins in the House and Senate 391
No Consumer Protection 397
Americans are Getting Healthier—But the FDA Remains
    a Major Impediment 401
FDA Seeks to Destroy Alternative Health Websites. 413

1999

Encore! The FDA Suffers Another Legal Defeat 419
Cancer-Causing Drug Tamoxifen Approved for
    Healthy Women 421
The Plague of FDA Regulation. 433
The FDA Versus Folic Acid 437

1998

FDA Regulation:
    At Odds—*Again*—with Your Health Freedom. 443
Life Extension vs. the FDA a Hollow Victory: Why the
    Agency's Approval of Ribavirin is Inadequate 445
First Amendment Alert 451
An Archaic System. 457

1997

Twelve Angry Jurors. 463

1996

Ozone Clinic Raided 469

1995

The FDA's Vendetta Against Dr. Burzynski 473

Index 481

Why You Should Join the Life Extension Foundation 497

Preface

OUNDED IN 1980 BY WILLIAM FALOON AND SAUL KENT, THE
Life Extension Foundation (LEF) is a nonprofit research-
based organization dedicated to finding new scientific methods for eradicating old age, disease, and death. The largest organization of its kind in the world, the Life Extension Foundation
has been at the forefront of discovering new scientific breakthroughs to reduce, and ultimately eliminate, such age-related
killers as heart disease, stroke, cancer, and Alzheimer's disease.

The Life Extension Foundation is responsible for a long and
distinguished list of achievements in promoting optimal health.
It was the first to recommend the use of coenzyme Q10 and low-
dose aspirin therapy for heart health; the first to offer lycopene
as a cancer-preventative; the first to introduce melatonin to support immune function; and the first to introduce S-Adenosyl
methionine (SAMe) in the United States.

LEF commits its research dollars to projects that are difficult
or impossible to fund with government dollars, institutional
grants or through other funding sources. Life Extension has provided financial support to help fund scientific studies at major

universities and biotechnical companies in the United States including the Mayo Clinic.

LEF members are provided with the latest scientific breakthroughs, services, and information about products to empower them to make better health choices and live healthier, longer lives. They also receive the monthly *Life Extension* magazine, which reports current advances in health research and offers scientifically referenced articles on the use of nutritional supplements.

The Life Extension Foundation also plays an active role as consumer advocate. Its involvement in political and bureaucratic developments helps facilitate public access to health products and information faster and less expensively.

LEF has been a tireless advocate of health freedom—that is, the right of consumers to choose the treatment protocols which they and their medical practitioners believe will support their health. This might include therapies that are backed by solid scientific research but which, for one reason or another, are outside the mainstream of contemporary allopathic medical practice. And it would certainly include the use of nutritional supplements which are scientifically shown to have significant health benefits.

Unfortunately, this is where the US Food and Drug Administration comes in. According to their mission statement,*

> The FDA is responsible for protecting the public health by assuring the safety, efficacy, and security of human and veterinary drugs, biological products, medical devices, our nation's food supply, cosmetics, and products that emit radiation.
>
> The FDA is also responsible for advancing the public health by helping to speed innovations that make medicines and foods more effective, safer, and more affordable; and helping the public get the accurate,

---

* http://www.fda.gov/AboutFDA/WhatWeDo/default.htm; accessed 8/24/09.

science-based information they need to use medicines
and foods to improve their health.

As you will read in these essays, which are culled from the
past fourteen years of *Life Extension* magazine, the FDA's mission
and the FDA's actions are utterly at odds with one another. The
Agency has been responsible for injuring—not protecting—the
public health. It has approved drugs and medical devices that are
not safe or efficacious. It has impeded public health by censoring
scientific research and preventing the dissemination of information that would help the public make informed decisions. It has
interfered with the medical education of doctors, promoting the
information which their vested commercial interests prefer doctors to have, and censoring the research that a physician actually needs to make the best decisions for and with their patients.
For the FDA to say that it helps the public get "the accurate, science-based information they need to use medicines and foods to
improve their health" is, to be perfectly blunt, not just the half-
truth or white lie that we have come to expect from Washington.
It is an outright falsehood.

No one has sought to reveal the truth about the FDA's actions,
methods, and behind-the-scenes duplicity with more zeal and
persistence than the Life Extension Foundation. It has documented FDA aggression and harassment, and has demonstrated
time and time again the myriad ways the FDA has failed the
citizens of the United States. Whether by going through FDA-
approved channels like Citizen Petitions or by extensive legal
battles, LEF has proven itself to be—not to put too fine a point
on it—a warrior to the cause.

With one exception, we have arranged these essays in reverse
chronological order. Because each essay concerns the FDA, but
will often have several different emphases, we found an arrange-
ment by subject unsuitable. We decided on reverse chronological
order simply so that readers could get a more accurate picture of

the current state of affairs—so that they can see which issues have been resolved, which battles have been won (or lost), and which ones are still undecided.

We begin, however, with an essay from 1996, which forms the book's Introduction. "Victory Over the FDA" tells the story of how the FDA, for the first time in its 88-year history, was forced to give up on a criminal prosecution. The US Food and Drug Administration spent millions of taxpayer dollars, conducted violent raids on LEF's affiliated store, warehouse, and shipping centers, arrested and jailed LEF's leaders, threatened them with prison terms of up to twenty years, and harassed them in and out of court for eleven years, but in the end was forced to concede. The story demonstrates the FDA at its most abusive, relentlessly pushing an agenda that serves only Big Pharma and the Agency itself—certainly not the American public it is claiming to protect.

In a quiet way, this book is a call to action. It is not meant simply to stir the emotions. *FDA: Failure, Deception, Abuse* provides readers with the ammunition—the hard evidence and the scientific data—to become effective advocates for real healthcare change and reform.

CRAIG R. SMITH
Editorial Director
Praktikos Books

Introduction

Victory Over the FDA

by Saul Kent

A FTER AN ELEVEN-YEAR REIGN OF TERROR BY THE US FOOD & Drug Administration (FDA) against the Life Extension Foundation, the FDA has "thrown in the towel."

In November 1995, Federal Judge Daniel Hurley dismissed all but one of the 56 criminal charges filed against Foundation officers Saul Kent and William Faloon. In February 1996, Judge Hurley dismissed the final charge.

This is the first time in its 88-year history that the FDA has been forced to give up on a criminal prosecution. After spending millions of taxpayer dollars, the FDA has abandoned its crusade to destroy the Foundation and throw its leaders into prison.

The FDA's dismissal of the charges against me (and Bill Faloon) is an unprecedented victory against FDA tyranny that goes far beyond winning in court. The FDA's historic defeat is a victory for everyone who cherishes freedom in healthcare. Before we discuss the implications of this victory, let's take a look at the story behind it.

THE FDA RAIDS THE FOUNDATION

On Feb. 26, 1987, I was in California, meeting with anti-aging scientists whose research was being funded by the Foundation. Early in the day, I called Foundation headquarters in Florida and knew immediately that something was wrong when no one answered the phone. After an hour, I reached an employee at home, who told me that the Foundation had been raided by the FDA.

I didn't find out the details of the raid until later that evening when I finally reached Bill Faloon at his home in Florida. I was in shock all that day, assuming that the FDA had seized the Foundation's assets and shut it down. I wondered if Faloon had been arrested and whether he was in jail.

WHAT IT WAS LIKE AT THE FOUNDATION

At the Foundation, Faloon didn't have time to think about such things. He had his hands full dealing with the battalion of troops that had invaded the Foundation. Here's what Faloon had to confront that day, as noted in the April–May 1987 issue of *Life Extension Report*:

> On Feb. 26, 1987, an armed force of about 25 FDA agents and US Marshals smashed down the glass doors of our store . . . and stormed into our nearby warehouse with guns drawn.

> At 10 AM, Bill Faloon received a phone call telling him that the FDA was breaking into our store with a battering ram. As Bill started to leave the warehouse, he suddenly found himself staring down the barrel of a .45-caliber pistol, which belonged to one of a second group of FDA agents, who were simultaneously attacking our warehouse!

TERRORIZED EMPLOYEES

The reaction of the Foundation's employees to the raid was absolute terror. To get some idea of what is was like for them on that day, let's return to the same issue of *Life Extension Report*:

> When Helen Bishop walked to the back of the warehouse, she heard someone say "hello." She thought it was a delivery man, but the next thing she knew "cops were rushing in from both doors to surround us."
>
> One of them stopped her, showed her his badge, and forced her to line up against the wall with the other employees. A search was then conducted of the personal belongings of every employee.
>
> Al Wood, one of our advisors, was working on the upper level of the warehouse when a marshall came up the stairs with his gun drawn and said "Get up!" Wood immediately threw his arms up and was told to march down the stairs. "Everyone moved slowly," he recalls, "so they wouldn't excite the Marshal waving his gun. When we asked him what this was all about, he said he had a search warrant."

ILLEGAL SEARCH AND SEIZURE

We later discovered that the search warrant had been obtained with perjured testimony by FDA agent Martin Katz before Magistrate Lurana S. Snow. This pattern continued throughout the day as FDA agents engaged in continuous illegal and unconstitutional behavior.

When the authorities didn't find the items they were supposed to search for, they seized products, literature, documents, computers, and personal effects NOT on the search warrant! Evidence presented at a later hearing showed that more than 80% of the items seized by the FDA on the day of the raid was done so illegally . . . in direct violation of the 6th amendment to the Constitution! An FDA official testified at the hearing that the FDA's policy is to instruct its agents to seize anything they want! These agents are told, said the official, that "if it turns out that you've seized the wrong things, you can always return them later."

As it turned out, this blatantly illegal policy was further corrupted by the FDA's refusal to return the items they seized illegally from the Foundation. It took a court order from a federal judge to force the FDA to return the illegal fruits of their seizure.

Another court order had to be obtained (at considerable expense) by a tenant in our building who had nothing to do with us, to force the FDA to return his property, which the FDA had also seized illegally!

REPEATED VIOLATIONS OF THE FIRST AMENDMENT

The FDA's illegal actions on the day of the raid started a pattern of repeated violations of our first amendment (free speech) rights. One of the FDA's most outrageous acts was their seizure of 5,000 copies of our newsletter *Life Extension Report*, which were in sealed envelopes ready to be mailed to our members. Since each of these 5,000 copies was identical, the FDA's purpose in seizing them was to prevent our members from receiving their newsletters.

Interestingly, the 5,000 issues seized featured a report on the scientific research we were funding, which had nothing to do with promoting "unapproved" products.

Several years later we discovered that FDA agent Katz had called the producer of a South Florida radio show that Bill Faloon had appeared on in an attempt to persuade the producer to ban Bill from future shows. This blatant attempt to interfere with our first amendment rights backfired when the producer testified in court (at one of our hearings) about the FDA's attempt to "intimidate" him.

CONSEQUENCES OF THE FDA RAID

The immediate consequences of the FDA raid were daunting. The first problem we had was that most of our product inventory had been seized by the FDA. Next was the fact that they had taken many of the documents we needed to do business and most of our literature. Then there were the traumatic effects on our employees, who were afraid to come to work, suffered from nightmares, and found it difficult to concentrate.

The next wave of problems involved the vendors we were using to supply the products and services we needed to stay in business. Suddenly, nobody wanted to give us credit, and some companies didn't want to do business with us at all. Having to pay for everything up front was especially difficult because of the losses we had incurred. It didn't help that we were now targets for the media as well.

Finally, there was the reaction of our members. Many of them supported us in our time of need; but others began to look for other sources for their life extension products. They figured that any company raided by the government wouldn't be in business much longer.

"PLEAD GUILTY"

Every attorney we consulted said we could expect 5-to-20 years in prison and that our only hope of getting reasonable prison time was to "plead guilty."

Everyone we consulted, including attorneys who were FDA "experts," told us we had to submit to the FDA's authority to have any chance of surviving. They told us we had to stop promoting "unapproved" therapies to extend the human lifespan immediately!

We ignored all this advice and instead decided to wage all-out war against the FDA. We did this knowing that we would not only risk our livelihood, but our personal freedom as well.

This was a war that even our most avid supporters thought we could never win.

We were told again and again that the FDA had the unlimited resources of the federal government at its disposal, and that an organization with fewer than 5,000 members had no chance of winning an all-out war with them.

ENTERING THE POLITICAL ARENA

We knew our position was scientifically correct, and that the public would support us if we could expose the truth about FDA corruption and incompetence. But this was 1987, when the FDA still had the public's confidence and most people still "trusted" the government.

Nonetheless, we began an aggressive political campaign to attack the FDA's credibility. We began to work with health freedom advocates such as Clinton Ray Miller, who's been fighting for alternative medical causes for decades, as well as other freedom fighters around the country.

ESTABLISHING A POLITICAL BRANCH

Our next move was to establish the Political Coordinator's Office and hire a full-time advocate to lobby against the FDA.

Our first political victory was in 1991 when we helped defeat a bill that would have expanded the FDA's enforcement powers to the point of possibly destroying the supplement industry. Most people have short memories, or don't realize that we were responsible for initiating the public uprising against the FDA that began in 1991.

Our current Political Coordinator is John Hammell. John's in-your-face style of political battling has made the Foundation the nation's foremost advocate for healthcare freedom. While most groups focus on a single area, the Foundation fights for the rights of all Americans to have access to therapies of their choice.

The Foundation has been spending its political capital on a wide variety of causes. We've fought for citizens who want free access to dietary supplements, unapproved therapies from offshore countries, more rapid approval of drugs and devices, and the development of revolutionary anti-aging therapies.

OUR GREATEST WEAPON

Our greatest weapon is the willingness of our members to send letters, faxes, and phone calls to political leaders. The activism of our members has given us the political clout to exert major influence over the political process in this country.

A LEGAL ASSAULT ON THE SYSTEM

At the same time we were developing our political capability, we also began to enter the legal arena by filing lawsuits against the FDA. Some of these lawsuits dealt with the FDA's assault on us, but others were on behalf of the American people as a whole.

PROTECTING THE RIGHTS OF ALZHEIMER'S PATIENTS

A good example of our legal efforts was the Class Action lawsuit we filed in 1990 on behalf of millions of Alzheimer's patients who were denied access to Tacrine, an effective therapy whose approval had been blocked by an FDA smear campaign. The FDA tried to sabotage Tacrine and to destroy the career of Dr. William Summers, the scientist who discovered its benefits for Alzheimer's patients.

While the Foundation's lawsuit did not lead to a court decision to force the FDA to play fair with Alzheimer's victims, its filing (and the evidence it presented) played a major role in persuading the FDA to approve Tacrine as a treatment for Alzheimer's disease.

FIGHTING FOR INDIVIDUAL CITIZENS

Another example is our legal program to help companies, clinics, and individuals who have felt the brunt of a system that operates for the benefit of the large pharmaceutical companies.

The Foundation provides legal advice and services, and political and psychological support for the victims of FDA tyranny. We know better than anyone how utterly devastating an FDA raid can be, and do everything we can to help the victims of this kind of abuse.

INFORMING THE PUBLIC AT ALL COSTS

The final tactic in our war against the FDA was to stand our ground on the actions that caused the FDA to attack us in the first place. These include making claims (based upon scientific evidence) for therapies that have yet to be approved by the FDA, and telling people how, where, and for how much they can obtain these therapies.

THE CRITICAL DECISION

Our decision to continue providing accurate information about therapies for health and longevity was at the core of our struggle with the FDA. By refusing to back down on the principles that the FDA attacked us over, we made it clear that nothing could sway us from the pursuit of health, longevity, and physical immortality.

This stand is at the heart of what, ultimately, turned the tide against the powerful and wealthy forces we were up against.

THE FDA STRIKES BACK

In the summer of 1989, an ex-employee told us she had received a subpoena, which would force her to testify before a Grand Jury in Florida. She had been told that the Grand Jury was investigating Saul Kent, William Faloon and the Life Extension Foundation. We soon found that the FDA had referred our case to the

US Attorney's Office, which had convened a Grand Jury to seek a criminal indictment against us!

During the rest of the year, subpoenas were sent far and wide in a massive "fishing expedition" for witnesses who might provide testimony that could be used against us. The search for such witnesses even led to scientists whose research we had funded.

The vast majority of these witnesses had little or nothing to tell the Grand Jury, but the FDA continued to send a parade of witnesses to the stand in the hope that they would, eventually, strike paydirt against us.

THE SECOND GRAND JURY

When the Grand Jury ran its course (18 months) without indicting us, the case was transferred to a second Grand Jury, which began to call witnesses all over again.

Many of these witnesses, which included current Foundation employees, were terrorized by the Grand Jury process, which forced them to testify without counsel, and in some cases, subjected them to verbal abuse and fear that they might be a target of the "investigation."

For example, one of our longtime employees, Ursula Arias, was called a liar repeatedly by US attorney Alan Sullivan because she wouldn't admit that the purpose of her vacation trip to Europe was to further some nefarious mission that we had put her up to. Ursula was not only abused verbally for her entirely truthful testimony, but she also had her passport seized! She has yet to get it back!

The enormity of the tax-dollar waste of these multiple grand jury sessions is hard to imagine. The federal government spent enormous sums of money interrogating everyone we had ever had contact with. There was no limit to what the government would spend to get us indicted on "something."

THE RAID IN ARIZONA

While the FDA was squandering huge financial resources to find a "crime" to indict us on, they simultaneously raided the company in Arizona that was selling many of the products we were recommending to our members.

At the beginning of 1991, the FDA deceived the Arizona Board of Pharmacy into thinking the nutrients you use every day are "unapproved new drugs," and that the sale of these "drugs" had to be stopped immediately!

So on Jan. 9, 1991, Pharmacy Board officials and FDA agents from California raided LEF without a search warrant and imposed an embargo on 42 of our most popular products.

EFFECTS OF THE EMBARGO

The immediate effect of the embargo was to paralyze our overall activities. Since the embargo was on highly popular products representing about 70% of the company's business, it was essentially shut down.

LIFE EXTENSION TAKES ACTION

As soon as we heard about the embargo, we began to take steps to fight it. I flew to Arizona to help retain a local law firm to work with the Foundation's attorneys in Washington, DC in an attempt to obtain a court order to overturn the FDA's actions. What follows is a quote from the April 1991 issue of *Life Extension Report*, which describes the systematic defense that was mounted against the FDA.

> A thick, well documented lawsuit was prepared to block the FDA-imposed embargo.... The research, investigation, and writing that went into this lawsuit involved 7 attorneys and a private investigator in 3 different states working for 12 straight days. It was an unprecedented effort.

While the attorneys worked on the legal basis to challenge the FDA's gestapo-like action, the Life Extension Foundation gathered medical testimony to prove that these nutrient products were safe and effective. Because of our close ties to the scientific community, we were able to obtain sworn Affidavits from first-rate doctors and researchers about the value of the embargoed products. Hundreds of pages of scientific evidence were attached to the lawsuit to document the safety of the products and the mechanisms by which they improve health and prevent disease.

VICTORY IN ARIZONA!

Fifteen days after the embargo had been imposed, one of our attorneys strolled into the Arizona Attorney General's Office with a 300-page lawsuit in hand. He told the Attorney General about the illegal actions taken to impose the embargo, and warned that—if action wasn't taken immediately—he would be filing the lawsuit that afternoon.

The Attorney General's reaction was swift and definitive. He ordered the Pharmacy Board to lift the embargo and decreed that any further action by the Board would require adequate notice to the company. In a later discussion, the Pharmacy Board Director acknowledged that his agents had been duped by the FDA, and that they would never again take action against any company without first investigating the matter themselves.

After our victory in Arizona, no civil enforcement action was ever again taken against the Life Extension Foundation, or any of its affiliated companies!

TERRORISM AGAINST KENT AND FALOON

Instead, the FDA threatened to indict Kent and Faloon on "criminal charges" and to throw them in jail without bail on Oct. 1, 1991!

Kent and Faloon were told—in no uncertain terms—that on Oct. 1st, they would be hit with a massive, multicount criminal indictment that would be followed by other multicount indictments, which would, in effect, "destroy their lives forever" and that their only hope of avoiding lifelong imprisonment would be to plead guilty to "crimes against the state" and voluntarily go out of business!

LIFE EXTENSION HITS BACK

In response, we filed a lawsuit against the FDA in US District Court in Florida seeking a declaratory judgment and injunction prohibiting the FDA from selectively prosecuting us in a discriminatory manner. By filing this lawsuit, we served notice that nothing the FDA could do would intimidate us! Our resolve to continue our war against the FDA was discussed in the November 1991 issue of *Life Extension Report*:

> The Life Extension Foundation will not back down from FDA pressure of any kind because we are motivated by far more than our right to make a living. The Foundation has more ambitious goals and higher principles than the FDA and the medical establishment for which it stands. The Foundation will win its war against the FDA because we are right; because the American people are behind us, and because the FDA is guided by political expediency.

The lawsuits we filed against the FDA involved hundreds of thousands of dollars in legal fees and thousands of hours of work. They included lawsuits to force the FDA to return our illegally seized property, to grant us our due process rights, to answer our freedom of information requests, to stop treating foods as "drugs," to stop selectively prosecuting us, to stop violating our constitutional rights, to protect the right of Americans to import unapproved drugs, and to force the FDA to approve Tacrine for Alzheimer's disease. As we put it in our newsletter:

> The Foundation's lawsuits against the FDA represent the most ambitious attempt in history to challenge an oppressive government agency in the courts. The lawsuits are unprecedented in their scope, legal analysis, philosophic content, and moral authority. Collectively, they represent a critical challenge to the US legal system, which is being asked to stand up for the principles upon which this nation was founded.

THE ARREST AND THE INDICTMENT

On the morning of Nov. 7, 1991, we were arrested and taken into custody at the federal court building in Fort Lauderdale. We were photographed, fingerprinted, and taken to a jail cell to await arraignment. The jail was a fenced-in, 8-by-8-foot cubicle that contained two hard benches, a toilet (without a seat), and a small sink. We shared the cell with several men charged with drug-related offenses who were also facing arraignment that day.

THE ARRAIGNMENT

At 2:30 p.m., we were brought into court (handcuffed to other prisoners). A few minutes later we stood before magistrate Snow. She told us we had been indicted on 28 criminal counts including engaging in a "conspiracy" to sell "unapproved drugs," "prescription drugs," and "misbranded drugs."

Bail was set at $825,000 each. A bail bondsman who we had secured earlier was present to work with our attorneys to execute a bond that would enable us to go free that day.

Magistrate Snow set the following conditions on our release. We would have to report by phone to Pretrial Services every two weeks and pay a visit in person once a month. We were permitted to travel in the US, but only if we informed Pretrial Services (at least 24 hours prior to leaving) where we were going and how long we would be away from home. We were not permitted to travel outside the continental United States.

After the arraignment, we were led back to our cell (again in handcuffs chained to other prisoners), where we were kept another two hours until we were finally released from custody at 5 p.m.

WHAT WE WERE UP AGAINST

After we left the building, our attorneys told us that if we were convicted on all 28 counts in the indictment, our maximum penalty would be 84 years in prison and a seven million dollar fine! They also told us the FDA's "investigation" of our activities would continue indefinitely, and that we could expect additional multicount criminal indictments in the future!

WE REFUSE TO BACK DOWN

The indictment dealt with the fact that in the mid 1980s we told Americans how to obtain unapproved drugs from two overseas companies: The Longevity Institute in Panama and The Hauptmann Institute in Austria. We offered this information because of evidence that the drugs could help people live longer, and because the FDA had (and still has) a policy permitting the importation of unapproved drugs for personal use.

After the indictment, we continued to provide Americans with information about therapies from around the world. We weren't about to back down from the very real threats we were now faced with!

LIFE EXTENSION FIGHTS BACK

Since we had now been branded "criminals" by the government (and had to face the prospect of additional criminal indictments), it was clear that we truly had the fight of our lives on our hands!

First we stepped up our political activities by asking our members to protest the FDA's indictment against us to their congressional reps.

Then we placed full-page ads in South Florida newspapers, attacking the FDA for restricting the flow of information about health and longevity, and accusing them of contributing to the deaths of millions of Americans.

Finally, we started filing Motions to attack the legal and constitutional foundations of the indictment.

MOTIONS TO DISMISS THE INDICTMENT

In the Spring of 1992, we filed a Motion asking for dismissal of the indictment on the grounds that the FDA had illegally obtained their search warrant, and had then illegally seized vast numbers of items not on the search warrant.

We then filed another Motion to dismiss the indictment on the grounds that we were being prosecuted selectively because the FDA was openly permitting organizations such as AIDS Buyers Clubs to engage in acts far more violative of the Food, Drug and Cosmetic Act than anything we were alleged to have done.

THE FDA REVEALS ITS ILLEGAL ACTIONS

We were granted hearings before magistrate Snow on both these Motions. At these hearings, we presented powerful evidence of illegal and unconstitutional actions on the part of the FDA, and revealed the ignorance and shockingly immoral behavior of one FDA employee after another.

FDA enforcement officer Martin Katz admitted he had committed perjury in writing up the search warrant, and that he had tried to intimidate a radio talk show producer into keeping us off the air. Katz' partner, Roy Rinc, admitted he had threatened to put our printer out of business if he didn't "cooperate" with the agency, and that he believed he could seize anything at all from us, whether it was on the search warrant or not.

Higher FDA officials testified that the FDA actively encourages its agents to ignore search warrants during raids, and that the FDA deliberately avoids defining any of its "rules," "regulations," or "policies," so that it can interpret them in any way it wishes, or ignore them completely if it suits their purpose.

BEATING UP ON THE FDA

Although magistrate Snow ultimately ruled against us on both Motions, the two hearings helped us immensely in our struggle against the FDA.

They forced us to begin constructing a powerful defense that could be used at trial. They enabled us to obtain hard evidence of the corruption and immorality of the FDA. And they helped us buy precious time to search for key witnesses, while the FDA's case gradually began to wither away.

The most valuable benefit, however, may have been the opportunity to beat up on the FDA. During both hearings, our attorneys hammered away at one FDA witness after another with difficult, spirit-sapping questions that must have been quite demoralizing for the agency. It was exhilarating for us to able to give the "bully boys" a taste of their own medicine!

UNRELENTING INTIMIDATION

During this period, rumors of new FDA raids were heard every week. The FDA constantly threatened to bring waves of new indictments against us that would bankrupt the Foundation and result in us spending the rest of our lives in prison. And our printer was threatened with the seizure of his presses if he printed any more "illegal literature" for us.

The FDA was involved in a vicious campaign of psychological state-sponsored terrorism. The fact that such acts continue to this very day against other innocent Americans is a flagrant violation of basic human rights.

Despite the ongoing threats, we continued to make our products available to our membership, with our attorneys saying it would only aggravate our already hopeless legal position.

In 1992, we introduced the synthetic pineal hormone melatonin in the United States. Our supporters were shocked that we would openly sell a hormone when the FDA was already seeking to destroy us in every way possible. The supplement industry was convinced that the FDA would never allow melatonin to be sold, and we were the only ones who had the courage to sell melatonin in the United States!

THE TIDE BEGINS TO TURN

One of the first signs that the tide was beginning to turn came in 1992 when we won our lawsuit to have the items seized illegally by the FDA returned to us. While the nutrient products the FDA had been storing at a warehouse since 1987 (at taxpayer expense) were spoiled by then, it was very encouraging to win a victory over the FDA in court.

Even more encouraging was the fact that the judge ordered the FDA to pay our attorneys' fees for unreasonably holding on to our property. This made it more than just a symbolic victory. Our spirits were buoyed considerably by this award, which further demoralized the agency.

THE FDA STARTS TO CRACK

An even greater sign that things were beginning to turn our way also occurred in 1992, when the FDA offered us a deal to settle our case. We were told that most of the charges against us would be dropped, and that we might avoid going to prison entirely, if we would just plead guilty to one or two of the charges against us and agree to submit totally to FDA authority. Moreover, we were told that—if we refused the deal—we would be prosecuted to the full extent of the law, and that we would have to face waves of new criminal indictments.

Although the proposed deal was a major concession that would have tempted most defendants, we didn't hesitate. We replied that we had no intention of giving in to the FDA, that we were totally innocent of any wrongdoing, and that we would continue to provide Americans with lifesaving information, even at the risk of being thrown into prison for life!

This was the first of several "deals" proposed by the FDA, each one followed by a threat that never materialized. Every new deal was better than the previous one, which told us that the FDA was beginning to crack under the pressure we had been submitting them to.

THE FDA HOLOCAUST MUSEUM

In 1994, we established the FDA Holocaust Museum where we documented the 70-year reign of terror that the FDA had perpetrated against Americans. We showed the FDA's corrupt practices were causing needless suffering and the deaths of millions of Americans every year. We received international media coverage on the museum showing that even the prospect of lifetime incarceration couldn't stop us from telling the truth about the FDA!

MORE FDA THREATS

In 1995, the FDA made even more serious threats against us. They said they had new evidence that would enable them to incarcerate us for life, and that they were on the verge of seizing every penny we had!

It is hard to describe the psychological effect of this unrelenting government pressure. Historically, the FDA has destroyed its opponents through this type of illegal intimidation, thereby maintaining a dictatorial grip on the practice of medicine in the United States.

We knew that capitulation was the easy way out, but that it would mean an end to our lifelong goal of extending the human lifespan. We vowed to continue the battle no matter what. Contingency plans were made to continue publishing our newsletters from prison if necessary.

THE REALITIES OF GOING TO TRIAL

We were confident we could win our case in court, but dreaded the time and expense of going to trial. By then, the Foundation was rapidly growing, we were again funding life extension research, and it was hard to get into the mindset of preparing for a trial that we knew was an absolute farce.

THE TRIAL APPROACHES

In mid-1995, the FDA was pushing to bring the case to trial. We had a trial date that might not be possible to postpone, and the FDA had an 88-year history of never giving up on any enforcement action, especially a criminal indictment against a political opponent!

We were then offered a deal to guarantee that we would not go to prison, and that it might even be possible for us to remain in business in some limited capacity. But, by then, we had come to the conclusion that any admission of guilt would irreparably compromise our principles, which would significantly hamper our quest for an extended human lifespan.

So we dug our in our heels and went after the FDA again by having our attorneys file a battery of new legal motions, by escalating our political attacks on the agency, and by spending more and more of our time preparing for a trial that would require our total concentration for months as well a great deal of our money.

THE FDA CAVES IN

As it turned out, our "dread" at going to trial was mild compared to the FDA's horror at facing us in court! By the end of 1995, the FDA and the US Attorney's Office no longer had the stomach to fight us. In short, they figured they would lose and that the process of losing would be an extremely unpleasant experience!

But they still weren't ready to give up completely. In November 1995, the FDA asked Judge Hurley to drop every charge against us, except one. They still intended to prosecute me for "obstruction of justice"—a charge that had absolutely no merit, but had the apparent virtue of being easy to prosecute.

We then concentrated our efforts on this charge. We interviewed the witnesses the FDA planned to bring against me, and it turned out that the FDA had no case, but was holding on to this charge in the hope that I might be convicted of "something."

In February 1996—exactly 9 years after the FDA launched its brutal attack on the Life Extension Foundation—the US Attorney's Office filed a motion to dismiss this final count.

It is difficult to calculate the total cost of the FDA's war against the Life Extension Foundation because the costs have been so high and so many of the them have been hidden from view.

The first and most obvious costs have been the millions of dollars spent by both sides in fighting the war. In 9 years of combat, we were forced to spend about 1.3 million dollars for legal fees, private investigator fees, expert consultant fees, and travel.

There's no telling how much the government spent on our case, but everything points to the fact that they spent much more than we did. In fact, the raids themselves (against the Foundation and Life Extension International) were extremely costly, involving months of preparation and dozens of law enforcement personnel from different agencies.

OTHER ENFORCEMENT AGENCIES

At various stages of the "investigation," almost every US law enforcement agency was involved, including the Federal Bureau of Investigation (FBI), the Drug Enforcement Agency (DEA), the Justice Department and its prosecutorial arm the US Attorneys Office, and the Internal Revenue Service (IRS). These costs have to be added to the large ongoing costs (salary, support staff, and expenses) of FDA agents such as Martin Katz, who worked on the case for nine long years!

THE GRAND JURY INVESTIGATIONS

Then there were the costs of carrying out the two Grand Jury Investigations, each of which lasted about 18 months. Among these costs were: funding for several government prosecutors and their staff, funding for FDA attorneys and agents, payment and transportation costs for 22 grand jurors for almost 36 months, and the huge costs of finding, interviewing, and paying for the travel expenses of a large number of witnesses from the US and abroad, most of whom had absolutely nothing to tell the Grand Jury.

THE HEARINGS

There were two major hearings on Motions we filed to get the case dismissed as well as other shorter hearings—all of which involved the time and expenses of dozens of FDA attorneys, agents, officers, and their support staff, as well as the prosecutorial costs of the US Attorney's office.

Perhaps the single largest cost came from the efforts of FDA Commissioner David Kessler to avoid testifying at our Selective Prosecution hearing. Kessler was a material witness whose testimony could have provided critical evidence that the FDA was prosecuting us unfairly. Kessler ordered FDA attorneys to file numerous legal briefs on his behalf (at taxpayer expense), including an emergency appeal (flown down by private jet) to the Court of Appeals in Atlanta, which saved Kessler from having to testify at the eleventh hour.

DERAILING LIFE EXTENSION RESEARCH

As large as the above costs were, they were minuscule in comparison to the much larger costs of the life extension research that remained unfunded and the life extension therapies that remained undeveloped because of the FDA's war against the Foundation.

The FDA raid in February 1987 forced us to stop our PROJECT 2000 program to achieve a major breakthrough in aging by the year 2000 just as it was gaining momentum. The March 1987 issue of *Life Extension Report*, which was seized in the FDA raid, featured an in depth report on the life extension scientists we were funding at the time.

THE RESEARCH WE WERE FUNDING

At the time of the raid, we had already donated $790,000.00 to the PROJECT 2000 Research Fund, and had awarded a total of $380,000.00 in grants to research projects conducted by eminent scientists. Among these were the following:

- *The effect of fetal thymus gland extract on immune function and lifespan in mice*—Roy L. Walford, MD, UCLA Medical Center.
- *The development of the genetically-engineered SOD transgenic mouse to determine whether extra superoxide dismutase can slow down the aging process*—Richard Cutler, PhD, National Institute on Aging.
- *The effect on aging of the transplantation of brain tissue from young animals into old animals*—Don Ingram, PhD, National Institute on Aging.
- *The effects of thymus hormones on aging*—Allan Goldstein, PhD, George Washington University Medical School, Washington, DC

- *The effect of tryptophan restriction on neuroendocrine aging*—Paul Segall, PhD, and Paola Timiras, PhD, University of California at Berkeley
- *Analysis of the chemical responsible for the loss of protein synthesis with advancing age*—George C. Webster, PhD, Florida Institute of Technology

The Foundation had donated the money to fund these projects and others over a period of fourteen months, with the fund growing at an ever-increasing rate as the Foundation grew in size. We had every reason to believe that our funding for research would continue to accelerate indefinitely—when we were suddenly stopped cold by the FDA raid!

TIME LOST

It wasn't just the money needed to fight the FDA that derailed our research program, but the enormous amount of time we spent—month after month, year after year—for nine interminable years, fighting for survival against a powerful government agency backed by the medical establishment. There is no adequate way to measure the thousands of hours we spent on this case: going through files, writing memos, doing legal research, going to conferences, reading briefs and motions, attending court hearings, speaking with expert witnesses, and preparing to testify.

The enormous time we had to spend fighting for our lives had severely detrimental effects on our business. It was extremely difficult to manage our affairs, find and develop new products and therapies, and attend to the myriad details of running an organization.

WHAT WAS LOST

It's hard to calculate how much was lost because of the FDA war against us, but it's safe to say it was a great deal. We feel that— by now—we would have been investing millions, perhaps tens of millions, or even hundreds of millions of dollars a year in break-through life extension research; that we would have already succeeded in achieving our PROJECT 2000 goal of a major lifespan-extending advance; and that we'd now be well on the way to our PROJECT 2020 goal of total control over aging by the year 2020.

This is an enormous loss . . . far greater than the mere money expended in fighting the FDA. It is a loss that will be felt by millions of people worldwide, who will die prematurely because of delays in developing the kind of breakthrough life extension therapies destined to have a revolutionary impact on human life in the 21st century!

2009

The Unscientific Bioidentical Hormone Debate

by William Faloon

I HAVE SYMPATHY FOR THE LAY PUBLIC WHO TRY TO STAY informed about life-and-death medical issues. With doctors making so many contradictory claims, it is no wonder that confused consumers die from lethal ignorance!

When the media attempts to sort out fact from fiction, the public hears biased doctors proclaim that their opposition's position is reckless and risks killing those who implement it. The tragic result of these kinds of sound bite debates is that most people do nothing, and miss out on proven methods to reverse premature aging.

DRUG PROPAGANDA WARS

Today's battleground is over who will derive the most economic benefit from the sale of female hormone drugs. All sides seem to have spokespersons to emphatically state that their product is the safest and most effective.

We at *Life Extension* are in the unique position of arguing against what is in our economic interests. For the past two decades, we have advised women needing estrogen drugs to use individualized combinations of estriol and estradiol topical creams.

The problem is the FDA has effectively forbidden the sale of estriol.[1] This ban is in direct response to pressure from a pharmaceutical company[2] that wanted the FDA to censor your right to obtain estriol, which we consider a safer[3] form of estrogen.

DANGEROUS ESTROGEN DRUGS STILL SELL BRISKLY

The market for female hormone replacement drugs is gargantuan. The lethal side effects of Premarin® (horse urine-derived estrogens) and Prempro® (horse urine-derived estrogens and a synthetic progestin) were revealed in the Women's Health Study in 2002 and 2004.[4,5] These drugs, however, continue to be sold to unsuspecting female patients.[6]

The fact that medical doctors continue to prescribe horse urine-derived estrogens and synthetic progestins with proven risks is a testament to mainstream medicine's apathy and ignorance.

That the FDA allows the continued sale of horse urine-derived estrogens and synthetic progestin, under the guise that the agency is not sure if plant-derived estrogens and progesterone are safer reveals how much political influence pharmaceutical companies wield in government.

That the maker of Premarin® and Prempro® doesn't even make the effort to bring out "new and improved" versions of their brand-name drugs (using plant-derived estrogen and natural progesterone) shows how little pharmaceutical companies care about the public's health.

I see innovation in the natural products industry virtually every day, yet the same formulas for Premarin® (horse urine-derived estrogens) and Prempro® (horse urine-derived estrogens and a synthetic progestin) have been used for decades.

Premarin®, in fact, was approved by the FDA way back in 1942.[7] What else do you know that was brought out 67 years ago that still sells briskly today? The only answer is antiquated drugs protected by a federal regulatory agency called the FDA.

PLENTY OF PLANT-DERIVED ESTROGEN DRUGS TO CHOOSE FROM

There is no shortage of drug companies that sell estrogen drugs that cost them virtually nothing to make. For example, pharmaceutical manufacturers will produce tens of millions of tablets at a time containing 1 mg of a potent estrogen called estradiol.

These drug companies (and the Life Extension Pharmacy) make money when women buy these 1 mg estradiol tablets. The scientific literature, however, indicates that it is safer and more effective if aging women are prescribed individualized doses of topical creams that provide about 80% estriol and only 20% estradiol.

To reiterate, while it is in Life Extension's economic interest to sell mass-produced estradiol and/or conjugated estrogen tablets, we instead recommend that women in need of estrogen drugs obtain them from compounding pharmacies that provide the more scientifically substantiated estriol. (Our pharmacy does provide compounding services, but we can't offer estriol because of the FDA's ban.)

WHY DRUG COMPANIES ATTACK ESTRIOL

Pharmaceutical companies make their money in an assembly line style which involves selling you the same drug as everyone else. The problem is that you are not like everyone else as far as your individual hormone needs are concerned.

In order to deceive the public into believing they need to be "protected" against compounded estriol-based creams, drug company shills proclaim that compounding pharmacies are "unregulated" and lack the quality control found in FDA-approved manufacturing facilities. These deceptions frighten most of the public into using toxic mass-produced drugs in lieu of safer compounded versions.

The bottom line is that there are billions of dollars to be made if American women can be deceived into using dangerous mass-produced estrogen and synthetic progestin drugs. You can believe pharmaceutical giants will leave no stone unturned to sic regulatory agencies against those who sell natural forms of these hormones. An even more sinister tactic is to pay doctors to attack those who seek to alert the public about the suffering and deaths caused by these unnatural and toxic hormone drugs.

CORRUPT FDA ACTIONS CAUSE CONSUMERS TO BE FINANCIALLY RAPED

There is a financial downside for women seeking compounded estriol-based creams.

Since the FDA was so kind (to Big Pharma) to ban the sale of estriol, its gray market price has sharply increased. The FDA's biased action causes US consumers to now pay grossly inflated prices for estriol.

In order to protect the economic interests of the pharmaceutical industry, the FDA has no qualms about bankrupting the healthcare system of the United States. Life Extension exposed this back in the early 1980s, and little has changed since then—except that the medical system is facing virtual insolvency because of unrelenting corrupt FDA practices.

A study this year in fact revealed that more than 60% of personal bankruptcies are caused not by lavish spending, but by medical bills![8]

OPRAH WINFREY CRITICIZED FOR AIRING
SCIENTIFIC TRUTHS

On January 29, 2009, Oprah Winfrey dedicated an entire one-hour program to the bioidentical hormone debate. Oprah did her research and identified numerous maturing women who suffered horrendous quality-of-life deficits that were reversed by bioidentical hormones.

Oprah assigned one of the most prestigious medical doctors in the United States (Dr. Mehmet Oz) to go inside a compounding pharmacy to show the audience how much quality control goes into making a compounded natural hormone cream.

Suzanne Somers was the featured guest, along with doctors who urged aging women to have their blood tested and their hormones naturally restored.

In her O magazine, Oprah Winfrey stated:

> After one day on bioidentical estrogen, I felt the veil lift. After three days, the sky was bluer, my brain was no longer fuzzy, my memory was sharper. I was literally singing and had a skip in my step.[9]

Unfortunately, Oprah Winfrey tried to air a "balanced" report on her TV show , in which the opposition got to torpedo scientific reality with sound bite scare tactics that have no basis in fact. Oprah found mainstream doctors who supported the FDA's biased position against bioidentical hormones. These doctors attacked the safety of biodentical hormones and suggested that aging women should do virtually nothing to restore youthful hormone balance, or rely only on FDA-approved hormone drugs.

After the program, some media sources were critical that Oprah favored the bioidentical side of the debate, and claimed that Oprah was "damaging" women's health by suggesting women could benefit from bioidentical hormones.

NEWS MEDIA DISSEMINATES BLATANTLY FALSE INFORMATION

Drug companies appear to be terrified of Oprah Winfrey. Many months after Oprah's bioidentical hormone show aired, the news media was still finding doctors to criticize her. Drug companies spend huge amounts of money on public relations firms for the purpose of influencing the public, as well as the FDA and Congress.

One prominent news magazine quoted a doctor as stating:

> Despite (Suzanne) Somers's claim that her specially made, non-FDA-approved bioidenticals are "natural" and safer, they are actually synthetic, just like conventional hormones and FDA-approved bioidenticals from pharmacies—and there are no conclusive clinical studies showing they are less risky.[10]

Numerous clinical studies substantiate the safety and efficacy of these "natural to the human body" hormones[3] extolled by Oprah Winfrey, Suzanne Somers, and tens of thousands of anti-aging doctors and their patients.

Most appalling are the innuendos that bioidentical hormones are no different than FDA-approved Premarin® and Prempro®. Both Premarin® and Prempro® contain horse estrogen extracted from pregnant mares' urine. Unlike bioidentical estrogen creams that provide the hormones found naturally in the human female body, horse estrogen contains equilin and other equine estrogens found exclusively in horses![11,12]

The human female body contains enzymes to metabolize the natural proportion of estriol, estradiol, and estrone, but not horse estrogens such as equilin. These horse estrogens produce estrogenic effects that are much more potent and longer-lasting than those produced by natural human estrogens.[13]

As two leading reproductive physiologists point out, when women take Premarin®:

Levels [of equilin] can remain elevated for 13 weeks or more post-treatment due to storage and slow release from adipose [fat] tissue. In addition metabolism of equilin to equilenin and 17-hydroxyequilenin may contribute to the estrogen stimulatory effect of [conjugated estrogen] therapy.[14]

Another metabolite of equilin, 17-dihydroequilin has been found to be eight times more potent than equilin for inducing endometrial growth, a possible precursor to cancer.[14]

The drug Prempro® consist of conjugated equine estrogens and medroxyprogesterone acetate, a synthetic progestin that has been implicated in many of the adverse effects uncovered in the Women's Health Initiative study.[4] Medroxyprogesterone acetate is not the same as natural progesterone found in bioidentical hormone creams, yet establishment doctors are telling the news media that there is no difference.

There are other FDA-approved estrogen drugs that provide too much estrone and estradiol (and no estriol). These so-called "natural estrogen" drugs are also not the same as bioidentical hormone creams that can be obtained from compounding pharmacies.[15]

On her January 29, 2009, show, Oprah Winfrey warned the medical establishment:

We have the right to demand a better quality of life for ourselves, and that's what doctors have got to learn to start respecting.[10]

Profit-driven pharmaceutical companies don't want patients to revolt and seem willing to disseminate egregiously falsified propganda to protect their multibillion dollar assembly line franchise of dangerous estrogen/synthetic progestin drugs.

FOLLOW THE MONEY AND YE SHALL FIND THE TRUTH

The Oprah Winfrey Show strongly supported the anti-aging benefits women could attain from bioidentical hormones. Regrettably, the conventional doctors Oprah used to "balance" the program served their purpose, i.e., they cast doubt on the safety of natural hormones. These sound-bite scare tactics (often used by those running for political office), will cause most aging women to do nothing to restore their hormones based on imaginary fears.

A simple method to discern the truth is to see who economically benefits from the hormone debate.

Pharmaceutical companies lavish conventional doctors with enormous financial rewards in exchange for these doctors' support of FDA-approved drugs. The economic incentive for mainstream doctors is thus to toe the pharmaceutical industry's party line and attack those who offer natural alternatives.

But what are the financial motivations of Oprah Winfrey, Suzanne Somers, and the numerous beneficiaries of bioidentical hormones that appeared on Oprah's show? The fact is that *none* of them sells bioidentical hormones. They represent the uncompensated majority who only seeks out the truth, without money influencing their decision-making process.

When listening to future debates about whether women should use FDA-approved hormone drugs that are proven to kill, as opposed to bioidentical hormones whose safety and efficacy are strongly supported, follow the money and you will see who has your best interests at heart.

Pharmaceutical Company Pays Ghostwriters to Push Dangerous Hormone Drugs

Drug company Wyeth faces 8,400 lawsuits from women who claim Premarin® or Prempro® caused them to become ill.

Newly released court documents from these cases reveal that Wyeth paid ghostwriters to produce 26 "scientific" papers supporting the use of their dangerous hormone drugs.

The Wyeth-funded articles extolled purported benefits of these unnatural hormone drugs while downplaying their lethal risks. Nowhere in these articles was Wyeth's role in initiating and paying for them disclosed.

Court documents show how Wyeth contracted with private companies to outline articles, draft them and then solicit top physicians to sign their names, even though many of the doctors contributed little or no writing to them.

Physician prescribing practices are strongly influenced by what they read in peer-reviewed scientific publications. these tainted articles were published in medical journals between 1998 and 2005, and helped generate billions of dollars of sales for Wyeth.

These revelations substantiate allegations that LifeExtension® made decades ago that drug companies manipulate scientific data to enable dangerous drugs to be prescribed.

References

1. http://www.fda.gov/NewsEvents/ Newsroom/PressAnnouncements/ 2008/ucm116832.htm.

2. http://www.fda.gov/ohrms/DOCKETS/ dockets/05p0411/05p-0411-cp0000101-vol1.pdf.

3. *Postgrad Med.* 2009 Jan;121(1):73–85.

4. *JAMA.* 2002 Jul 17;288(3):321–33.

5. *JAMA.* 2004 Apr 14;291(14):1701–12.

6. http://www.slideshare.net/finance12/ wyeth-4q-2008-net-revenue-report.

7. http://www.fda.gov/Drugs/DrugSafety/ InformationbyDrugClass/ucm168838.htm.

8. *Am J Med.* 2009 Jun 4.

9. http://www.oprah.com/article/omagazine/200902_omag _oprah_for_sure.

10. http://www.newsweek.com/id/200025.

11. *Br J Clin Pharmacol.* 2000 May; 49(5):489–90.

12. *J Am Soc Mass Spectrom.* 2005 Feb;16(2):271–9.

13. *J Steroid Biochem Mol Biol.* 2003 Jun;85(2–5):473–82.

14. Barnes R, Lobo R. Pharmacology of Estrogens. In: Mishell D, ed. *Menopause: Physiology and Pharmacology.* Chicago, IL: Year Book Medical Publishers, Inc; 1986.

15. http://www.drnorthrup.com/ womenshealth/healthcenter/ topic_details. php?topic_id=129.

Why American Healthcare is Headed for Collapse

by William Faloon

WHILE POLITICIANS DEBATE A WIDE RANGE OF FINANCIAL issues, the most dangerous threat to the United States economy is ignored as if it did not exist. The reason you don't hear about this problem is that no one seems to know how to solve it.

I will briefly review this impending disaster and then provide some real world solutions. For the benefit of new members, the Life Extension Foundation predicted today's healthcare cost crisis back in the early 1980s. Our prophetic warnings were ridiculed at the time, but events over the past decade document the financial train wreck we fought so hard to prevent.

Discussions rage today about how to provide universal healthcare. Overlooked is the fact that the government will soon be unable to pay the medical costs it is already on the hook for.

Not only do 40 million Americans depend on these government-funded programs, but these individuals have already paid for them with their Medicare tax dollars.

THE MAGNITUDE OF THIS ISSUE

Very soon, Medicare will start paying out more in hospital bills than the premiums (taxes) it will collect. When that time arrives, the federal government will have to tap some other source to cover this gargantuan unfunded liability. One obstacle is that the federal government is over $11 trillion in debt and is projected to run trillion dollar deficits for the next several years. If these numbers sound high, they pale in comparison to Medicare's unfunded liability of $34 trillion.

To put this in perspective, the government collects only about $2 trillion each year in total tax revenue (including Medicare premium taxes).[1] There are virtually no reserve funds left to pay promised Medicare (and Medicaid) benefits. The government is relying on the money it takes in each day to cover its enormous Medicare cost burden.

As the country ages, Medicare will devour huge chunks of US economic output and eventually overwhelm every other item on the federal budget. While politicians stick their heads in the sand and disregard this issue, no one can argue against the math showing a financial disaster of unprecedented magnitude.

MEDICARE SCAMS

The government points to rampant fraud as one reason behind Medicare problems. It is estimated that 20% of every dollar Medicare pays out goes to criminals who submit claims for nonexistent or bogus services. For example, it was recently discovered that Medicare paid out $100 million for wheelchairs, canes, prescription drugs, and other items prescribed by dead doctors.[2] In other words, people working at doctor's offices pretended their doctors never died and falsely billed Medicare for medical treatments that were never rendered.

The government brags when it cracks down on Medicare fraud, but they only catch a fraction of the crimes perpetrated. The reality is that the living con artists defraud Medicare out of far more than dead doctors do.

MEDICARE SCAMS

What the government does not like to admit is that another 20% of Medicare dollars are paid out in the form of overpayments to those with political connections. What companies do is lobby Congress to enact legislation mandating that Medicare pay inflated prices for certain products and services that can be obtained for a fraction of the price on the free market. This enables those who are politically connected to grossly overcharge Medicare because Congress mandates the inflated expenditures.

How inflated are the monies Medicare pays out? Take for example, an oxygen concentrator, a device that delivers oxygen through a tube to patients with respiratory illness. You can buy one new on the open market for $600. By law, Medicare is only allowed to rent these devices at a price that winds up costing $7,142 over a 36-month period. Medicare covers 80%, so it spends $5,714, while the patient has to pay the other 20%, or $1,428.[3] Under this absurd system, Medicare and patients can pay ten times the free market price it would cost to buy the device new! (Think how much money would be saved if the devices were bought used?)

Perhaps the most expensive politically-induced overcharge is for prescription drugs. Under the Medicare Prescription Drug Act that *Life Extension* vehemently battled against, Medicare is required by law to pay full retail drug prices.[4]

The Medicare Prescription Drug Act was largely written by pharmaceutical companies and passed under intense pressure by pharmaceutical lobbyists (refer to the August 2007 issue of *Life*

Extension magazine for the sordid details).[5] Medicare will pay out hundreds of billions of dollars for drugs that could be obtained for far less in a competitive-bidding system, something that the Medicare Prescription Drug Act prohibits.

THE GENERIC DRUG RIP OFF

Once a brand drug comes off patent, generic equivalents emerge, but they cost far more than they need to because of FDA overregulation.

Take the drug finasteride (Proscar®), for example. It came off patent in the year 2006, but at the end of 2008 chain pharmacies were charging about $90 for 30 tablets (a one-month supply). All it takes to make this drug is to put 5 mg of finasteride into a tablet that dissolves in the stomach. Vitamin companies do this every day with nutrients, but the FDA does not allow them to freely do the same thing with drugs.

We checked on the cost of buying finasteride and making it into tablets. The free market price for 30 tablets is only $10.25, which includes independent assay of the ingredient quality, potency and tablet dissolution—and a reasonable profit margin. It is against the law, however, for GMP-certified (Good Manufacturing Practices) vitamin manufacturers to be able to offer low-cost generic drugs. This prohibition must be lifted as America can no longer afford to subsidize those who are politically connected while the country is driven into insolvency.

Finasteride is a drug that not only helps relieve benign prostate enlargement, but that may also reduce the risk prostate cancer.[7–9] Widespread use could save Medicare lots of money in expensive prostate treatments. Those who follow *Life Extension*'s other recommendations would be expected to reduce prostate cancer risk even more.

As evidence mounts about the prostate cancer risk reduction associated with drugs like finasteride, more companies are competing to make it, but its average price at chain pharmacies is around $86 a month—a staggering eight times higher than what its free market price would be!

Please note that generic prices tend to wildly fluctuate. In this case, as more competitors entered the market, chain pharmacies did not substantially lower the price of finasteride. In some cases, the opposite occurred, and by the time you read this, the price could be different.

MEDICARE PAYS FOR HIV TREATMENTS NEVER DELIVERED

It is remarkable how creative people get when a bloated government bureaucracy such as Medicare/Medicaid pays out almost $500 billion each year with few questions asked.

According to the federal government, hundreds of Medicare-licensed clinics in South Florida defraud Medicare with fake HIV-drug claims. The scam is not hard to pull off. Clinics find indigent HIV-infected drug users who agree to "sell" their cards to the clinics and pretend they are receiving outrageously expensive HIV infusion treatments. These kinds of therapies were long ago abandoned in favor of more effective antiviral drugs, but Medicare pays for them anyway.

To give you an idea of the magnitude of the problem, just one drug addict enabled one clinic to file more than $1.1 million in false Medicare claims for these fabricated anti-HIV infusions.[6]

Even if these treatments were medically necessary, they would only be needed once or twice a month. In one instance, scammers billed Medicare three times a day for each patient—and Medicare paid these bills! According to the federal officials, Medicare continued to pay these clinics for multiple HIV infusion treatments (costing $1,500 to $3,000 per therapy) because Medicare allows them.

THE REAL PROBLEM

Despite inappropriate disbursements that Medicare makes based on private sector fraud and political corruption, the main culprit behind Medicare's eminent collapse is the demographics.

Like Social Security (which is nowhere near as broke as Medicare), the federal government forced workers to pay premiums (taxes) for their Medicare "insurance." Private insurance companies are required by law to maintain reserves in order to pay out future claims. The federal government, on the other hand, has been running a Ponzi scheme and has exhausted virtually every penny. The government is now on the hook for $34 trillion of liabilities. No one knows where the money will come from for these future Medicare/Medicaid disbursements.

A VERY RADICAL APPROACH

I am as libertarian in my thinking as anyone I know, but there are radical approaches that could not only spare Medicare, but protect future generations as well.

Cigarettes officially kill 440,000 people in the US each year, but the real number is higher. When tabulating cigarette smoking-induced deaths, many cancers related to cigarette smoking (such as pancreatic and esophageal cancers) are not usually counted.[23]

The fact that 18-year-olds are allowed to buy something as addictive as cigarettes is obscene. What is worse is that even if a person stops smoking in their 20s, the DNA gene damage inflicted in their early years predisposes them to lifelong increased cancer risks.

I am personally livid over the amount of secondhand smoke I was forced to inhale throughout my early life. It could very well be the cause of my death.

While outright prohibition would not work in the long term, the federal government could impose a three-month moratorium on all tobacco sales. This would enable a huge number of smokers to quit. Financial penalties for anyone caught selling cigarettes during this proposed three-month ban could be so large that it might conceivably work.

If just 30% of all smokers stopped as a result of this three-month moratorium, that alone might save Medicare. Just debating it in Congress may remind smokers of what they are doing to their bodies and motivate them to break their addiction.

I realize this proposal is draconian and would be still another government intrusion on individual liberty. The facts, however, are that smoking-related illnesses are responsible for a huge portion of Medicare/Medicaid outlays—and this country can no longer afford it.

PARTIAL SOLUTIONS

If you are curious as to why Congress has failed so miserably in overseeing Medicare, look no further than the political contributions and lobbying efforts made by those who benefit by scamming the Medicare system. Partial reform will happen when free market forces are allowed to compete for Medicare dollars, as opposed to the bureaucratic albatross that now exists.

One problem is that Medicare will only pay for FDA-approved medical devices and drugs. As we know, this means that Medicare recipients are forced into overpriced therapies that are laden with side effects. Treating drug-induced side effects results in the expenditure of even more healthcare dollars. To make matters worse, the efficacy of certain FDA-approved drugs is so mediocre that patients sometimes live only a few months longer by taking them. The cost to Medicare for these drugs can easily exceed $50,000 per patient. Complementary physicians who prescribe unapproved cancer therapies that cost a fraction of FDA-approved drugs are subject to criminal prosecution.

So we have a system in place today in which progressive doctors are persecuted, while those who sell dangerous and often ineffective therapies receive protection and payment from the federal government. People without the financial wherewithal have no choice, since Medicare will only pay for what the FDA claims is safe and effective. Conventional medicine's goldmine will end when Medicare exhausts its ability to pay.

A group of FDA scientists recently revolted against their superiors and went directly to Congress.[10] The reason was that they were told by their superiors to certify new medical devices as safe and effective, when the clinical testing data showed the opposite. This is just one example of how the FDA contributes to today's healthcare cost crisis by allowing dangerous products on to the market that Medicare then pays for.

ONE WAY TO SLASH MEDICARE OUTLAYS

Low blood levels of vitamin D are associated with increased incidences of virtually every human disease.[11-14]

In 2007, I petitioned the federal government to mandate vitamin D supplementation in Medicare-eligible individuals in order for them to be eligible to receive benefits.[15] I proposed that the government require that people must have a minimum blood level of 32 ng/mL of vitamin D or they would be denied coverage. This would force aging people to take this ultra-low-cost supplement, which in turn would drastically slash the incidences of the most common aging-related disorders.

Optimal vitamin D blood levels are over 50 ng/mL, yet most Americans' levels test far below 30.[16-19] By mandating basic vitamin D supplementation, Medicare might regain some of its solvency, as it would be paying out far fewer medical expenses.

A study published in the *New England Journal of Medicine* evaluated blood levels for vitamin D in intensive care unit (ICU) patients.[20] The average serum vitamin D level was only 16 ng/mL. All patients with undetectable levels of vitamin D died.

Patients with the lowest vitamin D blood levels had the most severe organ dysfunction and the most adverse outcomes. The predicted mortality (death) rate was:

Vitamin D Status	Mortality Percentage
ICU patients with sufficient vitamin D	16%
ICU patients with insufficient vitamin D	35%
ICU patients with deficient vitamin D	45%

It costs Medicare about $2,674 a day to care for ICU patients, and some of them linger for weeks or months in this expensive hospital setting.[21] Mandating optimal vitamin D levels could slash the number of Medicare patients requiring ICU care.

HARSH REALITIES

While common sense solutions exist, the aging population will challenge the solvency of Medicare unless something radical is done to keep humans healthy.

Mainstream medicine bases its financial projections on lots of aging people contracting cancer, vascular disease, and dementia. Today's medicinal "industry" does not want any interference with their income stream and have no incentive to institute preventive programs.

The public is more health conscious today than ever. The problem is that too many people continue to abuse their bodies with excess intake of dangerous calories, cigarette smoking, and physical inactivity. Add to this the insufficient intake of nutrients such as magnesium, vitamin D, omega-3s, and it is no wonder that healthcare expenditures are bankrupting this country.[22]

GOVERNMENT HAS TO FESS UP TO THE PROBLEM

To shock the public into a pro-active state, the federal government has to admit that they are not able to pay future Medicare claims unless aggressive steps are taken to prevent age-related disease. The public needs to know that if they don't take personal responsibility for their healthcare, there may be no Medicare dollars available to cover their sick care.

The government needs to initiate mandatory warnings (that I would be happy to write) on the labels of all dangerous foods. People would be less likely to buy toxic foods if they were reminded about the risks associated with eating them. The government should encourage food companies to state truthful claims about healthy foods such as "eating broccoli reduces cancer risk."

The main reason Medicare is facing insolvency is that too many aging people are getting sick. These diseases of aging are preventable via a wide variety of lifestyle alterations. It will require a sustained governmental public relations campaign to hammer in the need for Americans to follow healthier lifestyles.

Alternatively, lifting the ban currently in place that precludes the dissemination of truthful health information about a wide variety of foods, hormones, nutrients, and even certain drugs would make a significant positive impact on the aging population, which in turn would help resolve the catastrophic Medicare cost crisis we now face.

References

1. http://www.taxpolicycenter.org/taxfacts/displayafact. cfm?Docid=407.
2. http://online.wsj.com/article/SB121556119847437537.html.
3. http://online.wsj.com/article/SB121556116413437535.html.
4. http://www.ustreas.gov/offices/public-affairs/hsa/pdf/pl108-173.pdf.
5. *Life Extension.* 2007 Aug; 13(8):7-9.
6. http://www.miamiherald.com/428/v-print/story/628288. html.
7. *Rev Urol.* 2003;5 Suppl 5:S12-21.

8. *Urology.* 2009 May; 73(5):935-9; discussion 939.

9. *Prostate.* 2009 Jun 1; 69(8):895-907.

10. http://energycommerce.house.gov/Press_110/110nr383.shtml.

11. *Am J Clin Nutr.* 2008 Apr; 87(4):1080S-6S.

12. *Drugs Aging.* 2007; 24(12):1017-29.

13. *J Nutr.* 2005 Nov; 135(11):2739S-48S.

14. *QJM.* 1996 Aug; 89(8):579-89.

15. *Life Extension.* 2007 Oct; 13(10): 7-17.

16. *Am J Clin Nutr.* 2006 Jul; 84(1):18-28.

17. *J Nutr.* 2005 Nov; 135(11):2739S-48S.

18. *Med J Aust.* 2002 Aug 5; 177(3):149-52.

19. *Mayo Clin Proc.* 2003 Dec; 78(12):1457-9.

20. *N Engl J Med.* 2009 Apr 30; 360(18):1912-4.

21. *Crit Care Med.* 2004 Jun; 32(6):1254-9.

22. http://www.cms.hhs.gov/NationalHealthExpendData/02_NationalHealthAccountsHistorical.asp.

23. http://www.cancer.org/docroot/PED/content/PED_10_2X_Cigarette_Smoking_and_Cancer.asp

The Generic Drug Rip-off

by William Faloon

I DID EVERYTHING I COULD—INCLUDING RISKING LIFE IN PRISON. Back in the 1980s–1990s, the Life Extension Foundation crusaded to enlighten Americans about the economic ruination that would occur if this country's corrupt drug regulatory structure was not abolished. At the behest of pharmaceutical interests, the FDA brutally retaliated against us.

What I am about to divulge is a shocking revelation about why prescription drugs cost so much. Before I describe this pervasive fraud, I want to remind readers what happens when an apathetic public allows archaic government regulations to rule the marketplace.

THE ECONOMIC COLLAPSE OF ARGENTINA

In the 1940s, Argentina was the ninth wealthiest country in the world. At one point it was richer than France and boasted a higher standard of living than Canada. It was considered one of the best countries in which to live.[1]

After an endless series of reckless governmental actions including uncontrolled borrowing and economic mismanagement, Argentina's standard of living ranking has plummeted to 46th.[2] If you had money in an Argentinean bank in 1999, it vanished. If you owned Argentinean government bonds, you lost most of your principal as the central government defaulted on its obligations.

Other countries have faced worse problems, including the mass murder of their citizens in one form or another by the central government.

The reason I mention Argentina is that its economic collapse has similarities to what the United States is facing.

Misguided and corrupt government policies, combined with citizen apathy, allowed financial ruination to happen in Argentina. We in the United States are not immune to the same calamity.

If what I expose in this article does not motivate citizens to take action, I don't know what will. It is beyond my comprehension that the common-sense free market solution I propose will be ignored by the American citizenry.

HEALTHCARE COSTS BANKRUPTING UNITED STATES

Everything Life Extension predicted about the healthcare cost crisis is happening before our eyes. Major corporations, individuals, and the government are being bankrupted by out-of-control medical costs. Some say the economic challenges facing the United States will result in substantially reduced standards of living. This does not have to happen.

As we long ago identified, the cause behind spiraling medical costs is a crooked and ludicrous regulatory structure.

Today's healthcare cost crisis is widely acknowledged and feared. No one, however, has yet proposed a practical solution to resolve it.

OVERPRICED DRUGS

The reason for high-priced generics is not because the active ingredients are expensive. On the contrary, compared with complicated nutrient extracts, the ingredients in drugs are usually synthetic chemicals that cost only pennies a day.

The culprit behind overpriced generic drugs is an archaic regulatory environment that functions to protect pharmaceutical financial interests, forcing consumers to pay artificially inflated prices for their generic medications.

If our proposal to overhaul today's inefficient regulatory system succeeds, at least part of the healthcare cost crisis will disappear quickly. A side benefit to lower-priced generic drugs is that it will force pharmaceutical companies to bring out life-saving medications faster, since almost-as-good generics will cost virtually nothing.

AN EXAMPLE OF A GROSSLY INFLATED GENERIC PRICE

Once a brand drug comes off patent, generic equivalents emerge, but they cost far more than they need to because of FDA over-regulation.

Take the drug finasteride (Proscar®) for example. It came off patent in 2006, but at the end of 2008, chain pharmacies were charging about $90 for 30 tablets (a one-month supply). All it takes to make this drug is to put 5 mg of finasteride into a tablet that dissolves in the stomach. Vitamin companies do this every day with nutrients, but the FDA does not allow them to freely do the same thing with drugs.

We checked on the cost of buying finasteride and making it into tablets. The free market price for 30 tablets is only $10.25, which includes an independent assay of the ingredient quality, potency, and tablet dissolution—and a reasonable profit margin. It is against the law, however, for GMP-certified (Good Manufacturing Practices) vitamin manufacturers to offer low-cost generic drugs. This prohibition must be lifted as America can no longer afford to subsidize those who are politically connected while the country is driven into insolvency.

Finasteride is a drug that not only helps relieve benign prostate enlargement, but may also reduce the risk of prostate cancer.[3–5] Widespread use could save Medicare lots of money in expensive prostate treatments.

As evidence mounts about the prostate cancer risk reduction associated with drugs like finasteride, more companies are competing to make it, but its average price at chain pharmacies is around $86 a month—a staggering eight times higher than what its free market price would be!

Please note that generic prices tend to wildly fluctuate. In this case, as more competitors entered the market, chain pharmacies did not substantially lower the price of finasteride. In some cases, the opposite occurs, and by the time you read this, the price could vary.

HOW THE "GENERIC" REGULATORY SYSTEM WORKS

If a company wants to manufacture a generic drug, be it a prescription drug like finasteride or an over-the-counter (OTC) drug like ibuprofen, it must file an Abbreviated New Drug Application (ANDA) with the FDA, even if it is manufactured by others already.

While the company does not have to perform clinical trials for an ANDA, it does have to show its bioequivalence to the original drug. For drugs that are difficult to synthesize, this requirement is important. For most drugs, however, the raw material can be purchased, often from the identical supplier that provides it for the branded drug.

To show bioequivalence, the company typically needs to perform human studies that take 1.5–2 years, unless a sufficient number have already been performed successfully, in which case it might be able to use those prior studies to support the

ANDA. But the FDA could reject the ANDA and require the company to perform studies anyway.

The cost and time involved in the ANDA process varies, depending on the drug, its safety, how long it has been on the market, etc.

To have an ANDA approved, it typically requires an investment of about $2 million, and it takes a total of two to three years to get the drug to market.

To manufacture a common drug like ibuprofen (the active ingredient in Advil® and numerous other OTCs) might cost about $1 million and take 1.5 years, because the company would not have to do its own studies, and because it is a drug with a known safety profile.

In addition to these costs, a company should budget 15% for legal fees, because wherever there is a big manufacturer with a sizable market share involved, they will sue, just to try to eliminate more competition from the market.

One's political connections with the FDA are critically important. Those who are not in the FDA's good graces might find it more difficult to get an ANDA approved. The company should have experience with this bureaucratic process to know when and how to object to unreasonable FDA requirements.

So as you can see, what should be a straightforward process to manufacture drugs like finasteride instead turns into a bureaucratic quagmire that results in generic drugs costing far more than they need to. If a person was to take 5 mg finasteride tablets made by a vitamin manufacturer, all they would need to do to document its efficacy would be to test their blood levels of dihydrotestosterone (DHT). Finasteride alleviates benign prostate enlargement symptoms by inhibiting the 5-alpha-reductase enzyme that converts testosterone into DHT. Properly made finasteride will lower DHT.

Under a free market system, consumers would have the choice of paying $86 for a one-month supply of FDA-approved generic

finasteride, or $10.25 for a one-month supply of generic finas-
teride made by a GMP-certified (Good Manufacturing Practices)
vitamin manufacturer.

HOW MUCH ARE YOU OVERPAYING?

Life Extension investigators have spent an enormous amount of
time identifying what it really costs to make a generic drug. The
price of the active ingredient for most drugs is remarkably low.
A greater expense involves GMP manufacturing and the kinds
of quality control measures that we at Life Extension mandate
for the supplements that carry our label.

The chart opposite reveals the shocking numbers. Compared
with what chain pharmacies are charging today, the free market
prices are an astounding 51% to 94% lower!

On average, Americans are paying 837% more at chain pharmacies compared with what the free market price would be for
the identical medications.

When looking at the ultra-low free market prices, it becomes
evidently clear that there is no real prescription drug cost crisis.
A month's supply of some of the most commonly used drugs
could be obtained for the price of a box of cereal.

There never was a need for Congress to pass the thoroughly
corrupt Medicare Prescription Drug Act that involves the massive expenditure of tax dollars to pay full retail prices for these
hyper-inflated drugs.

The free market price of generics would be so low, in fact, that
even those with medical insurance will save money on most drugs
compared with what their co-pays are now.

If these free market medications became available, medical
insurance premiums will be lowered, Medicare's day of insolvency
postponed, and many businesses and consumers spared from
bankruptcy. The chart on the next page reveals how little free
market generic drugs would cost.

GENERIC DRUG COMPARISON CHART

Brand Name	Generic Name	Average Price at Chain Drugstores	Free Market Price
Proscar®	Finasteride 5 mg	$ 86	$ 10.25
Zocor®	Simvastatin 20 mg	$ 27.99	$ 3.20
Norvasc®	Amlodipine 10 mg	$ 39.99	$ 4.41
Depakote®	Divalproex 500 mg	$ 129.99	$ 9.59
Lopressor®	Metoprolol 50 mg	$ 12.99	$ 2.21
Trileptal®	Oxcarbazepine 300 mg	$ 109.99	$ 15.50
Pravachol®	Pravastatin 40 mg	$ 51.99	$ 6.68
Altace®	Ramipril 10 mg	$ 61.99	$ 4.25
Lamictal®	Lamotrigine 100 mg	$ 119.99	$ 7.50
Neurontin®	Gabapentin 400 mg	$ 54.99	$ 5.85
Lotensin®	Benazepril 20 mg	$ 31.99	$ 4.40
Wellbutrin SR®	Bupropion 150 mg	$ 49.99	$ 17.99
Pamelor®	Nortriptyline 50 mg	$ 36.99	$ 4.39
Sonata®	Zaleplon 10 mg	$ 61.99	$ 12.43
Prilosec®	Omeprazole 20 mg (Rx)	$ 25.99	$ 12.70

The Free Market Prices listed on this chart are based on what an efficiently run pharmacy could sell these non-FDA-approved generics for. These prices would be lower if non-pharmacies were allowed to sell them. There are many expensive bureaucratic regulations that pharmacies have to adhere to, and the price of any drug you buy reflects the costs of complying with over-regulation of pharmacies, as well as over-regulation of generic drug manufacturing. The Free Market Prices on this chart would drop even further if large quantities of these non-FDA-approved generics were manufactured.

DOUBLE-DIGIT DRUG PRICE INCREASES SO FAR IN 2009

Despite inflation remaining at near zero this year, pharmaceutical companies are jacking up the prices they charge for patented drugs to even more exorbitant levels.

Since the Medicare Prescription Drug Act[6] requires the federal government to pay full retail price, pharmaceutical companies can literally name their price and receive guaranteed payment courtesy of taxpayers. Drug companies receive a substantial percentage of the retail price from private health insurers also, so the more they raise the prices, the more money they make.

Consumers are the ultimate victims. They face higher Medicare premiums and taxes, higher private insurance premiums, more exclusions and higher co-pays, and higher taxes to cover the $600 billion Medicare Prescription Drug Act.

Proposed legislation calls for the FDA to get more funding, so taxpayers may also be contributing to the bureaucracy that serves to protect drug companies against lower-priced competition.

The growing number of Americans without medical insurance and who don't qualify for government aid are priced out of the market for patented medications unless they are economically well-endowed. The federal government recognizes this problem and is proposing that even more tax dollars now be used to subsidize prescription drugs, though not at full retail price.

In fact, one reason pharmaceutical companies are increasing prices is that they fear the federal government will soon require they "discount" their patented medications. So the more they jack up the prices now, the greater amount they will receive after they are forced to lower them via government-mandated "discounts."

The chart on the next page shows the double-digit price increases that occurred on popular drugs in the beginning of 2009.

Rising Drug Costs

Price of selected drugs, and change from previous year

Drug	Disease Treated	Dosage	Price (1Q 2009)	% change
Sprycel®	Leukemia	60 20-mg pills	$ 3,763.98	32.7%
Viagra®	Erectile dysfunction	30 25-mg pills	$ 519.46	20.7%
Strattera®	ADHD	30 10-mg pills	$ 159.28	15.6%
Sutent®	Kidney cancer	28 25-mg pills	$ 4,997.81	14.3%
Cialis®	Erectile dysfunction	30 20-mg pills	$ 551.17	14.2%

Source: Credit Suisse analysis based on Wolters, Kluwer, Price, Rx Pricing Database. This chart is reproduced from the *Wall Street Journal*, April 15, 2009. Reprinted with permission.

HOW CONSUMERS WILL BE PROTECTED

We are proposing that the law be amended to allow GMP-certified manufacturing facilities to produce generic prescription drugs that do not undergo the excessive regulatory hurdles that force consumers to pay egregiously inflated prices.

To alert consumers when they are getting a generic whose manufacturing is not as heavily regulated as it is currently, the law should mandate that the label of these less-regulated generic drugs clearly states:

> This is not an FDA-approved manufactured generic drug and may be ineffective and potentially dangerous. This drug is NOT manufactured under the same standards required for an FDA-approved generic drug. Purchase this drug at your own risk.

By allowing the sale of these less costly generics, consumers will have a choice as to what companies they choose to trust.

The inevitable concern raised by this free market solution is safety. Who will protect consumers from poorly made generic drugs?

First of all, there will be the same regulation of these drugs as there are with GMP-certified supplement makers. FDA inspectors will visit facilities, take sample products, and assay to ensure potency of active ingredient, dissolution, etc. Laboratories that fail to make products that meet label claims would face civil and criminal penalties from the government.

Secondly, there is no incentive not to provide the full potency of active ingredient in these less-regulated generic drugs. The price of the active ingredients makes up such a small percentage of the overall cost that a manufacturer would be idiotic to scrimp on potency.

Companies that foolishly make inferior generics will be viciously exposed by the media, along with the FDA, consumer protection groups, and even prescribing physicians who will be suspicious if a drug was not working as it is supposed to.

Companies producing inferior products will be quickly driven from the marketplace as consumers who choose to purchase these lower-cost generics will seek out laboratories that have reputations for making flawless products.

These substandard companies would not only be castigated in the public's eye, but face civil litigation from customers who bought the defective generics. When one considers that GMP-certified manufacturing plants can cost hundreds of millions to set up, a company would be committing suicide if it failed to consistently produce generic drugs that at least met minimum standards.

MOLLIFYING THE CYNICS

No matter how many facts I list showing that these free market drugs will be safe, there are alarmists who believe that even if

The Secret About Compounding Pharmacies the FDA Does Not Want You to Know!

If you're like most people, you think prescription drugs are only made by pharmaceutical companies. This myth causes Americans to pay outrageous prices for drugs that can be bought for a fraction of the price from compounding pharmacies.

For example, the price of a particular drug made by a major pharmaceutical company is $245 a month. You can obtain the identical quantity of this natural substance from a compounding pharmacy for as low as $29 a month! Since many insurance companies do not reimburse for this item, you would save over $2,592 a year by purchasing the compounded version of this drug as opposed one made by a pharmaceutical company. By law, I am not even allowed to mention the name of this drug. How's that for press freedom!

Pharmaceutical companies would prefer that you don't find out how to obtain your prescription drugs for 92% less than what you may now pay. That's why pharmaceutical giants lobby the FDA to incite the agency to censor compounding pharmacy advertising.

In a landmark legal case, the US Supreme Court ruled that the FDA violates the First Amendment's free speech provisions when it seeks to restrict advertising or promotion of compounded drugs. As a result of this Constitutional victory, you are now allowed to at least find out that there are compounded prescription medications available at a fraction of the price you have been paying. In fact, the cost for some compounded drugs is lower than co-pays for pharmaceutical company-manufactured ones.

one person suffers a serious adverse event because of a defective generic drug, then the law should not be amended to allow the sale of these less-regulated products.

What few understand is that enabling lower-cost drugs to be sold might reduce the number of poorly made drugs. The reason is that prescription drug counterfeiting is a major issue today. Drugs are counterfeited because they are so expensive. With a month's supply of free market simvastatin selling for only $3.20, it is difficult to imagine anyone profiting by counterfeiting it. So amending the law to enable these super-low-cost drugs to be sold might reduce the counterfeiting that exists right now.

Another reason these less-regulated generics will do far more good than harm is that people who need them to live will be able to afford them. The media has reported on heart-wrenching stories of destitute people who cannot afford even generic prescription drugs. They either do without, or take a less-than-optimal dose. The availability of these free market generics will enable virtually anyone to be able to afford their medications.

PRESERVING OUR COUNTRY'S FINANCIAL FUTURE

The cost of prescription drugs is a significant factor in today's healthcare cost crisis, a problem that threatens to bankrupt consumers and this nation's medical system. Passage of common-sense legislation would quickly slash the cost of generic drugs so low that consumers could obtain them for less than what their co-pays currently are. Enormous amounts of money would be saved by public and private insurance programs, and ultimately consumers.

According to the Government Accountability Office (GAO), all federal revenue will be eaten up by government outlays for Medicare, Medicaid, Social Security, and public debt interest by 2025[7]—just 16 years from now!

We as a nation can no longer afford to be bound by today's inefficient regulatory system that artificially inflates the cost of our prescription medications. The money is no longer there to support this bureaucratic morass.

References

1. www.wikipedia.org/wiki/Argentina.
2. www.hdrstats.undp.org/en/2008/countries/country_fact_sheets/cty_fs_ARG.html.
3. *Rev Urol.* 2003;5(Suppl 5):S12–21.
4. *Urology.* 2009 May;73(5):935–9; discussion 939.

5. *Prostate.* 2009 Jun 1;69(8):895–907.

6. www.citizen.org/congress/reform/rx_benefits/drug_benefit/.

7. www.house.gov/budget_republicans/entitlement/roadmap_detailed_entirereport.pdf.

Ending the Atrocities

by William Faloon

TODAY'S POPULATION LIVES ON A RAILROAD TRACK. EVERY-
thing may be fine for the moment—until a freight train
comes along and wipes us out.

We at Life Extension have pled for 29 years to get off the track
before the train comes.

A startling number of reports reveal the FDA is in far worse
shape than originally thought. Few people comprehend that
they are likely to suffer and die prematurely as a result of FDA's
failures.

The media does a decent job reporting on FDA disasters. The
apathetic public, however, often forgets what they read the next
day. That is, until they are diagnosed with a serious illness. Then
they go into a panic mode to find an effective treatment. All too
often, however, the cure does not exist because of FDA bureaucratic roadblocks. In other cases, the FDA-approved drugs available induce horrific side effects.

It is our mission to memorialize these tragedies to demonstrate the urgent need to radically reform the FDA. This "state-sponsored" carnage of the American citizenry must be stopped!

FDA DISSEMINATES FRAUDULENT SAFETY DATA

Ketek® is a drug the FDA approved to treat mild to moderate pneumonia. Ketek® can also cause sudden and serious liver damage. In some cases complete liver failure develops necessitating the need for a liver transplant. Some patients die before a liver transplant can be performed.[1]

The risks of liver failure (and other toxic side effects) were known *before* the FDA approved Ketek®. In order to convince an outside scientific advisory committee to recommend that Ketek® be approved, the FDA knowingly allowed a *fraudulent* safety study to be presented. Here is what the Senate Investigative Committee uncovered:[2]

- FDA accepted the resubmission of a new drug application that included safety data that was fraudulent, in whole or in part.

- FDA instructed its employees preparing to appear before the advisory committee that they should present this fraudulent safety data.

- FDA employees presented the fraudulent study data to the advisory committee tasked with recommending Ketek's approval or disapproval.

- FDA approved a pediatric clinical trial of Ketek®, involving infants as young as six months old, despite concerns related to known toxicities affecting the heart, eyes, liver and vascular system.

- FDA continued to knowingly cite the fraudulent study data in publically released safety information on Ketek®.

How fraudulent was this data? While the FDA was presenting this fake data, a criminal investigation was simultaneously being conducted that found the clinic where the "safety" study allegedly occurred was *closed* during the time the study was supposed to have taken place. It was also determined that documents relating to the safety study had date modifications and signature inconsistencies.

Shortly after the advisory committee meeting where the fake safety data was presented by FDA employees, the person who conducted the study was criminally indicted, pled guilty, and sentenced to almost five years in jail.

It is even more shocking that the FDA continued to cite this safety study long after the principal investigator admitted it was fraudulent. While the perpetrator of this "safety" study was in prison for falsifying the data, the FDA used the very same study to issue a Public Health Announcement stating:

> Based on the pre-marketing clinical data it appeared that the risk of liver injury with telithrmycin (Ketek®) was similar to that of other marketed antibiotics.[3]

The "pre-marketing clinical data" FDA cited to tell the public that Ketek® was safe was the fraudulent study, a study that may never have actually occurred. According to the Senate Investigative Committee report, "it defies explanation why the FDA would continue to cite" this fraudulent study to the American public to imply that Ketek® is safe.[3]

The Senate Committee report concluded by stating that

> Retaliation against these individuals, or any other FDA employees who communicate with the committee with reference to Ketek® will not be tolerated.[4]

Based on the tone of the Senate investigative report, it would appear that the FDA functioned as a continuous criminal enterprise in this instance.[5, 6]

THE REVOLVING DOOR

You may wonder why certain officials in the FDA would go to such extreme lengths to get a lethal drug like Ketek® approved.

Look no further than the gargantuan economic benefits drug companies reap when a patented compound like Ketek® receives the FDA seal of approval.

When we first exposed the revolving door of FDA employees going to work for companies they regulate, virtually no one believed us. Back in the 1980s, most Americans were deceived by FDA propaganda stating that the agency "is responsible for protecting the public health by assuring the safety . . . of human drugs."[9]

The harsh reality is that the FDA functions primarily to protect the financial interests of the pharmaceutical industry, not the public's health. If anyone ever questioned this, look no further than the FDA's attempts last year to ban the safest form of estrogen (estriol). The FDA has no qualms about publically stating their ban on estriol was based on a petition filed by Wyeth, the maker of dangerous estrogen drugs like Premarin® and PremPro®.

There are a number of estrogen drugs that have not been shown to increase stroke and breast cancer risk.[10] The FDA, however, has done nothing to remove Premarin® or PremPro®. Instead, the FDA openly seeks to protect Wyeth's market share by denying American women access to natural estriol.

According to the FDA, "bioidentical hormone products are unsupported by medical evidence and are considered false and misleading by the agency."[11] The truth is that bioidentical hormones are far less expensive and pose a major competitive threat to Wyeth, ergo the FDA's aggressive attempts to disallow them.

In a report issued by the Associated Press just last year, it was revealed that a record number of FDA employees are leaving the agency to go to work for pharmaceutical companies. According to the Associated Press, these FDA staffers are resigning in order to go into "the more lucrative side of the business."[12]

THE FDA'S BRAIN DRAIN

As experienced FDA scientists leave the agency to work for Big Pharma, the remaining staff is leaner and less competent to approve new lifesaving medications. As reported by the Associated Press, a consequence of FDA employees going to work for pharmaceutical companies is a clogging of the drug approval pipeline.

As long time Life Extension members know, the FDA drug approval process has always been a bureaucratic quagmire, where lifesaving medications languish for years, decades and sometimes forever. The drug pipeline has been "clogged" for almost 50 years. We are deeply disturbed that it is now taking even longer for lifesaving medications to become available to those in need.

The *Wall Street Journal* continues to support our position with blistering exposes on human beings who suffer horrendously and die while potential lifesaving therapies languish in the FDA approval process. An article published last year titled "Sick Patients Need Cutting-Edge Drugs," disclosed heart-wrenching reports of young cancer patients who were denied compassionate-use access to experimental drugs. The *Wall Street Journal* article raised the logical questions:

> Why do terminally ill patients have to wait so long to get access to the only treatments that hold any promise of saving their lives? And why is it not their right to decide?[13]

These very issues have been discussed in Life Extension's publications for nearly 30 years. We have analogized in previous articles how it is perfectly legal to engage in all kinds of risky activities, such as parachuting off of high bridges, but it *illegal* to make experimental medications available to terminally ill people without the FDA's permission.

According to the *Wall Street Journal*, the drug delay problem is getting much worse. The problem has been magnified in recent years as the number of new drug approvals has fallen dramatically. The FDA approved just 16 new drugs in 2007 and only 17 in 2008.[14,15] That's down from 53 in 1996 and 39 in 1997.

With the approval of lifesaving drugs grinding to a snail's pace, the moronic cruelty of denying experimental drugs to terminal patients must stop. Each day a life saving drug is delayed, human beings perish. The case for radical reform of the Food, Drug, and Cosmetic Act and the FDA itself has never been stronger.

FDA BUNGLES NEW SYSTEM TO TRACK SIDE EFFECTS

Even when data used to approve a new drug is *not* fraudulent, there are inherent limitations in assessing toxic side effects in the clinical study setting. Reasons for this include the relatively short time period the drugs are evaluated in a clinical study compared to how long patients use them in the real world. Another problem is that clinical studies are often tightly controlled by doctors with specialized expertise in the particular drug they are evaluating. Practicing physicians, on the other hand, see dozens of patients a day and may not be familiar with the proper way to prescribe drugs that have a narrow safety window. Still another issue is the relatively small number of patients taking the drugs in a clinical study compared to the millions who may eventually be prescribed it.

Due to these serious limitations, post-approval surveillance is critical to identifying lethal side effects of prescription drugs that were not detected in the clinical trials.

According to a report by an independent auditing institute, the FDA squandered $25 million on a bungled computer system to track side effects of approved drugs.[16, 17] As a result, the FDA will have to rely on a dysfunctional system to track what are record breaking numbers of adverse reports being made about drugs the agency previously approved as safe.

After this report showing that FDA errors and mismanagement caused this system to not be available, the FDA asked that most of the findings of the report be deleted. The independent institute who put the report together refused to capitulate to the FDA's attempts to obstruct the report's findings.[17, 18]

DRUG PRICES SURGE

In today's upside down regulatory system, Americans are prescribed drugs whose approval may be based on fraudulent or insufficient research data. Experimental therapies that could save their lives are routinely denied. The *cost* of existing medications meanwhile is skyrocketing.

Drug price increases often exceed the inflation rate. The average increase for the top 50 best selling drugs was 7.82% in 2007, 6.73% in 2006, and 6.22% in 2005.[19]

Some very popular drugs are increasing at astronomical rates. The antidepressant Wellbutrin XL® went up by 44.5% from 2005 to 2007. The attention-deficit drug Adderall XR® went up by 33.5%. The price of the sleep-aid drug Ambien® shot up 70.1% during this period.[19]

On less popular drugs, the price surges are worse than obscene. A drug used to treat heart problems in premature babies went from $136.10 to $1,875.00 in one year. A drug used to treat a certain cancer (Cosmegen) increased from $16.79 to $593.75 in one year. A drug used to treat spasms in babies (Acthar) was increased from about $1,650.00 to more than $23,000.00 in one year. Just imagine your baby suffering spasms and being asked to fork over $23,000.00 for one drug![20]

Whether you use these drugs or not, you still suffer. The thoroughly corrupt Medicare Prescription Drug Act passed at the behest of pharmaceutical lobbyists mandates that taxpayers pay full retail prices for these drugs.[21] Taxpayers will fork over $600 billion for these egregiously overpriced drugs in the first ten years.[22]

Where consumers are really hurt is in their ever-increasing health insurance premiums. If you are fortunate enough to have someone else paying your premiums, you cannot help but note the higher deductibles and greater exclusions.

The FDA enables drug companies to financially rape the American consumer by stifling competition. There are so many regulatory hurdles to getting FDA approval for even a competitive generic drug that consumers often pay eight times more than they need to.

Under the guise of "consumer protection," the FDA has been manipulated by pharmaceutical interests to restrict free market forces that would drive down drug costs.

Do Drug Companies have *Any* Decency?

It is beyond my comprehension to understand how pharmaceutical companies can look themselves in the mirror when they know they are selling drugs proven to kill.

Back in 1994, our best selling product was shark cartilage. The problem we uncovered was that it was not curing cancer patients. We immediately notified our customers that a survey we conducted of those who bought shark cartilage showed it to be ineffective. We urged these people to seek other therapies.

The supplement industry was shocked at our findings, but most stopped promoting shark cartilage as anti-cancer therapy. Our findings about shark cartilage's lack of efficacy were confirmed several years later in a controlled study.

We were a relatively small organization in 1994 and losing our best selling product was financially challenging. In no way, however, could we continue telling cancer patients that shark cartilage might help them when are own findings showed it did not work.

The fact the multibillion dollar pharmaceutical companies have no qualms about using fraudulent data to support the approval and continued sale of lethal drugs is an atrocity. That certain people within the FDA collude with pharmaceutical companies to allow dangerous and ineffective drugs on the market is an act so heinous that words to not exist to describe it.

FDA BOTCHES PUBLIC RELATIONS CAMPAIGN

The FDA has been pummeled by Congress and the media about its many scandals, including poor inspections of tainted foods, drugs and other products it regulates.

Needless to say, this has created a severe image problem. So FDA officials decided to hire a public relations agency that would "create and foster a lasting positive public image of the agency for the American public," according to agency documents.[23]

When taxpayer dollars are involved, the law mandates a bidding process be used to insure that the contract go to the lowest cost contractor. According to an exposé published by the *Washington Post*, the propaganda contract went instead to a public relations firm with ties to the FDA official who arranged the deal. A loophole was used to avoid putting the contract up for bid.[24]

After being made aware of this apparent corrupt act, an FDA deputy commissioner suspended the public relations contract and ordered an independent investigation.

Congress responded by launching still another investigation into the FDA. According to the chairman of the House committee that oversees the FDA, "The agency chose to use its limited resources to save face instead of saving the public health."[25]

The FDA retains the power to make life and death decisions that affect all of us. When it comes to analyzing new therapies to extend human longevity, this involves the scientific and common sense ability to understand complex biochemical interactions that occur within living organisms. The FDA's botched attempt to launch a misinformation campaign to cover up its inadequacies further calls into question its competency and moral legitimacy.

FIGHTING BACK

In 1994, we established the FDA Museum to document how the FDA's failings were responsible for the needless deaths of millions of Americans.

Sadly, every assertion we made about the FDA back then has been validated by third parties and the FDA itself. I lament that we were proven correct, because this means that millions more Americans perished unnecessarily over the past 15 years . . . and the cost of today's corrupt healthcare system threatens to financially decimate our country.

The FDA's credibility is at an all-time low. There has never been a better time to enact legislation to reform the way healthcare is regulated in this country. With a new Congress in session, health freedom activists are aggressively seeking to have the law changed to allow free market forces to tear down the corrupt wall of bureaucracy that causes the needless death of thousands of Americans each day.

We at Life Extension are working with the American Association for Health Freedom (AAHF)* to make our voices heard in Congress. AAHF is a coalition of integrative physicians, healthcare consumers, and health freedom activists committed to a complete reform of the FDA. Its Reform FDA Petition is available for signing at www.ReformFDA.org.

More scientific innovation is occurring in the medical field than at any time in human history. This progress is irrelevant, however, if a regulatory barrier denies the fruits of this research to people in need, or allows drugs to be sold with lethal side effects, or renders the cost of medications unaffordable.

The Life Extension Foundation has been battling FDA ineptitude for three decades. Your support enables us to continue this ongoing struggle to convince Congress to radically reform the way healthcare is controlled in this country.

---

* AAHF is now the Alliance for Natural Health USA (ANH–USA). Their website is http://www.ANH-USA.org.

How Many Drug-Induced Suicides?

The same Senate committee investigating the Ketek® scandal uncovered another study with falsified data. This fake data was used to support the approval of a popular antidepressant drug used by millions of human beings.

According to a report authored by a Harvard medical doctor, when the Paxil® application was submitted to an FDA advisory committee in 1991, the drug company improperly counted those taking the real drug as placebo subjects. This was done to make it appear there to be no difference in the risk of suicidal behavior in those taking Paxil® compared to placebo.

It took until year 2006 for the manufacturer to send a letter to doctors admitting the risk of suicidal behavior was 6.7 times higher in study subjects taking Paxil® as compared to placebo.[7]

Suicide is the 11th leading cause of death in the United States.[8] It killed over 34,000 people in year 2004. The number of suicides attributed to drugs like Paxil® (select serotonin reuptake inhibitors) could be in the hundreds of thousands during the 13 years it was fraudulently marketed.[4, 5]

References

1. Available at: http://www.drug-injury.com/druginjurycom/2007/12/ketek-case-repo.html. Accessed December 5, 2008.

2. Available at: http://www.druginjuryblog.com/2008/06/11/ketek-fraudulent-clinical-trials-prove-fda-not-doing-its-job-congress-says/. Accessed December 5, 2008.

3. Available at: http://www.fda.gov/ora/about/enf_story2006_archive/ch3/default.pdf. Accessed December 5, 2008.

4. Available at: http://www.ketekliverinjury.com/liver_failure/study.html. Accessed December 5, 2008.

5. Available at: http://finance.senate.gov/press/Gpress/2007/prg122007a.pdf. Accessed December 5, 2008.

6. Available at: http://www.senate.gov/~finance/press/Gpress/2008/prg061208.pdf. Accessed December 5, 2008.

7. Available at: http://us.gsk.com/docs-pdf/media-news/ Paxil-CR-and-Paxil-Adult-Suicide.pdf. Accessed December 5, 2008.

8. Available at: http://www.cdc.gov/ncipc/dvp/suicide/ SuicideDataSheet.pdf. Accessed December 5, 2008.

9. Available at: http://www.fda.gov/opacom/morechoices/mission. html. Accessed December 5, 2008.

10. Available at: http://www.mayoclinic.com/health/breast-cancer/ WO00092. Accessed December 5, 2008.

11. Available at: http://www.fda.gov/bbs/topics/NEWS/2008/ NEW01772.html. Accessed December 5, 2008.

12. Available at: http://www.msnbc.msn.com/id/24953413/ wid/7279844/. Accessed December 5, 2008

13. Available at: http://cei.org/articles/sick-patients-need-cutting-edge-drugs.

14. Available at: http://www.pharmacistsletter.com/pl/newdrugs/ FDA2007.pdf?cs=&s=PL. Accessed December 5, 2008.

15. Available at: http://pharmacytechniciansletter.com/pl/new-drugs/FDA2008.pdf?cs=&s=PTL. Accessed December 5, 2008.

16. Available at: http://www.ahrp.org/cms/content/view/ 476/28/. Accessed December 5, 2008.

17. Available at: http://www.ahrp.org/cms/index2.php?option= com_content&do_pdf=1&id=476.

18. Available at: http://finance.senate.gov/press/Bpress/2007press/ prb030707a.pdf. Accessed December 5, 2008.

19. Available at: http://online.wsj.com/article/ SB120355185318681367.html. Accessed December 5, 2008.

20. Available at: http://assets.aarp.org/rgcenter/post-import/ dd113_generic_drugs.pdf. Accessed December 5, 2008.

21. Available at: http://www.ustreas.gov/offices/public-affairs/hsa/ pdf/pl108–173.pdf. Accessed December 5, 2008.

22. Available at: http://www.aafp.org/fpm/20050300/49what. html. Accessed December 5, 2008.

23. Available at: http://www.nytimes.com/2008/10/05/ opinion/05sun4.html?ref=opinion. Accessed December 5, 2008.

24. Available at: http://www.washingtonpost.com/wp-dyn/
content/article/2008/10/01/AR2008100103061_pf.html.
Accessed December 5, 2008.

25. Available at: http://energycommerce.house.gov/
Press_110/110nr362.shtml. Accessed December 5, 2008.

Millions of Needless Deaths

by William Faloon

I T IS HARD TO IMAGINE, BUT IT WAS NOT UNTIL **1867** THAT **JOSEPH** Lister published his findings about the critical need of using sterile procedures in the surgical setting. Back then, doctors seldom washed their hands prior to surgery, let alone sterilize the instruments they had used on the previous patient.

Before Dr. Lister's sterile techniques were adopted, patients frequently died from infections introduced during surgery.

Joseph Lister had little interest in financial or social success. These traits enabled him to endure the criticisms hurled by the medical establishment about the extra steps he took to ensure his surgical environments were clean.

One of Dr. Lister's greatest challenges was to persuade his colleagues that germs did in fact exist. Back then, most doctors still believed in the theory of spontaneous generation.[1]

Convincing today's medical establishment about proven methods to save lives may be less daunting than what Dr. Lister encountered, but it is still nonetheless challenging.

TODAY'S BODY COUNT

Back in 2007, I urged the federal government to declare a national emergency. My rationale was that millions of Americans were going to needlessly die if the epidemic of vitamin D insufficiency was not immediately corrected. My article was based on irrefutable scientific evidence documenting how vast numbers of lives could be spared if everyone took at least 1,000 IU of vitamin D3 each day.[2]

I went a step further and showed how mandatory vitamin D supplementation could resolve today's healthcare cost crisis by slashing the need for expensive prescription drugs and hospitalizations.[2]

I took it two steps further and offered to donate 50,000 one-year-supply bottles of vitamin D3 so the government could give these away to those who could not afford this ultra-low cost supplement.[2]

It is now 16 months later. The federal government has done nothing to inform the public of the opportunity to radically reduce their risk of dying by taking a supplement that costs less than six cents a day!

VITAMIN D MORE EFFECTIVE THAN PREVIOUSLY KNOWN

A large number of new vitamin D studies have appeared in the scientific literature since I wrote my plea to the federal government. These studies don't just confirm what we knew 16 months ago—they show that optimizing vitamin D intake will save even more lives than we projected.

For instance, a study published in June 2008 showed that men with low vitamin D levels suffer 2.42 times more heart attacks. Now look what this means in actual body counts.[3]

Each year, about 157,000 Americans die from coronary artery disease-related heart attacks.[4] Based on this most recent study, if every American optimized their vitamin D status, the number of deaths prevented from this kind of heart attack would be 92,500.

To put the number of lives saved in context, tens of millions of dollars are being spent to advertise that Lipitor® reduces heart attacks by 37%. This is certainly a decent number, but not when compared with how many lives could be saved by vitamin D. According to the latest study, men with the higher vitamin D levels had a 142% reduction in heart attacks.[3]

This does not mean that you should stop taking medications if you can't get your cardiac risk factors under control by natural methods. It does mean that you should make certain you are not vitamin D-insufficient.

Please note that all forms of heart disease kill over 869,700 Americans each year.[4] These lethal forms of heart disease include cardiomyopathy, valvular insufficiency, congestive heart failure, arrhythmia, coronary thrombosis (blood clot in coronary artery), and coronary atherosclerosis (narrowing or blockage of coronary arteries). There is reason to believe that vitamin D could help protect against most of these forms of cardiac-induced death.

BILLIONS OF DOLLARS IN HEALTHCARE SAVINGS

There are 920,000 heart attacks suffered in the United States every year.[4] According to the American Heart Association, the annual cost of healthcare services, medications, and lost productivity related to these heart attacks is over $156 billion.[4]

The annual retail cost of all 300 million Americans (including children) supplementing with 1,000 IU of vitamin D per day is $6.6 billion.

So if vitamin D's only benefit was to reduce coronary heart attack rates by 142%, the net savings (after deducting the cost of the vitamin D) if every American supplemented properly would be around $84 billion each year. That's enough to put a major dent in the healthcare cost crisis that is forecast to bankrupt Medicare and many private insurance plans.

SPARING COUNTLESS NUMBERS FROM THE AGONIES OF CANCER

The evidence supporting the role of vitamin D in preventing common forms of cancer is now overwhelming.[2]

Vitamin D-deficient women, for example, have a 253% increased risk of colon cancer.[6] Colon cancer strikes 145,000 Americans each year and 53,580 die from it.[7] Based on these studies, if everyone obtained enough vitamin D, 38,578 lives could be saved and medical costs would be reduced by $3.89 billion.[8,9]

A study published in January 2008 showed that women with the lowest level of vitamin D were at a 222% increased risk for developing breast cancer.[10] Most studies show that higher levels of vitamin D can reduce breast cancer incidence by around 30–50%.[11–14]

Each year, approximately 186,800 women are diagnosed with breast cancer and 40,950 perish from it in the United States.[15] This needless toll of suffering and death caused by insufficient intake of vitamin D is unconscionable.

Prostate cancer will be diagnosed in an estimated 189,000 American men this year. Almost 30,000 will die from it.[16] Men with higher levels of vitamin D have a 52% reduced incidence of prostate cancer.[17]

The first-year costs of prostate cancer treatment are approximately $14,540.[18] If all aging men achieved sufficient vitamin D status, about $1.4 billion could be saved each year.

So as you can see, there is no real healthcare cost crisis. What the population suffers from is frighteningly low blood levels of vitamin D. During winter months in Canada, for instance, an estimated 97% of the population is vitamin D-deficient.[19]

VITAMIN D PROTECTS AGAINST STROKE

Stroke is the number three cause of death in the United States.[20] It is also one of the most feared diseases because of its high incidence of permanent disability.

In a study published in September 2008, blood indicators of vitamin D status were measured in 3,316 patients with suspected coronary artery disease. The subjects were followed for 7.75 years. For every small decrease in blood indicators of vitamin D status, there was a startling 86% increase in the number of fatal strokes.[21]

The doctors who conducted this study concluded:

> Low levels of 25(OH)D* and 1,25(OH)2D* are independently predictive for fatal strokes, suggesting that vitamin D supplementation is a promising approach in the prevention of strokes.[21]

If all that vitamin D did was to reduce stroke risk, it would be critically important for every American to ensure optimal blood levels.

LOW VITAMIN D DOUBLES DEATH RATE

Vitamin D deficiency is a worldwide problem. Yet no conventional medical organization or governmental body has declared a health emergency to warn the public about the urgent need of achieving sufficient vitamin D blood levels.

According to John Jacob Cannell, MD, founder of the nonprofit Vitamin D Counsel:

> Current research indicates vitamin D deficiency plays a role in causing seventeen varieties of cancer as well as heart disease, stroke, hypertension, autoimmune diseases, diabetes, depression, chronic pain, osteoarthritis, osteoporosis, muscle weakness, muscle wasting, birth defects, and periodontal disease.

---

* 25[OH]D and 1,25[OH]2D are blood markers that measure vitamin D status in one's body.

This does not mean that vitamin D deficiency is the only cause of these diseases, or that you will not get them if you take vitamin D. What it does mean is that vitamin D, and the many ways in which it affects a person's health, can no longer be overlooked by the healthcare industry nor by individuals striving to achieve and maintain a greater state of health.[22]

Vitamin D seems to reduce the risk of almost every killer disease of aging. In fact, a recent study shows that humans with low vitamin D status are twice as likely to die over a seven-year time period![5]

Each year, the federal government spends $1 billion in research aimed at finding ways to prevent or cure the killer diseases of aging.[23] Yet the government is oblivious to the most medically effective and cost-effective way of preventing needless death. This is analogous to how the establishment ignored Joseph Lister's pleas for a sterile environment in the surgical arena.

DIFFERENCE BETWEEN "DEFICIENCY" AND "INSUFFICIENCY"

Doctors are not trained to recognize a vitamin D deficiency until rickets develop in children or osteomalacia (softening of the bones) develops in adults. Clinical vitamin D deficiency is diagnosed when blood levels of a vitamin D metabolite (25-hydroxyvitamin D) drop below 12 ng/mL.

According to the world's foremost experts, however, optimal blood levels of vitamin D are between 30 and 50 ng/mL and higher.[24,25] Those with blood levels below 30 ng/mL are considered to have insufficient vitamin D.

These widely varying numbers explain why mainstream medicine is at a loss to understand the widespread health problem created by less than optimal vitamin D levels. If physicians view a patient's medical chart and see a vitamin D blood level of 18 ng/mL, they will think this person has adequate vitamin D. The reality is that a vitamin D blood level this low predisposes this patient to virtually every killer disease of aging and may in fact be the reason that individual has become a "patient" instead of remaining healthy.

There clearly is a need for a new consensus in the medical community to redefine vitamin D deficiency as a blood reading below 30 ng/mL. As we at *Life Extension* long ago learned, it can take decades for the establishment to change its reference ranges to reflect scientific reality.

WHAT CAN BE DONE?

Despite the startling number of needless deaths, the federal government has done nothing to warn the public of the lethal dangers associated with vitamin D insufficiency.

We will distribute my original 2007 article along with this editorial to every member of the new Congress and the President in January 2009. Hopefully someone will understand the urgency of declaring a health emergency and advise that every American maintain a vitamin D blood level of at least 30 ng/mL (and preferably above 50 ng/mL).

If the government continues to ignore our pleas, perhaps private insurance companies will consider sending free bottles of vitamin D supplements to all of their subscribers. The outlays for medical procedures and prescription drugs would be expected to plummet in groups who took their vitamin D supplement each day.

The media has done a good job in reporting on the numerous positive findings about vitamin D over the past two years. Sales of vitamin D supplements have been increasing, so at least some Americans are getting the message and taking steps to guard against vitamin D insufficiency.

In the meantime, *Life Extension* will continue to report on new findings about vitamin D. We have found that if we repeat a message long enough, much of the public will wake up to scientific reality and the desire for self-preservation.

All Hospitalized Patients Should be Tested for Vitamin D

The pioneer of antiseptic procedures in the hospital setting was a Hungarian physician named Ignaz Semmelweis. In one of the world's great detective stories, Dr. Semmelweis went back 100 years to find out why there was such an increase in puerperal fever (child-bed fever) that had killed thousands of mothers in obstetric units.

Dr. Semmelweis correlated increases in autopsies performed at hospitals with greater incidences of lethal puerperal fever. It turned out that doctors would leave an autopsy room with their hands covered in decomposing human tissues (and lots of bacteria) and deliver babies with their fetid hands.

Semmelweis instructed his interns to wash their hands with chlorinated lime solutions and documented an immediate reduction in puerperal fever incidence.

Despite the logic of his arguments and concrete proof shown by the reduction in mortality when handwashing procedures were followed, Semmelweis faced a wall of opposition. Back in those days, maternity hospitals had horrendous reputations and were sometimes referred to as deathtraps. Some suggested that lives could be saved simply by closing the clinics where people went in with minor problems and ended up dying agonizing deaths. Doctors of the day refused to accept that they were the ones responsible for the deaths of thousands of young woman. Semmelweis was eventually committed to an insane asylum where he died.

Move forward to 2009, and hospitals are still places to avoid. Medical errors, antibiotic-resistant infections, sleep interruption, pneumonia, and malnutrition continue to ravage those confined to the hospital setting.

An overlooked problem with institutional confinement is that patients admitted with insufficient vitamin D can rapidly develop severe vitamin D deficiency due to complete lack of sunlight and malnutrition caused by commotion in the hospital environment.

A strong argument could be made that every patient admitted to a hospital should have their blood tested for vitamin D and supplements administered to ensure that blood levels remain considerably above 30 ng/mL. The improvement in immune function along with reduced inflammatory responses alone could result in many more patients leaving via the hospital lobby rather than its morgue.

There are respected medical authorities today advocating universal vitamin D supplementation, but their pleas are all but ignored by most practicing doctors. Unlike the plight of women in childbirth exposed to puerperal fever by ignorant doctors in the past, no informed person has to suffer from lack of vitamin D. More and more people are taking their supplements with them when they go to the hospital because they know they will need them there more than in any other place.

WHERE TO PURCHASE VITAMIN D

Fortunately, the patent for synthesizing vitamin D expired long ago. It is an ultra-low-cost supplement available at any health food store, pharmacy, and most grocery stores. There is no economic impediment precluding immediate widespread supplementation.

Please know we remain relentless in tearing down the walls of medical ignorance that are by far the leading causes of disability and death in the United States.

References

1. Available at: http://en.wikipedia.org/wiki/Abiogenesis. Accessed September 4, 2008.
2. Faloon W. Should the president declare a national emergency? *Life Extension.* 2007 Oct;13(10):7–17.
3. Giovannucci E, Liu Y, Hollis BW, Rimm EB. 25-hydroxyvitamin D and risk of myocardial infarction in men: a prospective study. *Arch Intern Med.* 2008 Jun 9;168(11):1174–80.
4. Available at: www.americanheart.org/downloadable/heart/1200082005246HS_Stats%202008.final.pdf. Accessed October 29, 2008.
5. Dobnig H, Pilz S, Scharnagl H, et al. Independent association of low serum 25-hydroxyvitamin d and 1,25-dihydroxyvitamin d levels with all-cause and cardiovascular mortality. *Arch Intern Med.* 2008 Jun 23;168(12):1340–9.

6. Holick MF. Vitamin D and sunlight: strategies for cancer prevention and other health benefits. *Clin J Am Soc Nephrol.* 2008 Sep;3(5):1548–54.

7. Available at: www.cdc.gov/cancer/colorectal/statistics/. Accessed September 4, 2008.

8. Lappe JM, Travers-Gustafson D, Davies KM, Recker RR, Heaney RP. Vitamin D and calcium supplementation reduces cancer risk: results of a randomized trial. *Am J Clin Nutr.* 2007 Jun;85(6):1586–91.

9. Brown ML, Lipscomb J, Snyder C. The burden of illness and cancer: economic cost and quality of life. *Annu Rev Public Health.* 2001;22:91–113.

10. Abbas S, Linseisen J, Slanger T, et al. Serum 25-hydroxyvitamin D and risk of post-menopausal breast cancer—results of a large case-control study. *Carcinogenesis.* 2008 Jan;29(1):93–9.

11. Rossi M, McLaughlin JK, Lagiou P, et al. Vitamin D intake and breast cancer risk: a case-control study in Italy. *Ann Oncol.* 2008 Aug 18.

12. Giovannucci E. Vitamin D and cancer incidence in the Harvard Cohorts. *Ann Epidemiol.* 2008 Feb 19.

13. Abbas S, Linseisen J, Chang-Claude J. Dietary vitamin D and calcium intake and premenopausal breast cancer risk in a German case-control study. *Nutr Cancer.* 2007;59(1):54–61.

14. Robien K, Cutler GJ, Lazovich D. Vitamin D intake and breast cancer risk in postmenopausal women: the Iowa Women's Health Study. *Cancer Causes Control.* 2007 Sep;18(7):775–82.

15. Available at: www.cdc.gov/cancer/breast/statistics/. Accessed October 28, 2008.

16. Available at: www.cdc.gov/cancer/prostate/statistics/. Accessed October 28, 2008.

17. Li H, Stampfer MJ, Hollis JB, et al. A prospective study of plasma vitamin D metabolites, vitamin D receptor polymorphisms, and prostate cancer. *PLoS Med.* 2007 Mar;4(3):e103.

18. Wilson LS, Tesoro R, Elkin EP, et al. Cumulative cost pattern comparison of prostate cancer treatments. *Cancer.* 2007 Feb 1;109(3):518–27.

19. Available at: http://vitamins-minerals.suite101.com/article. cfm/the_sunshine_vitamin; http://www.vitamindsociety.org/. Accessed September 4, 2008.

20. Available at: www.cdc.gov/nchs/fastats/deaths.htm. Accessed September 4, 2008.

21. Pilz S, Dobnig H, Fischer JE, et al. Low vitamin D levels predict stroke in patients referred to coronary angiography. *Stroke.* 2008 Sep;39(9):2611–3.

22. Available at: http://74.125.45.104/search?q=cache:fgZo6Q5-SO8J:www.vitamindcouncil.org /+Current+research+indicate s+vitamin+D+deficiency+plays+a+role+in+causing+seventeen &hl=en&ct= clnk&cd=1&gl=us. Accessed September 4, 2008.

23. Available at: www.nia.nih.gov/AboutNIA/NACA/MeetingInformation/DirStatusReportMay2007.htm. Accessed September 4, 2008.

24. Vieth R. Vitamin D supplementation, 25-hydroxyvitamin D concentrations, and safety. *Am J Clin Nutr.* 1999 May;69(5):842–56.

25. Holick MF. The role of vitamin D for bone health and fracture prevention. *Curr Osteoporos Rep.* 2006 Sep;4(3):96–102.

2008

Would You Tolerate This Abuse?

by William Faloon

AMERICANS NEEDLESSLY DIE WHILE SCIENTIFIC DISCOVERIES that could save their lives remain trapped in bureaucratic red tape.

There is a solution to this travesty. Allow free market innovation into the healthcare arena, and the development of new medical therapies will progress as rapidly as other technologies.

Do you remember how expensive long distance phone calling used to be?

Back in 1980, archaic federal rules enabled the original AT&T to control national long distance dialing. You could recognize a long distance call by the hissing and crackling noise heard before the caller spoke. High-speed Internet and mobile phone connections were not available.

CONSUMERS FOUGHT BACK

There was quite a debate around 1980 as to whether consumers would benefit if other companies were allowed to compete in offering long distance services. AT&T heavily lobbied Congress arguing that all kinds of terrible problems would occur if it lost its monopoly.

AT&T pointed to its stellar record of scientific advances and threatened that if it could not charge its monopolistic rates, then further improvements in communications technology would be hindered. AT&T's track record for scientific prowess gave them a strong argument.

Fortunately, free market theory prevailed and AT&T was forced to relinquish its stranglehold over long distance calling in the United States. The transition was by no means smooth. The initial long distance competitors' services were clearly inferior to AT&T. One newspaper columnist complained that he was tired of being solicited by these substandard discount carriers and wanted the government to reinstate AT&T's monopoly.

HOW TIMES HAVE CHANGED

Anyone who has paid attention to long distance rates over the past 28 years appreciates the enormity of the benefit brought about by abolishing AT&T's monopoly.

Consumers used to pay over 60 cents per minute for daytime long distance calls (equal to $1.39 per minute in today's depreciated dollars).[1] Can you imagine if you had to pay $250 for three hours of long distance calling? This would be unthinkable today where for under $40 a month, you can have an unlimited long distance service that usually includes local connection charges.

Consumers today save a whopping 84% compared with 1980, even if they only make three hours of long distance calls a month. Unlike AT&T's threats of technological stagnation, the quality, reliability, and speed of today's long distance phone service are vastly superior.

WHY DO AMERICANS TOLERATE PHARMACEUTICAL MONOPOLIES?

What if the federal government outlawed long distance competition and returned to the monopolistic ways of the past? If this were to occur, every elected politician who voted for this would be thrown out of office.

Yet the public today tolerates federal and state laws that enable pharmaceutical companies to conduct business as a virtual monopoly. The result is that Americans pay outlandish prices for mediocre drugs that are often laden with side effects.

As AT&T did in 1980, drug companies seek to deceive Congress and the public by stating their high prices are needed in order to discover better technologies. The reality is that after decades of exorbitant drug pricing, one's odds of surviving a serious disease using conventional methods are not substantially improving. Yet drug prices are exponentially higher.

Citizen apathy has allowed this economic and medical bloodbath to occur. One of Life Extension's missions is to provide the hard facts so that today's antiquated regulatory system can be eradicated. We believe that in a free market environment, technological breakthroughs that occurred in telecommunications will also happen in medicine.

UNREGULATED SUPPLEMENT PRICES PLUMMET

Unlike regulated prescription drugs, the cost of dietary supplements has plummeted over the past three decades.

For example, when coenzyme Q10 (CoQ10) was first introduced to Americans in 1983, a bottle containing 1,000 mg (100 10-mg capsules) retailed for $30. In 2008, the retail price of a bottle containing 5,000 mg (100 50-mg capsules) of a superior form of CoQ10 (ubiquinol) is $58. Based on milligram potency alone, the cost in inflation-adjusted dollars for CoQ10 has come down by 83%.

If the FDA had succeeded in turning CoQ10 into a drug as it tried to do in the early 1980s, you might be paying $337.50 for what retails now for $58.

Under the FDA's regulatory stranglehold, it is unlikely that the superior ubiquinol form of CoQ10 would have been "approved" any time soon. This would force Americans to pay the inflated price ($337.50 per bottle) for a less-than-optimal product. This illogic is what monopolies are all about, and why they cannot be allowed to exist.

If one looks at the price history of dietary supplements, costs are substantially lower now than when they were originally brought out. When SAMe was first introduced to Americans in 1996, it cost $45 for 4,000 mg (twenty 200 mg tablets). This was the European-regulated "drug" price. Soon after it became an *unregulated* supplement, the price went down a great deal. As more manufacturers competed to make SAMe, the price plummeted to where Life Extension members can obtain 8,000 mg (twenty 400 mg tablets) for only $21. Thus SAMe now costs 77% less than when it was originally introduced.

Prescription drug costs, on the other hand, have skyrocketed at a rate that far exceeds inflation. The difference is that prescription drugs are heavily regulated, as opposed to dietary supplements that are sold under free market conditions.

TODAY'S HEALTHCARE CATASTROPHE

Today's healthcare calamities are so numerous it is not possible to fit them into one issue of *Life Extension* magazine. To remind you of recent findings, we have reprinted a few of the appalling headlines.[2-10]

As you can clearly see by these reports, unless radical legal changes are made, Americans will continue to pay high prices for dangerous drugs that have limited efficacy.

More frightening is the suffocating effect that regulation has on the discovery of life-saving therapies. Just imagine if advancement in clinical medicine progressed at the same rapid rate as telecommunications. If it did, we would probably have cures for most killer diseases today!

For example, the first direct-dial transcontinental telephone call occurred in 1951.[11] That first call took 18 seconds to complete, had lots of static in the background, and most consumers could not readily afford it. Move forward to 2008, and we all have access to clear phone connections across the country instantly at minimal cost.

Now look at the dire prognosis for pancreatic cancer patients today. A patient diagnosed with pancreatic cancer in 2008 typically lives just a few months longer compared with 1951.[12-14] Yet the price for these additional months of life can be thousands of times higher than that in 1951.[15]

We need to swiftly improve medical science at a speed analogous to telecommunications, computers, and other unregulated technologies.

SCATHING FDA REPORT PROVIDES BASIS TO REVOLUTIONIZE MEDICINE

The FDA has provided a rare opportunity to enact legislation that can enable Americans to quickly gain access to life-saving medical therapies.

The FDA recently did a study of itself and its findings revealed that it is scientifically incompetent and incapable of doing its job.[16,17] These are not mere allegations from outside critics, but are instead the FDA itself admitting that it cannot carry out its mission.

There has never been a better time for a comprehensive overhaul of the FDA. Everything about it—from its mission to its management—needs to be taken apart, reviewed, redefined, and recreated so that it helps support, rather than obstruct, a vibrant free market in healthcare science.

CAN LOGIC PREVAIL OVER LETHAL DOGMA?

There are pessimists who think Americans will not be able to achieve true health freedom in the immediate future. Naysayers complain that if free market principles are extended to healthcare, some terminally ill patients will die sooner if experimental therapies fail.

Again, review what happened when long distance phone calling was deregulated. Sure, there were problems in the beginning, but look at where we are today with a dependable low-cost phone service affordable to all. Even more impressive are the incredible advancements in high-speed internet access and mobile phone connectivity that would have been unthinkable in the early 1980s.

Life Extension's enthusiasm for a free market approach to healthcare is based on its confidence in judging which novel medical therapies are truly safe and effective. A look at *Life Extension's* 28-year track record shows that it has been able to identify life-saving approaches to combating disease long before they are approved by the FDA.

Has LEF made mistakes? Yes, we have fallen victim to a few fraudulent studies that caused us to recommend products that we later found did not work. We have not, however, recommended products that killed anyone. Contrast this to regulated FDA-approved drugs that have collectively killed millions of Americans over the past three decades.

The logic of letting the free market determine what therapies Americans may use to prevent and treat disease will defeat the cynics who fear changing the regulatory quagmire that exists today. Existing laws that protect against real health fraud will still enable charlatans to be stopped and prosecuted.

Headline Quotes Reveal Just A Few Examples of Today's Healthcare Crisis

THE $34 TRILLION PROBLEM

Medicare is poised to wreak havoc on the economy. And our politicians are avoiding the issue.[2]

ELI LILLY SETTLES ZYPREXA® LAWSUIT

$15 million settlement announced; state of Alaska alleged the drug caused health problems that cost Medicaid program hundreds of millions.[3]

STUDY: DRUG ERRORS HURT ONE IN FIFTEEN HOSPITALIZED KIDS

Medicine errors, overdoses, bad reactions harm one in 15 hospitalized kids. This estimate translates to 7.3% of hospitalized children, or 540,000 kids annually. Patient safety experts say that the problem is most likely even bigger than the study suggests.[4]

US LAGS BEHIND FORTY-ONE NATIONS IN LIFE SPAN

For decades, the United States has been slipping in international rankings of life expectancy, as other countries improve healthcare, nutrition, and lifestyles.[5]

FDA BLAMED FOR DIP IN NEW DRUGS

New drug approvals down 31% so far this year: report; FDA still stinging from Vioxx® approval.[6]

BUREAUCRATIC OBSTACLES SHOULDN'T STAND IN THE WAY OF THE TERMINALLY ILL

Back in 2001, a vivacious, 21-year-old student at the University of Virginia—Abigail Burroughs—died of cancer. Her death was particularly heart-wrenching because, in the final weeks of her life, she was denied access to two investigational anticancer drugs recommended by her oncologist. The FDA later approved the drugs.[7]

US REPORTS OF DEATH, SIDE EFFECTS FROM PRESCRIPTION DRUGS TRIPLE

Reports of dangerous side effects and deaths from widely used medicines almost tripled between 1998 and 2005, an analysis of US drug data found.[8]

WOMAN LEFT IN CT SCANNER AFTER CLINIC CLOSES

A cancer patient says she was left alone in a CT scanner for hours after a technician apparently forgot about her. She finally crawled out of the device, only to find herself locked in the closed clinic. Doctor says it has happened before.[9]

BREAST CANCER PATIENTS MAY FACE MORE HEART RISK

Breast cancer survivors may face increased risk of heart disease. Doctors are debating if it is time to largely abandon a chemotherapy mainstay that is one reason for the problem.[10]

References

1. *Consumer Reports*. 1983. Nov;48(11): 618–20.

2. Available at: http://money.cnn.com/2008/03/03/news/economy/104239768.fortune/index.htm. Accessed June 23, 2008.

3. Available at: http://www.newsinferno.com/archives/1589. Accessed June 23, 2008.

4. Available at: http://www.cnn.com/2008/HEALTH/04/07/children.drug.errors.ap/index.html. Accessed June 23, 2008.

5. Available at: http://www.boston.com/news/education/higher/articles/ 2007/08/1 1/us_life_span_shorter/. Accessed June 23, 2008.

6. Available at: http://money.cnn.com/2007/08/15/news/companies/fda/index.htm. Accessed June 23, 2008.

7. Available at: http://blogs.usatoday.com/oped/2007/08/our-view-on-exp.html. Accessed June 23, 2008.

8. Available at: http://www.foxnews.com/story/0,2933,296427,00.html. Accessed June 23, 2008.

9. Available at: http://www.msnbc.msn.com/id/21033714/. Accessed June 23, 2008.

10. Available at:http://www.kmov.com/justposted/stories/kmov_health_071008_breastcancerheart.14e95c1d0.html. Accessed June 23, 2008.

11. Available at: http://www.corp.att.com/attlabs/reputation/timeline/51trans.html. Accessed June 23, 2008.

12. Stewart RJ, Stewart AW, Stewart JM, Ibister WH. Cancer of the pancreas in New Zealand 1970–1974. *Aust N Z J Surg.* 1982 Aug;52(4):379–84.

13. Available at: http://www.pancreatica.org/Pancreatica%20 Media%20Sheet.pdf. Accessed June 26, 2008.

14. Czernichow P, Lerebours E, Colin R. Epidemiology of cancer of the pancreas. Current data. *Presse Med.* 1986 Feb 22;15 (8):387–91.

15. Available at: http://www.medscape.com/viewarticle/409001_2. Accessed June 26, 2008. 16 Faloon W. The FDA indicts itself. *Life Extension.* 2008 July;14(7):7–11.

16. Available at: http://www.fda.gov/ohrms/dockets/AC/07/ briefing/2007-4329b_02_01_FDA%20Report%20on%20 Science%20and%20Technology.pdf. Accessed June 23, 2008.

17. Available at: http://www.apma.net/aahf/default.asp. Accessed June 23, 2008.

JULY 2008

The FDA Indicts Itself

by William Faloon

B ACK IN THE EARLY 1980S, LIFE EXTENSION PREDICTED HOR-rific tragedies if government control over healthcare was not abolished. The heartbreaking fact is that tens of millions of Americans have needlessly suffered and died because of FDA incompetence . . . and the FDA now admits its own incompetence!

These tens of millions of lives lost are not statistics of strangers. Virtually everyone has family or friends who have been victimized by dangerous drugs or denied access to life-saving ones.

FDA UNCOVERS ITS OWN INADEQUACIES

The FDA, in collusion with pharmaceutical giants and conventional medical orthodoxy, is the leading cause of suffering and death in the United States.

Back in the early days, the FDA would defend its position by proclaiming that it served to protect the public's health. An endless number of well-publicized scandals have caused the FDA itself to admit that it is incapable of carrying out its mission.[1-10]

If all the FDA did was act so cautiously that it almost never approved a dangerous drug, then at least the agency could point to some consumer value it provides. Instead, we are plagued by an antiquated regulatory agency that stifles the development of novel life-saving medications, while allowing a slew of drugs to be sold that have cumulatively cost millions of lives.

Americans thus suffer the "worst of both worlds" as they are poisoned by FDA-sanctioned prescription drugs, but denied the fruits of novel approaches to disease prevention and treatment.

FDA'S INDICTMENT OF ITSELF

In response to a barrage of criticisms, FDA commissioner Dr. Edward von Eschenbach requested that a special committee assess whether the FDA is capable of doing its job. The premise for the FDA's massive audit of itself was the fear that "the nation is at risk if FDA science is at risk."

Their sixty-page report, entitled "FDA Science and Mission at Risk,"[11] states that "the world of drug discovery and development has undergone revolutionary change," but the FDA's "evaluation methods have remained largely unchanged over the last half century. "

The following are exact quotes from the report:

- The FDA cannot fulfill its mission because its scientific base has eroded and its scientific organizational structure is weak.
- The FDA cannot fulfill its mission because its scientific work force does not have sufficient capacity and capability.
- The FDA cannot fulfill its mission because its information technology (IT) infrastructure is inadequate.
- The FDA does not have the capacity to ensure the safety of food for the nation.

- The development of medical products based on "new science" cannot be adequately regulated by the FDA.
- There is insufficient capacity in modeling, risk assessment, and analysis.
- The FDA science agenda lacks a coherent structure and vision, as well as effective coordination and prioritization.
- The FDA has substantial recruitment and retention challenges.
- The FDA has an inadequate and ineffective program for scientist performance.
- The FDA has not taken sufficient advantage of external and internal collaborations.
- The FDA lacks the information science capability and information infrastructure to fulfill its regulatory mandate.
- The FDA cannot provide the information infrastructure support to regulate products based on new science.

Most appalling is the FDA's own finding that it "cannot even keep up with the advances in science."[11] Said differently, this means that the FDA cannot keep up with scientific breakthroughs that could cumulatively save millions of human lives!

RESPONSES TO THE FDA'S DAMNING REPORT OF ITSELF

The *Wall Street Journal* wrote an editorial titled "The Real FDA Scandal" and quoted the following about the FDA's admitted statement:

> Particularly in complex and specialized fields like genomics and biotechnology medicine, the FDA lacks the basic competence "to understand the impact of product use, to maintain ongoing currency with their evolution or to evaluate the sophisticated products produced" and "to support innovation in the industries and markets that it regulates."[12]

The *Wall Street Journal* further wrote, "Think about that: We live amid a revolution in biology, but the FDA still thinks like it did when Sputnik launched."[12]

Dr. David Kessler was the most publicly recognized FDA commissioner of all time. Dr. Kessler is still sought out by the media as a proponent on FDA issues. In response to this horrific report, however, Dr. Kessler stated, "The problems are way bigger than one commissioner. . . . I'm not sure how anybody could do this job now."[13]

FDA commissioner Eschenbach stated, "I think to do what we need to do requires substantially more dollars than what has been invested in the FDA so far. . . . This is a systemic overhaul that must go on for years."[13]

PROBLEMS ARE WORSE THAN FDA ADMITS

Many recent reports from outside organizations have been harshly critical of the FDA. These reports made national news for a day or two and were then quickly forgotten.[14-24]

Our greatest impediment to saving human lives is an incompetent and corrupt federal bureaucracy that is strangling medical innovation, especially in the areas of genomics and biotechnology where breakthroughs in anti-aging medicine are most expected.

In discussions with scientists about methods to significantly extend our life spans, the problem with "the FDA" inevitably arises. If the FDA's bureaucratic roadblock is not torn down, we may all succumb to a disease that liberated scientists could readily prevent or cure.

There is not a magic immortality pill that the FDA is directly suppressing. Instead, the FDA is restraining the ability for medical science to progress. This is no longer just opinion. The FDA itself admits it cannot keep up with advances in science. So discoveries that could save human lives are not getting approved by the FDA and the cost is thousands of American lives being lost each day.

WHAT CAN BE DONE TO STOP THIS CARNAGE

There are a number of proposals to turn around this lethal barrier to medical progress called the Food and Drug Administration (FDA). Some politicians say throw more tax dollars at the problem, while other politicians refuse to reward an agency with so much documented incompetence.

The FDA's own report makes it clear that scientific innovation is suffocated by bureaucratic red tape and incompetency. Yet a medical renaissance is needed if our generation is to achieve dramatically extended life spans.

The only way to liberate scientific ingenuity is to allow Americans to obtain therapies that are clearly marked "Not approved by the FDA." Under this free market scenario, those who want the so-called "protection" the FDA previously pretended it provided could continue receiving it.

Enlightened individuals and their doctors, on the other hand, would be able to choose novel therapies that are clearly labeled "Not approved by the FDA."

Since it costs so much for a new drug to be approved, therapies that do not have to go through this arduous (and antiquated) approval process would cost less than outlandishly priced "approved" prescription drugs.

DON'T LET MEDICAL INNOVATION BE HELD HOSTAGE TO FDA BUREAUCRACY!

Back in 2003, *Life Extension* initiated a poll on a website that has about 400,000 new visitors each month.[25] The people visiting this site are not part of any anti-FDA group, nor were they exposed to anti-FDA teachings. These people were asked a simple question as to whether terminally ill cancer patients should have the right to any drug that might save their life. The results, after 22,506 votes were tabulated:

Terminally Ill Cancer Patients:

- Should have access to any drug that might save their life: **89%**
- Should only have access to drugs approved by the FDA: **11%**

We live in a constitutional republic where the people's wishes are supposed to be adhered to (so long as they don't infringe on the rights of others). If 89% of the American public thinks terminal cancer patients should have access to any drug that could save their life, then there is no reason for the law not to be changed to allow Americans to access therapies "Not approved by the FDA."

Companies that engage in fraud could be prosecuted under consumer protection laws that already exist. The FDA could post its opinion about the safety and efficacy of unapproved therapies on its website (www.fda.gov). The civil litigation risks to companies that knowingly sell bogus products would preclude large-scale unsavory activities that some are concerned with. The greater fear Americans face is being diagnosed with a lethal disease only to find out that a cure is nowhere in sight.

REACTIONS TO THE FDA'S CONFESSION

The FDA's admission that it cannot do its job has stirred up a hornet's nest of outrage from organizations who have long argued that the FDA is the greatest impediment to the advancement of medical science.

A new bill has been drafted that is being presented by health freedom activists to our friends in Congress. Passage of this bill into law will liberate Americans from the FDA's nearly 50-year tyrannical rule over what therapies an individual is allowed to choose to remain alive. A remarkable number of divergent health organizations are finally recognizing the lethal consequences of ignoring the FDA's ineptitudes and have committed to backing this legislation.

American citizens deserve the right to choose what goes into their bodies. Those who prefer therapies that are "Not approved by the FDA" should be allowed to do so, especially now that the FDA has come to the conclusion that it is too incapable and incompetent to keep up with scientific advances.

References

1. Available at: http://www.naturalnews.com/002157.html. Accessed March 19, 2008.

2. Available at: http://www.drugresearcher.com/news/ng.asp?id=58116-fda-in-the. Accessed March 19, 2008.

3. Available at: http://www.drugresearcher.com/news/ng.asp?id=60304-whistleblowers-reveal-fda. Accessed March 19, 2008.

4. Available at: http://www.lawyersandsettlements.com/articles/00680/ketek-scandal.html. Accessed March 19, 2008.

5. Available at: http://www.mises.org/story/1805. Accessed March 19, 2008. Accessed March 19, 2008.

6. Available at: http://www.ghchealth.com/the-aspartame-scandal.html. Accessed March 19, 2008.

7. Available at: http://healthcarescandals.wordpress.com/category/fda/. Accessed March 19, 2008.

8. Available at: http://www.twnside.org.sg/title2/health.info/twninfohealth034.htm. Accessed March 19, 2008.

9. Available at: http://www.naturalnews.com/002439.html. Accessed March 19, 2008.

10. Available at: http://query.nytimes.com/gst/fullpage.html?res=950DE4DD1E38F930A2575BC0A96F948260. Accessed March 19, 2008.

11. Available at: http://www.fda.gov/ohrms/dockets/AC/07/briefing/2007-4329b_02_01_FDA%20Report%20on%20Science%20and%20Technology.pdf. Accessed March 20, 2008.

12. Available at: http://online.wsj.com/article/SB120225742208745785.html?mod=opinion_main_review_and_outlooks. Accessed March 20, 2008.

13. Available at: http://online.wsj.com/article/SB1204075529255 95245.html?mod=distsmartbrief&apl=y&r=49040. Accessed March 20, 2008.

14. Available at: http://money.cnn.com/2007/08/15/news/ companies/fda/index.htm. Accessed March 21, 2008.

15. Available at: http://www.safecosmetics.org/your_health/index. cfm. Accessed March 21, 2008.

16. Available at: http://www.cspinet.org/foodsafety/. Accessed March 21, 2008

17. Available at: http://goliath.ecnext.com/coms2/gi_0199-5599197/ GAO-report-criticizes-FDA-drug.html. Accessed March 21, 2008.

18. Available at: http://ahrp.blogspot.com/2008/03/ gao-to-investigate-fda-review-process.html. Accessed March 21, 2008

19. Available at: http://www.newsinferno.com/archives/2585. Accessed March 21, 2008.

20. Available at: http://www.ahrp.org/cms/content/view/46/28/. Accessed March 21, 2008.

21. Available at: http://www.uspirg.org/uspirg.asp?id2=24595. Accessed March 21, 2008.

22. Available at: http://www.iom.edu/CMS/3793/26341/37329. aspx. Accessed March 21, 2008.

23. Available at: http://www.lifesitenews.com/ldn/2006/ aug/06082405.html. Accessed March 21, 2008.

24. Available at: http://www.psrast.org/bghsalmonella.htm. Accessed March 21, 2008.

25. Available at: www.deathclock.com. Accessed March 21, 2008.

The FDA's Cruel Hoax

by William Faloon

D O YOU REMEMBER HOW POPULAR TRYPTOPHAN WAS IN the 1980s? Back in those days, people seeking to lose weight, improve sleep, or alleviate depression used tryptophan to safely increase serotonin levels in their brain.

Serotonin is the natural compound that promotes feelings of wellbeing, satiety, and relaxation. A serotonin deficiency can result in sleep disturbance, anxiety, depression, and a propensity to overeat.

In 1989, the FDA restricted the importation of tryptophan. This forced American consumers to switch to expensive prescription drugs that produced only partial effects at best.

Tryptophan is an amino acid found naturally in the foods that we eat. The reason its sale was stopped was because of defective tryptophan made by a substandard company.

The FDA's prejudicial position against tryptophan caused Americans to suffer widespread deficiencies of serotonin in their brains. A result of serotonin deficiency may be reflected in today's epidemic of obesity, depression, anxiety, and insomnia.

TRYPTOPHAN IS BACK!

Despite intense lobbying efforts by pharmaceutical companies, the FDA could not rationally continue to block the sale of tryptophan. After all, tryptophan is not only found in food, but the very tryptophan that the FDA restricted is still used in infant formulas and intravenous feeding solutions. If there were any danger to tryptophan, we would have known about it long ago.

Pharmaceutical-pure tryptophan can now be imported for use in dietary supplements. This means that aging Americans may be able to discard certain prescription drugs and once again treat their serotonin deficiency disorder with what Mother Nature intended all along . . . the amino acid tryptophan itself!

A FINANCIAL WINDFALL FOR THE DRUG COMPANIES

At the time that the FDA restricted tryptophan, it was one the most popular dietary supplements sold in the United States. Perhaps it is a coincidence, but since 1989, the percentages of overweight and obese adult Americans have soared. Could it be that a nationwide serotonin deficiency has led to the high-carbohydrate overeating syndrome that so many Americans suffer from today?

The removal of tryptophan created an economic windfall for the drug companies. Sales of drugs that interfere with the brain's reuptake of serotonin (like Prozac®, and later Paxil® and Zoloft®) shot through the roof, earning tens of billions of dollars of profits for drug companies. While these drugs caused large numbers of unpleasant and possibly lethal side effects, the FDA withdrew none of them.

The ensuing epidemic of weight gain and sleeplessness resulted in dozens of anti-obesity and anti-insomnia drugs being approved by the FDA, some of which had horrendous side effects, and others that had virtually no efficacy.

Critics contend that the contaminated tryptophan coming from one substandard Japanese company provided a convenient excuse for the FDA to restrict the sale of all tryptophan dietary supplements. The FDA's actions guaranteed that Americans would become tryptophan-deficient, and therefore turn to prescription drugs for relief from a host of disorders related to insufficient serotonin in the brain.

PHARMACEUTICAL-PURE TRYPTOPHAN NOW AVAILABLE

Consumers now have access to pharmaceutical-pure tryptophan as an over-the-counter dietary supplement. According to the FDA, it is now the responsibility of the company who sells the tryptophan to ensure that it is not contaminated.

For 19 years, aging Americans have been forced to settle for less-than-optimal levels of tryptophan/serotonin in their bodies.

Based on what has been published in the peer-reviewed scientific literature, it would appear that consumers have suffered enormously from a host of disorders related to lack of serotonin in the brain.

Pharmaceutical companies, on the other hand, have accumulated exorbitant wealth, as depressed, overweight, and sleep-deprived consumers were forced to experiment with costly and side effect-laden drugs in order to combat the effects of serotonin deficiency.

If tryptophan dietary supplements provide relief to those suffering from common age-related disorders such as anxiety, depressed mood, sleeplessness, and unwanted weight gain, the FDA's nearly two-decade restriction on this natural agent may turn out to be one of the cruelest hoaxes of all time.

2007

The Little-Known Dangers of Acetaminophen

by Jay S. Cohen, MD

WHAT IF A DIETARY SUPPLEMENT WAS PROVEN TO CAUSE liver damage, liver failure and death? What if each year, this same supplement caused 100,000 calls to poison control centers, 56,000 emergency room visits, 26,000 hospitalizations, and more than 450 deaths from liver failure alone?

You know the answer. The FDA would immediately shut down the supplement company and seek to incarcerate the principals for life.

What if, on the other hand, a highly profitable drug caused this much disease and death? To no one's surprise, the FDA's response is to do the equivalent of nothing.

As we learned long ago, the FDA too often functions to protect the financial interests of pharmaceutical companies. The FDA's intentional inaction in this instance proves that this agency couldn't care less about how many Americans suffer and die each year.

Many people assume that over-the-counter medications are safe when taken as directed. Yet even at recommended doses, aspirin can cause ulcers, antihistamines can cause sedation, and acetaminophen can cause serious liver damage.

You can read about some of these risks in the product information that accompanies over-the-counter medicines. For example, the acetaminophen package insert warns about taking the drug if you consume three or more alcoholic drinks a day. The link between acetaminophen, alcohol, and an increased risk of liver damage was identified in the 1980s. This research identified another factor that can increase the risks associated with acetaminophen: fasting. This can refer to fasting due to abdominal upset or pain, nausea, vomiting, loss of appetite, anorexia, or malnutrition. Consider this case published in 1992:

> A 25-year-old, healthy Swedish man developed gastroenteritis while on holiday in Turkey. For a day and a half before flying home, the man experienced nausea and vomiting, and he was unable to keep food or liquid down. Noticeably ill during the flight, upon landing he was taken directly to a hospital. As his condition worsened, he was diagnosed with liver failure and transferred to await a liver transplant. Information from his brother, who had been with him in Turkey, indicated that the patient had taken 500 mg to 1,000 mg of acetaminophen two to three times each day, with a maximum total intake of 5,000–6,000 mg over two days. Unexpectedly, the patient's condition began to improve, liver transplantation was canceled, and he was discharged ten days later.[1]

What had the Swedish man done wrong to develop liver failure? Nothing. His use of acetaminophen was within the recommended dosage range. The maximum recommended dosage of acetamino-phen is 4,000 mg/day. The man took only 2,000 or 3,000 mg/day. He took acetaminophen merely to ease the pain of acute gastro-enteritis, as do thousands of people each day. He followed the rules but nearly died.

The doctors presenting this case concluded that liver toxicity "can occur after low, repeated doses of acetaminophen." They added, "The drug should not be used under conditions of star-vation, including acute gastroenteritis with nausea and vomit-ing."[1] Yet today, despite this report and many others, acetamino-phen products do not list a warning against using the drug when unable to eat.

A POWERFUL LIVER TOXIN

Many drugs can cause liver damage, liver failure, and death. Yet, acetaminophen prompts the most calls to poison control cen-ters—more than 100,000 per year. Each year, acetaminophen accounts for about 56,000 emergency room visits, 26,000 hos-pitalizations, and more than 450 deaths from liver failure.[2] Acet-aminophen causes more cases of acute liver failure than all other medications combined.[3]

In comparison to the millions of people who take acetamin-ophen each day without harm, the occurrence of liver failure and death is relatively rare. Still, many experts believe the num-bers are too high and must be reduced. Dr. William Lee, a highly respected expert on acetaminophen, wrote, "It still must be asked: Is this amount of injury and death really acceptable for an over-the-counter pain reliever?"[4]

UNINTENTIONAL OVERDOSES TAKE A HEAVY TOLL

Another daunting statistic about acetaminophen is that nearly half of all overdoses are unintentional.[5] These people do not intentionally take excessive amounts of acetaminophen; instead, they lose track of the amount they are taking and inadvertently take more than recommended.

Other individuals intentionally take 5,000–8,000 mg/day of acetaminophen because their pain is not relieved by the recommended doses. These people are not trying to harm themselves, but merely seeking relief from pain and are not aware that doses even slightly above the maximum therapeutic dose of 4,000 mg/day can be toxic.

REQUESTS FOR BETTER WARNINGS IGNORED

In addition to its alcohol warning, over-the-counter acetaminophen packaging also warns against use "with any other product containing acetaminophen."[6] Unfortunately, this weak warning does not convey the serious risks of acetaminophen overmedication, even at slightly elevated doses. Overuse can cause liver injury, liver failure, and death, but you would never know it by reading the information provided with acetaminophen products.

Despite calls for better warnings, nothing has changed. Over the years, the FDA has intermittently voiced a desire to reduce the number of cases of acetaminophen toxicity. In 2004, the agency launched an educational campaign on the safe use of over-the-counter medications.[7] This initiative appears to have had no impact on acetaminophen statistics. Since then, a large study has been published demonstrating that therapeutic doses of acetaminophen cause liver injuries in a substantial number of users,[8] and has raised serious questions about the safety of therapeutic doses of acetaminophen.

In 2007, an FDA medical officer revealed that the staff of the FDA's Office of Surveillance and Epidemiology (formerly Office of Drug Safety) had recommended initiating measures similar to those adopted in Great Britain to reduce acetaminophen toxicity. These measures include limiting the number of acetaminophen pills in a package and packing the pills individually in foil packs.

This recommendation never reached the FDA's Nonprescription Drugs Advisory Committee, where it could have been considered and approved.[9]

Recently, in response to a scathing report by the Institute of Medicine, the FDA has made a lot of noise about enhancing its efforts to promote drug safety. Until proven otherwise, the FDA's promises are hollow. The tilt of the FDA will continue to be in favor of the drug industry. For years, the FDA has understaffed and underfunded its safety divisions. It has not been unusual for high-ranking FDA officials to approve new drugs despite serious concerns of FDA medical officers about the drugs' safety. Indeed, just recently another article critical of the FDA was published in the *New England Journal of Medicine* (September 6, 2007), in which Dr. Sheila Weiss Smith concluded that the FDA's actions once again underscored "the low priority it assigns to its responsibility for arbitrating drug safety."[10]

FDA IGNORES ITS OWN GUIDELINES

With acetaminophen, FDA officials have long ignored their own regulations. FDA guidelines require drug companies to list adverse drug events if: 1) they are serious; 2) they occur in close proximity to using the drug; and 3) they are consistent with a drug's known effects.[11] Acetaminophen fits all of these requirements. In addition, animal studies provide ample evidence of a link between fasting, acetaminophen use, and liver failure.[12]

Moreover, a recent report demonstrated the link between acetaminophen, fasting, and liver toxicity. Doctors were at first puzzled why a nine-month-old child had developed liver toxicity after only two days of therapeutic doses of acetaminophen. Laboratory analysis revealed that the child had a genetically determined glutathione deficiency, causing her glutathione activity to be only 5% of normal. Without adequate glutathione, standard doses of acetaminophen were toxic in this child.[13] The case provides human evidence that markedly decreased glutathione activity, which can also be caused by fasting, increases the risk of acetaminophen liver toxicity in humans.

FDA guidelines also state that rare, serious adverse events should be listed in product information "even if there are only one or two reported events."[11] The first cases linking acetaminophen, fasting, and liver toxicity were reported in the 1980s. More than 20 years have passed, during which time many more cases have been published. Where is the warning? Where are the meaningful measures to improve acetaminophen safety?

Perhaps the FDA's inaction is related to resistance by the largest producer of acetaminophen products (McNeil Consumer Health, Tylenol® products) to implement a fasting warning and other safety measures. Acetaminophen is a widely used drug that generates more than two billion dollars per year in sales in the US. Additional warnings might undo acetaminophen's reputation as the safest over-the-counter pain and fever remedy, and safety packaging might depress sales.

Some argue that it has not been fully proven that fasting increases the risk of liver toxicity from acetaminophen. This is a specious argument. Experts know that absolute proof will be difficult to obtain. Liver toxicity from acetaminophen and fasting is a rare event. If it occurs in one in 100,000 users, a study demonstrating this would require at least 300,000 patients, and it would take years to accomplish. This is why FDA guidelines do not require absolute proof of causality. The FDA simply requires a close, plausible association between a drug and an adverse event. This is certainly the case with acetaminophen and fasting.

Jay S. Cohen, MD, is an associate professor of family and preventive medicine and psychiatry at the University of California, San Diego. Dr. Cohen is a nationally recognized expert on medications and their side effects. He has published books and medical journal articles and has spoken at major conferences and at the US Food and Drug Administration regarding the need for improved drug safety. Dr. Cohen also provides expert analyses and opinions in cases involving medication-induced injuries. His most recent book, *What You Must Know About Statin Drugs and Their Natural Alternatives* (Square One Publishers, 2006), explains who needs to reduce cholesterol or other risk factors for heart disease, and how they can do so safely.

References

1. Eriksson LS, Broome U, Kalin M, Lindholm M. Hepatotoxicity due to repeated intake of low doses of paracetamol. *J Intern Med*. 1992 May;231(5):567–70.

2. Nourjah P, Ahmad SR, Karwoski C, Willy M. Estimates of acetaminophen (Paracetamol)-associated overdoses in the United States. *Pharmacoepidemiol Drug Saf*. 2006 Jun;15(6):398–405.

3. Ostapowicz G, Fontana RJ, Schiodt FV, et al. Results of a prospective study of acute liver failure at 17 tertiary care centers in the United States. *Ann Intern Med*. 2002 Dec 17;137(12):947–54.

4. Lee WM. Acetaminophen and the US Acute Liver Failure Study Group: lowering the risks of hepatic failure. *Hepatology*. 2004 Jul;40(1):6–9.

5. Larson AM, Polson JS, Fontana RJ, et al. Acetaminophen-induced acute liver failure: results of a United States multicenter, prospective study. *Hepatology*. 2005;42(6):1364–72.

6. Tylenol® Extra Strength Acetaminophen. Warnings on package. *McNeil Consumer Healthcare*, 2006.

7. Available at: http://www.fda.gov/bbs/topics/NEWS/2004/NEW01008.html. Accessed September 20, 2007.

8. Watkins PB, Kaplowitz N, Slattery JT, et al. Aminotransferase elevations in healthy adults receiving 4 grams of acetaminophen daily: a randomized controlled trial. *JAMA*. 2006 Jul 5;296(1):87–93.

9. Ahmad SR. Safety of recommended doses of paracetamol. *Lancet*. 2007 Feb 10;369(9560):462–3.

10. Smith SW. Sidelining safety—the FDA's inadequate response to the IOM. *N Engl J Med*. 2007 Sep 6;357(10):960–3.

11. Center for Drug Evaluation and Research. *Guidance For Industry: Adverse Reactions Section of Labeling for Human Prescription Drug*

and Biological Product. US Food and Drug Administration, June 2006.

12. Price VF, Miller MG, Jollow DJ. Mechanisms of fasting-induced potentiation of acetaminophen hepatotoxicity in the rat. *Biochem Pharmacol*. 1987 Feb 15;36(4):427–33.

13. Tokatli A, Kalkanoglu-Sivri HS, Yuce A, Coskun T. Acetaminophen-induced hepatotoxicity in a glutathione synthetase-deficient patient. *Turk J Pediatr*. 2007 Jan;49(1):75–6.

SEPTEMBER 2007

The Abigail Alliance:
Motivated by Tragic Circumstances, Families Battle an Uncaring Bureaucracy

by Sue Kovach

OUNDED IN NOVEMBER 2001 AFTER THE TRAGIC CANCER death of its young namesake, Abigail Kathleen Burroughs, the Abigail Alliance is working for FDA regulatory changes that would allow patients with cancer and other life-threatening illnesses—and no other treatment options—to have access to promising investigational drugs.

The Abigail Alliance is seeking to have legislation passed that will remove the regulatory barriers currently preventing seriously ill patients from gaining early access to developmental drugs showing efficacy in clinical trials. The Alliance also aims to modernize the FDA's antiquated scientific approval process for drugs intended to treat life-threatening diseases, and seeks to place the decision to use experimental treatment options with patients and their physicians, rather than the FDA.

ABIGAIL BURROUGHS: INSPIRING CHANGE

Abigail Kathleen Burroughs was only 21 years old when she succumbed to squamous cell carcinoma that had invaded her neck and lungs. Her cancer diagnosis at age 19 was a tremendous shock, as the type of cancer she had is particularly rare in one so young. Typically, older men who smoked and drank for decades receive this devastating diagnosis. Abigail was an honor student and high school athlete, a confident yet humble person who was wise beyond her years, according to her family and friends. And she was compassionate, devoting much of her young life to charity work, making beds at homeless shelters and creating a free tutoring program for 50 families who couldn't afford tutors. Abigail had a great love of life and a deep respect for all beings.

Not long after her diagnosis, the Burroughs family learned of an investigational cancer drug, Erbitux®, that showed good response in early trials. Abigail's prominent oncologist at Johns Hopkins Hospital believed the drug had a significant chance of saving her life. But every effort on the part of her family, physician, and supporters to procure the drug for Abigail failed. She was ineligible for a clinical trial and the drug company couldn't provide her with Erbitux® for compassionate use. The FDA was unmoved by her life-and-death situation.

In November 2000, Abigail was recovering from a round of chemotherapy and radiation treatment when she said to father, Frank: "Dad, if I make it, I'd like you and I to devote our lives to helping people with cancer and other illnesses where there's an unmet need." After seven months of battling to acquire Erbitux® for Abigail, she died, her young life tragically cut short by an indifferent system that has cost an untold number of lives.

Hours after she died, through his tremendous grief, Frank Burroughs realized that the inability of seriously ill patients to obtain effective drugs still under study was a critical unmet need. His daughter had wanted to help not only herself, but others like her, and Burroughs knew then that he had to continue fighting the system.

Burroughs explained, "Hundreds of thousands of Americans die every year awaiting drug approval, a catastrophe of immense proportions. I said to myself, 'Why should I quit now? There are other people out there who are just as precious as Abigail.' She had planted the seed of an idea. She was the embodiment of the unmet need. But we certainly weren't the only ones."

After his daughter's death, Frank Burroughs formed a non-profit advocacy group, the Abigail Alliance for Better Access to Developmental Drugs. He gathered volunteers and supporters to raise awareness on Capitol Hill and in the general public of the issues surrounding compassionate use of developmental drugs, and to push for change in the FDA system that denies seriously ill patients access to possibly life-saving therapies.

In its short six years of existence, the Alliance has gained favorable media coverage for these issues and has presented the heartbreaking stories of the patients behind them. With the help of the Washington Legal Foundation, the Alliance has shown that it won't be ignored by filing a Citizen Petition and even taking the FDA to court. Its practical solutions to fix a flawed and deadly system are contained in the proposed legislation, which could save countless lives.

DRUG APPROVAL SYSTEM FAILS PATIENTS IN NEED

The problems inherent in the FDA clinical trial and drug approval system can be fully illustrated by looking at how it failed Abigail Burroughs and others, such as Jennifer McNellie, wife of Abigail Alliance co-founder Steve Walker. Jennifer was diagnosed with colon cancer at age 45 and ran out of treatment options after her first regimen. The couple, both scientists, did their own research and learned about several drugs under study that were found to be effective in trials. But they, too, discovered that the drugs were beyond their reach and that approvals could be years away. Jennifer McNellie died at age 47, another victim of the clinical trial system.

Says Steve Walker: "I delved into the regulations, trying to figure out why the system wasn't working. As scientists, Jennifer and I both understood how the trials were being conducted. It didn't take us long to determine that the FDA is an ineffective agency. I lobbied senators and representatives, and I lobbied the FDA, which was completely non-responsive."

The FDA's drug study and approval system is meant to protect patients, certainly, but shouldn't it also reap the benefits of billions of research dollars and years of drug development and testing by bringing medical progress to those who need it most? No seriously ill person should have to die merely because the FDA stamp of approval on a drug is years away. Yet that's exactly what is happening. The reason it's happening was a shock to Burroughs, Walker, and Abigail Alliance supporters.

NOVEL THERAPIES UNAVAILABLE TO MOST PATIENTS

Currently, drugs showing efficacy in clinical trials are completely unavailable to seriously ill patients who don't qualify for trials. The drugs often can't even be obtained on a compassionate use basis. But getting into clinical trials, no matter how ill you are, could be compared to winning a lottery because the odds of being selected can be almost as slim. This is due to the vast number of restrictive participant requirements imposed by the FDA, some of which demand that seriously ill patients with little time to waste first try—and fail—one or more other available treatments.

With no compassionate use program, Abigail's and Jennifer's only hope was to get into a clinical trial. In Abigail's case, Erbitux® was found to be effective in early trials against the type of cancer cell she had, one shared by both colon and head and neck cancer, among others. Cancer, however, is characterized in trials not by its cellular properties, but by the initial tumor site. So later trials were conducted according to where the cancer is located rather than the type of cancer cell—in this case, for colon cancer only. This restriction was the primary reason Abigail was kept out of the Erbitux® trials—though she had the right type of cancer cells, her cancer was in the wrong place. Economics also played a part, as the drug company would have had to spend twice as much money to put Erbitux® on two separate approval paths.

"Increasingly narrow trial participant restrictions—and more of them—leave most terminally ill people out of clinical trials, including Jennifer McNellie. Many of the restrictions are put in place purely for statistical reasons," says Walker. Of the patients who do qualify, only a few will be given the chance for a longer life. A Phase III clinical trial for a lung cancer drug, for example, might enroll only 700 patients, yet more than 150,000 die from lung cancer every year. Even worse, only half of those in trials will actually get the potentially life-saving drug because the FDA usually requires that 50% of trial patients—for statistical reasons—receive a sugar pill placebo. Seriously ill patients don't know if they're taking a new drug that could save them, or an empty placebo equal to a death sentence.

ACCOMPLISHMENTS AND CONTINUING EFFORTS OF THE ABIGAIL ALLIANCE

- Developed the Tier 1 Initial Approval (Tier 1) initiative that would greatly increase access to developmental drugs for tens of thousands of cancer patients and others with life-threatening illnesses. This effort resulted in the introduction of bills in the House and Senate known as the ACCESS (Access, Compassion, Care, and Ethics for Seriously Ill Patients) Act (S.1956 and H.R. 6303).

- Filed a Citizen Petition with the FDA in support of Tier 1, with the help of the Washington Legal Foundation, resulting in the FDA working on proposed policy changes. (Unfortunately, this is a very slow process at the FDA.)

- Filed a lawsuit effort in support of better access to new life-saving and life-extending therapies with the pro-bono help of the Washington Legal Foundation and the law firm of Latham and Watkins, LLP. Progress continues and in May 2007, the Abigail Alliance won a legal round in the US Appellate Court.

- Efforts led to an expanded access program for the colon cancer drug Erbitux®.

- Contributed to the effort to get thousands of multiple sclerosis patients back on the efficacious drug Tysabri®.

- Successful in having placebos removed from a clinical trial for kidney cancer, eventually resulting in all patients in the trial—and many who left the trial—receiving the efficacious cancer drug Nexavar®.

- Helped acquire trial drugs for several individuals who had to leave clinical trials on minor issues, but were responding well to their therapies. Additionally, helped other patients get compassionate use of promising investigational drugs.

- Along with others in the private sector, pushes the Critical Path Initiative (CPI), a US Department of Health and Human Services/FDA modernization project that would cut the costs of drug approvals, speed up the approval process, and reduce the use of placebos.

- Promotes ways to better inform the public about clinical trials. With the Lorenzen Cancer Foundation, the Alliance continues to work on an improved clinical trial database called Cancer Patients' Alliance for Clinical Trials (Cancer-PACT). Due to Alliance efforts, the NIH better promotes the vital website, www.clinicaltrials.gov.

- Continues to be the rallying point for individuals and organizations who agree with the need for change in the system, adding more friends and allies each year.

CLINICAL TRIALS RULED BY STATISTICS, NOT COMPASSION

According to Steve Walker,

> The clinical trial system is run by statistics—a branch of applied mathematics. It's caused millions of people to die sooner than they should have and it's all because of the FDA's single-minded focus on statistics as the only tool to use. In any other field of science, this is sacrilege. Statisticians are a support specialty. But in clinical research, it's considered sacrilege to question statistics. And statistics in no way reflect the reality of disease.

Specifically, the statistic so desired by the FDA is the probability value, or p-value—the mathematical probability that the data are the result of random chance. (Data with a low p-value of less than or equal to 0.05 are considered to be "statistically significant." A p-value of 0.05, for example, means there is a 1 in 20 probability that the data result from random chance.)

What many people don't realize is that the current drug approval system bases the decision to approve or not approve a new drug on average results. The way this drug approval process is designed, statistical analysis evaluates the probability that a drug will have a predefined desired outcome, such as a 50% reduction in tumor size and/or number, based upon an average result.

If a new cancer drug produced a dramatic improvement in 15% of the patients with a deadly form of cancer, yet the average of all patients achieving 50% reduction in tumor size failed to achieve statistical significance, this drug would be unlikely to be approved under today's outmoded system. But if the same drug did not produce a dramatic improvement in any patient, yet achieved statistical significance based upon an average response rate, the drug would be more likely to be approved in the current system.

Although the FDA is slowly and begrudgingly moving towards using active comparators rather than placebo in many studies, many drug approval studies in serious disease states like cancer still use placebo as a comparison. This raises significant ethical issues—why should a patient with deadly life-threatening cancer participate in a study when there is a high likelihood of receiving placebo for treatment?

Says Burroughs: "Essentially, they want people to die so they can see how many die. And that's the cruelty of all this. Cancer trials aren't like trials for toenail fungus cream. People's lives are at stake here."

The formal drug approval process needs to balance compassion with statistical analysis. The FDA's continued insistence on using placebo instead of active comparators of approved drugs raises significant ethical questions, since the lives of seriously ill patients are at stake.

It's not that the FDA doesn't know how to fix the broken system of cancer drug approval. The problem seems to be that it simply won't. The FDA is a stagnant agency existing in a constant state of institutional worry, says Burroughs. While the Abigail Alliance talks about the issues, the FDA talks about the status quo. "The resistance to change is so powerful. People want to hold on to the status quo," Burroughs says. "They say, 'This is how we've always done things.' They're concerned about how to handle the PR if someone dies during early access use. We are not trying to dismantle the clinical trial process—all we want to do is improve it."

PROMOTING CHANGE

The solutions proposed by the Abigail Alliance would indeed improve the process by modernizing the methods used to fit the current state of science, while relegating the use of statistics to its proper secondary role in the process. The Abigail Alliance has taken a hard stance in its fight against the FDA. Its first major effort, a 2003 white paper plan titled Tier 1 Initial Approval, became the basis for the legislative action. It described a three-tier approval process in which Tier 1 would allow early approval and provide developmental drugs to those abandoned by the current system. The Tier 1 white paper was presented to then-FDA commissioner Mark McClellan in person. The FDA's response was a letter to the Alliance that essentially said the agency would continue to do business as usual.

The Alliance then filed a Citizen Petition with the FDA in June 2003. To this day, they've received no response. Undeterred, the next step was a lawsuit filed on July 28, 2003 against McClellan and Tommy Thompson, then-Secretary of the Department of Health and Human Services (the FDA is an operational division of DHHS). The lawsuit seeks to stop the FDA from enforcing a policy that "violates the constitutional privacy and liberty rights of terminally ill patients, including numerous Abigail Alliance members, and their constitutional guarantee against deprivation of life without due process." The suit was dismissed in District Court in 2004, but the Alliance appealed and last May won the first round in Appellate Court, says Burroughs.

> The case was heard before a panel of three judges and we won in a two-to-one decision. The lawsuit was reinstated. But the FDA appealed and has requested that the US Appellate Court of DC re-hear the case en banc, meaning before all ten judges.

Legal watchers say the court is pretty evenly divided and they believe the appeal could go either way. But the Alliance is optimistic—when oral arguments were presented, observers say a third of the judges were hard on the Alliance, but a third were hard on the FDA, and the remainder were simply quiet. A decision is expected literally any day now.

Says Burroughs:

> We hope and pray that the patients win. One way or another, this will likely end up in the US Supreme Court, as the FDA will probably appeal if they lose, and if we lose, we'll definitely appeal. My guess is the Supreme Court will hear the case, as this is a landmark issue, and an important issue.

The Alliance believes that at its core, this is a major civil rights issue. While the FDA trembles at the word "risk," terminally ill patients can view the risks of taking developmental drugs as the only option they have left. The FDA greatly amplifies concerns about safety, and minimizes and contests evidence of efficacy, says Walker. "It's a risk-averse stance that the FDA routinely takes on all drug development and approval programs, and they use statistics to do it."

It's also a privacy issue in that the decision to take an investigational drug and the unknown risks associated with it should be the private decision of a patient in consultation with their doctor. The FDA shouldn't make the decision for others, a fundamental reason why the Alliance's fight can be viewed as patient and doctor versus paternalistic FDA.

Says Burroughs:

> One of our strengths is that we get the facts out there. We get a lot of good press, and when our issues are in the media, it resonates with the public. People understand that these are important issues. In poll after poll, we find that the public is willing to take risks, and the last time I checked this was a democracy,

but that's not what we're seeing. The FDA currently decides what the risk-benefit is, and they're sorry you have a terminal illness, but they don't want you having any side effects.

HOPE FOR THE FUTURE

The best evidence of the Alliance's effectiveness is that every drug they've pushed for has been approved. "Every drug for cancer and other serious life-threatening illnesses that the Abigail Alliance has pushed for earlier access to in our six year history is now approved by the FDA," Burroughs says. "Many lives could have been saved or extended, if there had been earlier access to these drugs."

PHASES OF CLINICAL TRIALS

- **Phase I:** An experimental drug or treatment is tested in a small group (e.g., 20 people) for the first time to evaluate preliminary short-term safety, determine a dosage range, study metabolism and pharmacologic actions in humans, and identify side effects with increasing dosages. Phase I trials may include healthy participants and/or patients.
- **Phase II:** The experimental study drug or treatment is tested in a larger group (e.g., 80 patients) to determine effectiveness for a particular indication or indications in patients with the disease or condition under study, for further safety evaluation and to continue to evaluate for side effects.
- **Phase III:** Performed after preliminary evidence suggesting effectiveness has been obtained, the experimental drug or treatment is given to larger groups of people (e.g., 1,000 patients) for longer periods of time. The overall risk-benefit relationship of the drug is evaluated and information is gathered for physician labeling.

- **Phase IV:** Post-marketing studies on the drug or treatment gather additional information on the risks, benefits, and optimal use.

References

Available at: www.clinicaltrials.gov. Accessed June 28, 2007.

Life-Saving Cancer Drugs Not Approved by the FDA

by William Faloon and Donna Pogliano

F OR THE PAST 27 YEARS, LIFE EXTENSION HAS IDENTIFIED LIFE-saving medications that languished too long in the FDA's archaic approval process.

When effective new drugs are delayed, the inevitable consequence is needless human suffering and death. An equally insidious problem is the chilling effect bureaucratic roadblocks have on the development of better drugs that might actually cure the disease.

Just imagine the difficulty of raising the tens of millions of dollars needed to get a new cancer drug into the approval pipeline when prospective investors see the FDA deny a drug with documented efficacy, as was done recently with Provenge®.

Another problem with the FDA's unpredictable approval pattern is the outrageous cost of the cancer drugs that actually make it to market. Even when classes of cancer drugs are finally approved, the out-of-pocket cost of these new drugs can exceed $12,000 per month. The media has reported on heart-wrenching stories of cancer patients who choose to die rather than send their families into bankruptcy from paying these costs.

It's easy to point fingers at drug companies for charging such extortionist prices, but the harsh reality is that getting these medications approved by the FDA is so costly and risky that the high prices can arguably be justified by the hideously inefficient drug approval process that now exists.

There are many drugs that have been shown to be effective against cancer, but are not yet approved by the FDA. While there are dozens of anti-cancer drugs in various stages of the approval process, the sad truth is that thousands of compounds with anti-cancer activity will never be submitted for FDA approval due to lack of patentability, lack of investor funding, or just plain unwillingness to deal with today's cancer bureaucracy.

Each day, about 1,500 Americans perish from cancer. Each day, over 3,000 Americans are diagnosed with this dreaded disease.[1] While the general population is relatively ignorant about medicine, virtually everyone knows that a cancer diagnosis means exposure to therapies that produce miserable—if not lethal—side effects. The public is also aware that in too many cases, government-approved therapies fail to cure the disease.

HOW THE FDA APPROVAL PROCESS WORKS

The clinical trial procedure depends on the ability of the pharmaceutical company to finance clinical trials and to recruit patients to participate in them. Many promising trials need to be halted due to lack of adequate funding or inability to recruit enough patients to make up an acceptable group of patients to form the study and/or control groups.

Patients can help bring new drugs and treatments to the marketplace by participating in clinical trials that fit their disease state, prior treatment profile, and eligibility status. Patients should ask questions to be certain that they are not sacrificing a proven treatment protocol for one which has little potential to help them, and they should ask questions until they thoroughly understand the details of the trial and how it will affect their disease management strategy. It is also important to verify that all patients in the study receive some form of active therapy and that no group will receive a worthless placebo.[2]

Clinical trials on promising anti-cancer drugs are done in three phases, with Phase I trials being conducted to establish dose-limiting toxicity, Phase II trials proceeding to establish effectiveness in a limited number of patients, and Phase III trials advancing to include widespread study populations and to gather data to make comparisons between the effectiveness of the new treatment versus current protocols.[2] Normally, application to the FDA (a New Drug Application, or NDA) for approval takes place after Phase III clinical trials have demonstrated that the new agent, procedure, or protocol is superior to the current standard of treatment in terms of effectiveness and/or tolerability. Only after FDA approval can the new drug or treatment be marketed and made available to the general public, even if such a treatment is approved in another country considered to have advanced medical care by our standards. Medicine clearly has geographical boundaries—drugs and devices approved in the USA may not be approved 10 feet beyond the US border into Canada, and vice versa. Drugs such as Taxotere®—considered to be the most active agent in breast, prostate, head and neck and lung cancer and an approved drug in Europe—were not made available to cancer patients in the USA until the FDA granted its approval. This "process" took approximately five additional years.

AN INTERIM PROPOSAL FOR FDA REFORM

Cancer patients should have access to drugs and technologies that have shown minimal toxicity, but that have shown efficacy based on peer-reviewed literature and formal presentations at recognized medical conferences. Such drugs and/or technologies could be granted a "semi-approval status" by the FDA with the implication that at some future date they could be granted full FDA approval.

The conditions for availability of such drugs and technologies would involve:

- Patient access to drugs with evidence of significant activity and safety.
- Pharmaceutical company ability to charge for agents without jeopardizing economic solvency, while agreeing to cost reductions of agents resulting from semi-approval status.
- Ongoing collection of complete and accurate data by designated physicians that is submitted for review.
- Physician reimbursement for services in delivering therapies.
- Legal counsel preparing documents to eliminate risk of litigious actions. Patients wanting access to agents must assume risks and waive access to liability.
- Creating task forces consisting of scientists, consumers, and other relevant individuals involved in a quarterly review process of clinical data.
- Access to state-of-the-art medicine is the birthright of all individuals. Included in that birthright is the option to use whatever alternative medicine or innovative medical procedure or pharmaceutical agent seems prudent, as it becomes available, without suppression by a politicized and bureaucratic governmental agency.

There is a revolution brewing, and FDA reform is the target. Every individual patient and all of those who are stakeholders—

and that's all of us—can be part of the solution, rather than passively accepting the status quo and remaining part of the problem. A government responsive to the needs of the people can't help but recognize the legions of cancer patients and their loved ones who are taking to the streets, carrying signs and demanding that their voices be heard.[3, 4] Other campaigns—such as the "Raise A Voice" movement being conducted by prostate cancer patients who are running out of time—are waging war on their cancer by confronting the myopic agency that prevents them from gaining access to the drugs and procedures that can prolong the length and improve the quality of their lives.[5]

References

1. Available at: www.cancer.org/docroot/stt/stt_0.asp. Accessed June 11, 2007.

2. Strum SB, Pogliano D. *A Primer on Prostate Cancer, The Empowered Patient's Guide*. 2nd ed. Hollywood, FL: the Life Extension Foundation; 2005.

3. Available at: http://www.nytimes.com/2007/06/04/health/04drug.html?ex=1181793600&en=8aadd4d94116b406&ei=5070. Accessed June 12, 2007.

4. Available at: http://psa-rising.com/blog/index.php/2007/06/02/washington-dc-june-4th-prostate-cancer-walk. Accessed June 12, 2007.

5. Available at: http://psa-rising.com/blog/index.php/2007/06/. Accessed June 12, 2007.

FDA Drops the Ball on Avandia® Warning

by Dale Kiefer

THE FDA CAME UNDER RENEWED CRITICISM RECENTLY, WHEN it was revealed that warnings by its own safety committee regarding a popular diabetes drug were ignored by the regulatory agency.* FDA safety staff had recommended that prescribing information for the type 2 diabetes drug, Avandia® (rosiglitazone), should include a so-called "black box" warning—the FDA's most dire alert—indicating that the drug might put some patients at increased risk of congestive heart failure. But the FDA ignored that recommendation.

Instead, the warning is buried on line 351 of the label, noted Senator Charles Grassley (R–IA), whose staff investigated the

---

* There are numerous other examples of FDA-approved drugs (like Vioxx® and Rezulin®) which were subsequently discovered to be dangerous or even to cause death. Please refer to the Index under "FDA-approved drugs, dangerous."

FDA's inaction. The investigation was prompted by the publication of an analysis of the drug's cardiovascular risk profile in the prestigious *New England Journal of Medicine* in May. In that analysis, researchers from the Cleveland Clinic concluded, "Rosiglitazone was associated with a significant increase in the risk of myocardial infarction and with an increase in the risk of death from cardiovascular causes."[1]

Reference

1. Nissen SE, Wolski K. Effect of rosiglitazone on the risk of myocardial infarction and death from cardiovascular causes. *N Engl J Med*. 2007 May 21; [Epub ahead of print]

The Untapped Healing Potential of DMSO

by Sue Kovach

DESPITE DECADES OF RESEARCH AND THOUSANDS OF STUDies attesting to its health-promoting properties, dimethyl sulfoxide (DMSO) remains virtually unknown to the medical professional and the public.

This inexpensive compound demonstrates potent anti-inflammatory and analgesic properties, has been shown to relieve painful musculoskeletal and urinary conditions, and may even fight Alzheimer's disease and cancer. Unfortunately, its widespread acceptance and use has been stymied by the FDA and their allies in the pharmaceutical industry.

DMSO: EXTENSIVELY RESEARCHED, CRIMINALLY IGNORED

Dimethyl sulfoxide (DMSO) is an anti-inflammatory and analgesic compound that holds promise in managing a wide range of debilitating health conditions. DMSO is an approved pharmacological agent in more than 125 countries, and its safety and therapeutic effects are backed by nearly 50 years of research and more than 10,000 scientific articles on its biological implications.

Unfortunately, the vast health-promoting potential of DMSO has gone unfulfilled in America, suppressed by a combination of bureaucratic ineptitude and pharmaceutical industry lobbying. In the United States today, DMSO is approved to treat only one medical condition: interstitial cystitis, or chronic inflammation of the bladder wall. Recent findings on DMSO's ability to help manage the effects of head injury have renewed interest in the many potential therapeutic applications of this versatile compound.

EARLY DMSO RESEARCH SHOWS PROMISE

Early studies in animals and humans showed that DMSO rapidly penetrates the skin and quickly relieves the pain and inflammation associated with injuries such as ankle sprains. Stanley Jacob, MD, and Robert Herschler, PhD, thought DMSO could effectively treat arthritis and possibly act as a drug-delivery system. Their first paper on DMSO's pharmacology, published in the journal *Current Therapeutic Research* in 1964, drew the attention of a number of pharmaceutical interests and made headlines in Oregon newspapers. It was quickly picked up by the *New York Times*.

"A front-page *Times* article that called DMSO the most exciting thing in medicine created a great deal of interest," Dr. Jacob recalls. "Six pharmaceutical firms were licensed by Crown Zellerbach to begin wide and well-funded evaluations of DMSO's safety and effectiveness. The studies primarily used DMSO applied topically to the skin."

According to Dr. Jacob, three companies—Merck, Centex, and Squibb—found DMSO to be safe and effective for a wide array of musculoskeletal problems like tendonitis and osteoarthritis. Minor side effects included a garlicky breath odor, temporary itching, flaking, and burning at the application site, and occasional nausea or drowsiness. While the companies submitted New Drug Applications to the FDA in 1965 stating that DMSO was safe and effective and ready to be a prescriptive agent, ongoing animal toxicity research revealed that DMSO caused changes in laboratory animals' eyes (myopia, or nearsightedness). Although no such problems were seen in humans, the FDA grew concerned. Then, on September 9, 1965, the *Wall Street Journal* reported the death of an Irish woman after undergoing DMSO treatment for a sprained wrist. Although no autopsy was conducted, drug company officials speculated the death was the result of an allergic reaction to DMSO.[2]

FDA OVERREACTS, HALTS DMSO RESEARCH

Dr. Jacob recalls that the FDA "halted all studies of DMSO on November 10, 1965, even though they had data in their files on more than 70,000 patients submitted by approximately 1,500 physicians in the US showing its safety and effectiveness."

FDA critics contend that the agency overreacted in halting the studies, considering how unconcerned the agency appears today with the number of deaths that occur from both trial and approved pharmaceuticals.

According to Jack de la Torre, MD, PhD, who has researched DMSO's role in treating central nervous system injuries, "Years ago the FDA had a sort of chip on its shoulder because it thought DMSO was some kind of snake-oil medicine. There were people there who were openly biased against the compound, even though they knew very little about it."[3]

Adding to the FDA's skepticism was that, in many ways, DMSO simply sounded too good to be true. Says Dr. Jacob, "In the 1890s, if someone had said, 'I have this little white pill and if you take it, it will relieve pain, reduce inflammation, protect you if you have a heart attack, and so on,' you'd say, 'Well, I don't believe it.' Yet aspirin does all those things. DMSO is similar in that it doesn't fit the 'one-pharmacologic-agent-for-one-indication' philosophy of the FDA."

Dr. Jacob resolutely continued his work on DMSO. In 1971, he and his colleagues brought so much pressure on the FDA that it commissioned the National Academy of Sciences (NAS) to evaluate the DMSO controversy. The NAS published its findings in 1972, concluding that DMSO was a promising and probably safe and effective agent. The FDA was unmoved. Dr. Jacob, however, finally achieved success and some vindication when the agency approved DMSO for treating interstitial cystitis in 1978.

TREATING HEAD TRAUMA

Traumatic brain injury is the most common injury of soldiers returning from the war in Iraq. In light of this, new clinical trials using DMSO to manage the elevated intracranial pressure common to such injuries are now being approved.

Dr. Jacob notes that in studies conducted from 1978 to 1982, "we observed that when the human brain was treated with intravenously administered DMSO after a head injury, the swelling could be reduced within five minutes. No other treatment comes close to acting that quickly. In patients given other commonly used therapeutic agents such as intravenous barbiturates, the brain continued to swell. We've known about DMSO's efficacy for this type of injury for a long time."

Astonishingly, however, the Food and Drug Administration (FDA) has not approved any new pharmacological agent of significance for the treatment of traumatic brain injury in more than three decades. With so much attention focused on the plight of severely injured soldiers returning home from war, Dr. Jacob is leading the charge to gain FDA approval of DMSO to treat this type of injury. He believes that DMSO would be more effective than some current therapies such as removing parts of the brain to reduce swelling.

Dr. Stanley Jacob currently serves as the Chairman of Abela Pharmaceuticals, Inc. Based in Orange County, California, Abela Pharmaceuticals was formed in 2005 for the purpose of developing and clinically testing DMSO and DMSO-related products. The company's mission is to bring DMSO to market for the treatment of injuries and conditions affecting the central nervous system, including traumatic brain injury, stroke, and Alzheimer's disease.

Dr. Jacob and his colleagues previously sponsored preliminary clinical trials of DMSO on traumatic brain injury patients in Europe. The results of the trial were remarkable, with an 80% survival rate (about twice the historical rate of 30–40%) and 70% of the patients experiencing a favorable outcome (far higher than the historical rate of less than 10%).[1]

Based primarily on these results, the FDA has given Abela's Investigational New Drug application "fast track" designation and will allow the company to clinically test DMSO on traumatic brain injury patients. The controlled, multicenter study is equivalent to a Phase 2b trial, and is expected to begin later this year.

References

1. Karaca M, Bilgin UY, Akar M, de la Torre JC. Dimethly sulphoxide lowers ICP after closed head trauma. *Eur J Clin Pharmacol.* 1991 ;40(1):113–4.

2. Carley W. DMSO may have caused death of woman, makers of "wonder" drug warn doctors. *Wall Street Journal.* September 9, 1965:6.

3. Argren R. *Arthritis: What Is It? Decades of Diagnosis and Management with an Exciting Future.* Lincoln, NE: iUniverse; 2004.

Does Green Tea Prevent Cardiovascular Disease?

by William Faloon

O N MAY 9, 2006, THE FDA STATED THAT THERE WAS NO credible evidence to support the claim that green tea reduces cardiovascular disease risk factors.[1]

The FDA's 21-page letter of denial was in response to a petition filed by a maker of green tea bags that sought to state a cardiovascular risk-reduction health claim on the label of its product.

Although the FDA identified dozens of published scientific studies suggesting that green tea might reduce heart attack and stroke risk, the agency decided that none of these studies met its criteria for allowing a health claim on the labels of green tea products.

On September 13, 2006, the *Journal of the American Medical Association* published a study that tracked the green tea consumption of 40,530 adults over an 11-year period. The study found that those who drank five or more cups of green tea a day cut their overall death rate by 16% compared to those who drank less than one cup of green tea a day.[2]

The most striking finding from this study was the reduction in cardiovascular death in those who consumed the most green tea. Women who drank five or more cups of green tea daily had a 31% reduced risk of dying from cardiovascular disease, whereas men who drank five or more cups had a 22% reduced risk of dying from cardiovascular disease.[2]

Stroke was the type of cardiovascular mortality against which green tea was shown to be most effective. Women who drank five or more cups of green teas had a 42% lower risk of stroke compared to those who drank less than one cup a day.[2]

WHY THE FDA DISAGREES WITH STUDY FINDINGS

The FDA's criteria for allowing a health claim on the label of a food or dietary supplement is quite archaic. For example, the FDA does not recognize low-density lipoprotein (LDL) oxidation as a validated cardiovascular disease risk factor. Therefore, scientific studies in humans showing that green tea extract inhibits LDL oxidation are excluded from the FDA's analysis of green tea's efficacy.

The FDA's antiquated position flies in the face of voluminous data showing that oxidized LDL severely damages the arterial wall and is a major contributor to atherosclerosis-induced heart attack and stroke.[3-22]

When choosing which studies of green tea to evaluate, the FDA excluded those that did not show significant reductions in total cholesterol, LDL, or blood pressure. According to the FDA's logic, if green tea does not lower cholesterol, LDL, or blood pressure, then a claim cannot be made on a green tea label that it reduces cardiovascular disease risk factors. The FDA did acknowledge studies in which people who consumed 10 cups of green tea a day showed a significant decrease in total cholesterol and LDL.

Completely overlooked by the FDA analysis are published studies showing that green tea protects against heart attack and stroke via mechanisms (such as inhibiting abnormal platelet aggregation)[23–32] that are different than the rudimentary measurements to which the FDA limited its green tea evaluation.

The FDA also made it clear that all in vivo animal studies are excluded from its analysis because these studies cannot mimic normal human physiological response to green tea ingestion. The FDA then found a reason to invalidate every human study that had ever shown a cardiovascular benefit in those who consumed green tea.

The FDA's conclusion was that no credible evidence existed to support a cardiovascular risk-reduction claim on the label of green tea products.[1] The recent study published by the American Medical Association, which included more study subjects and lasted far longer than any other previous study, did show a cardiovascular benefit to drinking greater amounts of green tea. Who then should consumers believe?[2]

MISCONCEPTIONS ABOUT GREEN TEA BEVERAGES

When green tea is consumed as a beverage, relatively little of its active polyphenols are absorbed into the bloodstream. This helps explain some inconsistent findings about how effective green tea may be in preventing common diseases.

The study published by the American Medical Association showed that daily ingestion of five or more cups of green tea reduced cardiovascular mortality and overall death rates. It also showed that those who drank two to four cups of green tea a day had less disease than those who drank less than one cup a day. This particular study failed to show a cancer risk reduction.[2]

The findings from another large human study, however, did show a 41% reduction in cancer incidence in those who consumed over 10 cups of green tea a day compared to those who consumed less than 3 cups a day. This same study showed a 28% reduction in cardiovascular disease incidence in those consuming 10 cups of green tea compared to those drinking less than 3 cups.[33]

Even the FDA's unfavorable report on green tea pointed to studies showing that daily intake of 10 cups of green tea lowered total cholesterol and LDL.[34]

It would appear from these studies that optimal benefits from green tea occur when one drinks 10 or more cups a day. The problem is that few people are ever going to ingest 10 or more cups of green tea every single day. The good news is that they don't have to.

GREEN TEA EXTRACTS VS. GREEN TEA BEVERAGES

Mainstream doctors often advocate obtaining nutrients from foods rather than supplements. A problem with certain nutrients, however, is that they are bound so tightly to food that less-than-optimal amounts of the active constituents are absorbed into the bloodstream.

Examples of nutrients that are better absorbed from supplements than from food include vitamin K, folic acid, and chlorophyll.[35-37] Lycopene, on the other hand, may be better absorbed from cooked tomato products[38] than from supplements.

In a recent study published in the *American Journal of Clinical Nutrition*, scientists sought to determine whether the active ingredients in green tea were better absorbed from green tea extract capsules or by drinking green tea. Thirty healthy test subjects were recruited and given either a specially prepared green tea beverage standardized for green tea's most active constituents (such as EGCG and ECG) or equally standardized green tea extract capsules.[39]

The results showed that subjects who received the green tea extract caps had a 60% greater increase in EGCG (epigallocatechin gallate) and a 90% greater increase in ECG (epicatechin gallate) compared to those who drank the identical amounts of these green tea constituents in standardized beverage form. The antioxidant effects in those who swallowed the green tea caps were also greater than in the green tea drinkers.[39]

The scientists concluded that when administered in the form of a green tea supplement, the active constituents (polyphenols) showed enhanced bioavailability compared to when identical amounts of polyphenols were provided in a green tea beverage.[39]

One reason for conducting this study was the previous findings that green tea polyphenols might be effective in preventing and treating cancer. By documenting that green tea extract supplements are superior to drinking green tea beverages, scientists now have a solid basis to test green tea extract capsules in human clinical studies.

NOT ALL GREEN TEA BEVERAGES ARE THE SAME

The amount of polyphenols contained in green tea beverages varies considerably, depending on where the tea is harvested and how it is processed. One study examined 19 commercial brands of green tea and found significant variation in the content of the polyphenols EGCG and ECG. The scientists who conducted this study recommended that the labels of green tea bags state the amount of the polyphenols (EGCG and ECG) contained in each cup so that consumers know how many milligrams of these active ingredients they are consuming each day.[40]

DID THE FDA ACTUALLY GET IT RIGHT THIS TIME?

The FDA's denial of a cardiovascular health claim was in response to a petition filed by a maker of green tea bags that sought to state that daily consumption of about one cup of green tea would reduce cardiovascular risk factors. The amount of polyphenols in this particular brand of green tea was 125 mg per cup.

Published scientific literature shows that it takes more than 125 mg a day of polyphenols to reduce cardiovascular risks. Although the FDA never mentioned this in its 21-page letter of denial, it would appear the FDA made the right scientific decision in disallowing this particular health claim on the label of green tea bags.

The good news for consumers is that green tea extract prices continue to plummet. This enables virtually everyone to ingest just two green tea extract capsules a day and obtain the amount of polyphenols (about 1250 mg) contained in 10 cups of green tea.

References

1. Qualified Health Claim Petition—Green Tea and Reduced Risk of Cardiovascular Disease (Docket No. 2005Q-0297) Letter of Denial.

2. Kuriyama S, Shimazu T, Ohmori K, et al. Green tea consumption and mortality due to cardiovascular disease, cancer, and all causes in Japan: the Ohsaki study. *JAMA*. 2006 Sep 13;296(10):1255–65.

3. Zhou ZX, Qiang H, Ma AQ, Chen H, Zhou P. Measurement peripheral blood index related to inflammation and ox-LDL, oxLDLAb in patients with coronary heart disease and its clinical significance. *Zhong Nan Da Xue Xue Bao Yi Xue Ban*. 2006 Apr;31 (2):258–62.

4. Naruko T, Ueda M, Ehara S, et al. Persistent high levels of plasma oxidized low-density lipoprotein after acute myocardial infarction predict stent restenosis. *Arterioscler Thromb Vasc Biol*. 2006 Apr;26(4):877–83.

5. Johnston N, Jernberg T, Lagerqvist B, Siegbahn A, Wallentin L. Oxidized low-density lipoprotein as a predictor of outcome in patients with unstable coronary artery disease. *Int J Cardiol*. 2005 Dec 7.

6. Shimada K, Mokuno H, Matsunaga E, et al. Circulating oxidized low-density lipoprotein is an independent predictor for cardiac event in patients with coronary artery disease. *Atherosclerosis*. 2004 Jun;174(2):343–7.

7. Holvoet P, Kritchevsky SB, Tracy RP, et al. The metabolic syndrome, circulating oxidized LDL, and risk of myocardial infarction in well-functioning elderly people in the health, aging, and body composition cohort. *Diabetes*. 2004 Apr;53(4):1068–73.

8. Doo YC, Han SJ, Lee JH, et al. Associations among oxidized low-density lipoprotein antibody, C-reactive protein, interleukin-6, and circulating cell adhesion molecules in patients with unstable angina pectoris. *Am J Cardiol*. 2004 Mar 1 ;93(5):554–8.

9. Nordin FG, Hedblad B, Berglund G, Nilsson J. Plasma oxidized LDL: a predictor for acute myocardial infarction? *J Intern Med*. 2003 Apr;253(4):425–9.

10. Tatsuguchi M, Furutani M, Hinagata J, et al. Oxidized LDL receptor gene (OLR1) is associated with the risk of myocardial infarction. *Biochem Biophys Res Commun*. 2003 Mar 28;303(1):247–50.

11. Tsai WC, Li YH, Chao TH, Chen JH. Relation between antibody against oxidized low-density lipoprotein and extent of coronary atherosclerosis. *J Formos Med Assoc*. 2002 Oct;101(10):681–4.

12. Wang TC, Hsu CC, Chin YP, Lin YL. The autoantibody expression against different source of oxidized low density lipoprotein in patients with acute myocardial infarction. *Thromb Res*. 2002 Aug 15;107(3–4):175–9.

13. Kelishadi R, Nadery GA, Asgary S. Oxidized LDL metabolites with high family risk for premature cardiovascular disease. *Indian J Pediatr*. 2002 Sep;69(9):755–9.

14. Dotevall A, Hulthe J, Rosengren A, Wiklund O, Wilhelmsen L. Autoantibodies against oxidized low-density lipoprotein and C-reactive protein are associated with diabetes and myocardial infarction in women. *Clin Sci* (Lond). 2001 Nov;101(5):523–31.

15. Ehara S, Ueda M, Naruko T, et al. Elevated levels of oxidized low density lipoprotein show a positive relationship with the severity of acute coronary syndromes. *Circulation*. 2001 Apr 17;103(15):1955–60.

16. Mustafa A, Nityanand S, Berglund L, Lithell H, Lefvert AK. Circulating immune complexes in 50-year-old men as a strong and independent risk factor for myocardial infarction. *Circulation*. 2000 Nov 21 ;102(21):2576–81.

17. Vaarala O. Antiphospholipid antibodies and myocardial infarction. *Lupus*. 1998;7 Suppl 2S132–4.

18. Holvoet P, Vanhaecke J, Janssens S, Van de WF, Collen D. Oxidized LDL and malondialdehyde-modified LDL in patients with acute coronary syndromes and stable coronary artery disease. *Circulation*. 1998 Oct 13;98(15):1487–94.

19. Ryan M, Owens D, Kilbride B, et al. Antibodies to oxidized lipoproteins and their relationship to myocardial infarction. *QJM*. 1998 Jun;91 (6):41 1–5.

20. Wu R, Nityanand S, Berglund L, et al. Antibodies against cardiolipin and oxidatively modified LDL in 50-year-old men predict myocardial infarction. *Arterioscler Thromb Vasc Biol*. 1997 Nov;17(1 1):3159–63.

21. Schumacher M, Eber B, Tatzber F, et al. Transient reduction of autoantibodies against oxidized LDL in patients with acute myocardial infarction. *Free Radic Biol Med*. 1995 Jun;18(6):1087–91.

22. Vaarala O, Manttari M, Manninen V, et al. Anti-cardiolipin antibodies and risk of myocardial infarction in a prospective cohort of middle-aged men. *Circulation*. 1995 Jan 1;91(1):23–7.

23. Hernandez Figueroa TT, Rodriguez-Rodriguez E, Sanchez-Muniz FJ. The green tea, a good choice for cardiovascular disease prevention? *Arch Latinoam Nutr*. 2004 Dec;54(4):380–94.

24. Neuhaus T, Voit S, Lill G, et al. Platelet aggregation induced by the C-terminal peptide of thrombospondin-1 (4N1-1) is inhibited by epigallocatechin gallate but not by prostaglandin E1. *Platelets*. 2004 Nov;15(7):455–7.

25. Son DJ, Cho MR, Jin YR, et al. Antiplatelet effect of green tea catechins: a possible mechanism through arachidonic acid pathway. *Prostaglandins Leukot Essent Fatty Acids*. 2004 Jul;71(1):25–31.

26. Lill G, Voit S, Schror K, Weber AA. Complex effects of different green tea catechins on human platelets. *FEBS Lett*. 2003 Jul 1 0;546(2–3):265–70.

27. Deana R, Turetta L, Donella-Deana A, et al. Green tea epigallocatechin-3-gallate inhibits platelet signalling pathways triggered by

both proteolytic and non-proteolytic agonists. *Thromb Haemost.* 2003 May;89(5):866–74.

28. Kang WS, Chung KH, Chung JH, et al. Antiplatelet activity of green tea catechins is mediated by inhibition of cytoplasmic calcium increase. *J Cardiovasc Pharmacol.* 2001 Dec;38(6):875–84.

29. de Maat MP. Effects of diet, drugs, and genes on plasma fibrinogen levels. *Ann NY Acad Sci.* 2001 ;936:509–21.

30. Kang WS, Lim IH, Yuk DY, et al. Antithrombotic activities of green tea catechins and (-)-epigallocatechin gallate. *Thromb Res.* 1999 Nov 1 ;96(3):229–37.

31. Yang JA, Choi JH, Rhee SJ. Effects of green tea catechin on phospholipase A2 activity and antithrombus in streptozotocin diabetic rats. *J Nutr Sci Vitaminol* (Tokyo). 1999 Jun;45(3):337–46.

32. Sagesaka-Mitane Y, Miwa M, Okada S. Platelet aggregation inhibitors in hot water extract of green tea. *Chem Pharm Bull* (Tokyo). 1990 Mar;38(3):790–3.

33. Nakachi K, Matsuyama S, Miyake S, Suganuma M, Imai K. Preventive effects of drinking green tea on cancer and cardiovascular disease: epidemiological evidence for multiple targeting prevention. *Biofactors.* 2000;13(1–4):49–54.

34. Kono S, Shinchi K, Wakabayashi K, et al. Relation of green tea consumption to serum lipids and lipoproteins in Japanese men. *J Epidemiol.* 1996 Sep;6(3):128–33.

35. Garber AK, Binkley NC, Krueger DC, Suttie JW. Comparison of phylloquinone bioavailability from food sources or a supplement in human subjects. *J Nutr.* 1999 Jun;129(6):1201–3.

36. Berg MJ. The importance of folic acid. *J Gend Specif Med.* 1999 May-Jun;2(3):24–8.

37. Ferruzzi MG, Schwartz SJ. Thermal degradation of commercial grade sodium copper chlorophyllin. *J Agric Food Chem.* 2005 Sep 7;53(1 8):7098–1 02.

38. van het Hof KH, de Boer BC, Tijburg LB, et al. Carotenoid bioavailability in humans from tomatoes processed in different ways determined from the carotenoid response in the triglyceride-rich lipoprotein fraction of plasma after a single

consumption and in plasma after four days of consumption. *J Nutr*. 2000 May;130(5):1 189–96.

39. Henning SM, Niu Y, Lee NH, et al. Bioavailability and antioxidant activity of tea flavanols after consumption of green tea, black tea, or a green tea extract supplement. *Am J Clin Nutr*. 2004 Dec;80(6):1558–64.

40. Seeram NP, Henning SM, Niu Y, et al. Catechin and caffeine content of green tea dietary supplements and correlation with antioxidant capacity. *J Agric Food Chem*. 2006 Mar 8;54(5):1599–603.

2006

OCTOBER 2006

Lifesaving Benefits of Storing Your Own Blood

by Sue Kovach

S AMERICA'S BLOOD SUPPLY SAFE? DESPITE FDA REGULATIONS, there are alarming risks associated with blood transfusions. Simply put, today's blood supply still is not guaranteed safe from a wide range of infectious diseases—many of them potentially fatal.

Autologous blood banking, or storing your own blood for future need, is the best way to guard against receiving tainted blood or experiencing adverse reactions to incompatible donated blood during a medical procedure.

New York physician Joseph Feldschuh, MD, learned this the hard way more than 40 years ago. His nightmare experience prompted him to devote his life's work to improving the safety of the nation's blood supply, and to open the nation's first autologous blood bank.

PERSONAL TRAGEDY FUELS A LIFE'S MISSION

In 1964, Dr. Joseph Feldschuh received a phone call. His father was ill and in precarious health, having suffered an allergic reaction to an incompatible blood transfusion for a bleeding ulcer. Another transfusion was required, but Dr. Feldschuh was told that a similar allergic response could be avoided if a close relative donated blood for the transfusion. Dr. Feldschuh rolled up his sleeve and contributed his own blood. His father later recovered and avoided any further complications due to Dr. Feldschuh's blood contribution.

Until this incident, Dr. Feldschuh was unaware that there are hundreds of blood subtypes beyond the basic groups and that compatibility is a critical issue in blood transfusions. To learn more, he embarked on what would become years of research into the chemistry of blood and the practice of blood banking.

Throughout his career, the specter of his father's terrible illness—and eventual contraction of deadly hepatitis from a blood transfusion—led Dr. Feldschuh to question the safety of the nation's blood supply. Like most Americans, he had trusted and believed that the blood supply was safe. However, what he learned as he studied the world of transfusions and blood banking led him to an opposite conclusion. He decided to do something about it, and was in a unique position to do so.

To help others avoid what he considered an unsafe blood supply, Dr. Feldschuh created the world's first autologous blood bank in 1985, where people could store their own blood over the long term for use if the need should arise. Far from being well received, his concept ran afoul of government regulators, was vilified by the blood-banking industry, and brought Dr. Feldschuh a world of professional trouble.

UNCOVERING PROBLEMS IN AMERICA'S BLOOD SUPPLY

In his 1990 book, *Safe Blood: Purifying the Nation's Blood Supply in the Age of AIDS*, Dr. Feldschuh documented his father's tragic 1988 death from transfusion-acquired hepatitis, how the blood industry can be made safer through increased screening for infectious diseases, and how individuals can ensure their personal safety by self-donating and storing their own blood. Since the book was published, a test for hepatitis C has been developed and is now used to test donated blood. Unfortunately, notes Dr. Feldschuh, not much else has changed in the last 16 years.

"I knew relatively little about blood banking and, like everyone else, assumed that everything that could be done to make blood safer was being done," he explains. "My first shocking revelation was that one out of ten people transfused was getting hepatitis. It wasn't just my father who had a problem. Blood banks always said their blood was safe, but one in ten is a very high figure."

Dr. Feldschuh examined statistics from the federal Centers for Disease Control and Prevention (CDC) for infections acquired through transfusions, and found that some of them made little sense. Incidents of hepatitis from transfusions are required to be reported. However, when he studied statistics from the 1970s and 1980s, curiously only 4,000–5,000 cases had been reported.

"During that time frame, about 4 million people each year received transfusions," he states. "If one in ten people transfused got hepatitis, that would have been about 400,000 cases. Yet the CDC got only 4,000 reports—meaning that about 99% of cases were never reported."

In the early 1980s, AIDS and the HIV virus brought blood safety and blood-banking practices into the public spotlight. Dr. Feldschuh felt there were far greater threats still being unaddressed. He maintains that there was no public outcry about the number of people contracting hepatitis from blood transfusions only because physicians and the public never knew about it.

However, the publicity surrounding AIDS did result in creation of the ELISA screening test for the HIV virus. Idant Laboratories, which had operated a sperm bank since the early 1970s, helped test the new screening procedure in 1984. In fact, the extreme level of testing done at the Idant semen bank provided what Dr. Feldschuh believed was a model for the blood-banking industry to follow:

> AIDS was never as big a problem as hepatitis. When the test for AIDS was developed, the blood-banking industry and organizations told the public that the blood supply was safe, but this was at a time when one of ten people still got hepatitis from transfusions.

FDA'S LAX ENFORCEMENT ENDANGERS PUBLIC HEALTH

The FDA is charged with ensuring the safety of the nation's blood supply by regulating the more than 3,000 centers that collect and process 14 million units of whole blood donated by volunteers each year.[1]

The FDA has developed and enforces quality standards, inspects facilities, and monitors reports of errors, accidents, and adverse clinical events. But is the current system working? The blood industry is often left to monitor itself, and reporting of errors and problems is more of an FDA suggestion than a requirement. The agency can propose solutions to problems in the system but then not follow through, as it did in June 2004 when it quietly dropped from its regulatory agenda an item that would have mandated a tracking and notification system to alert recipients of contaminated blood products.[2]

Congress has investigated blood banking in the past, but despite uncovering many flaws in the current system, it has made only recommendations. In 1996, for example, fully 15 years after the emergence of HIV as a threat to the nation's blood supply, the Committee on Government Reform and Oversight issued a report entitled "Protecting the Nation's Blood Supply from Infectious

Agents: The Need for New Standards to Meet New Threats."[3] Among many strong statements, the report declared,

> Current FDA and CDC regulatory systems are not adequate to meet the aggressive nature of emerging threats to blood safety. Product recalls and notification regarding possible exposure to blood-borne pathogens are not well communicated to physicians, pharmacists, patients, or the public. Regulation of blood collection, testing, and the production of blood-derived therapeutics is not well coordinated or consistently managed to minimize known risks.

The report also stated,

> The public is not well served if patients are permitted to believe there is no risk in blood transfusions or in the use of blood-derived therapies . . . greater efforts should be made to convey known risks to consumers who may wish to minimize even those risks through the use of alternative procedures or therapies.

Shockingly, the report drew little media attention. The FDA insisted that over the years, it had developed a compliance system with "five layers of overlapping safeguards."[1] The first, donor screening, requires donors to answer "specific and very direct questions" about their health, disease history, and high-risk behavior. Intravenous drug abusers are routinely deferred. Recently, donors who have lived in European countries with reported or suspected cases of "mad cow" disease have also been deferred. While the FDA claims this first line of screening weeds out 90% of unsuitable donors, it is entirely reliant on the truthfulness of the potential donor. Donors can answer the questions falsely if they so choose, and who is to know better?

Blood banks are required to keep a current list of deferred donors and not collect blood from them. Blood that is collected must then be quarantined until it can be tested for infectious agents. Currently, donor blood is required to be screened for hepatitis, human immunodeficiency virus (HIV), human T-cell lymphotropic virus (HTLV), and syphilis. Screening for West Nile virus was instituted in 2003.

The FDA takes the stance that maintaining a blood supply with zero risk of infectious disease transmission may not be possible, but claims that the blood supply is safer now than it ever has been. Dr. Feldschuh disagrees. "There's nothing that prevents further testing of blood," he says. "The sperm-banking industry does it routinely. It costs more, but once again, shouldn't that be the patient's choice?"

ADVANTAGES OF AUTOLOGOUS BLOOD BANKING

A blood transfusion is the most intimate contact you can have with another human being, says Dr. Feldschuh. Medically speaking, it is equivalent to an organ transplant.

"There are obvious benefits to donating blood to yourself," he explains. "You can't give yourself anything that you don't already have. Additionally, there's strong evidence that you heal more quickly when receiving your own blood."

There is no transfusion reaction with your own blood, he adds, whereas there is always at least a little transfusion reaction when receiving someone else's blood because there is never a perfect match. You avoid the risk of developing antibodies to one of the numerous human blood subtypes and suffering an allergic reaction, as Dr. Feldschuh's father did. Your own blood also carries your own antibodies, a significant advantage if you happen to be having cancer surgery.

"There's a fair amount of evidence that in colon cancer, for example, having a transfusion brings significantly higher risk of recurrence of the cancer, because someone else's blood lowers your immunity," Dr. Feldschuh says. "It's why we sometimes purposely give a transfusion to organ transplant patients, to lower immunity and decrease the chance of rejecting the transplanted organ."

ATTACKED BY THE BLOOD-BANKING INDUSTRY

With so many benefits to autologous blood storage, Dr. Feldschuh thought the concept would be well received. To his great surprise, the criticism was loud and strong, particularly from established blood banks. Idant Laboratories was attacked for being a for-profit entity, even though the company did not make any money from the venture. Blood groups termed the practice "speculative blood storage" and said it was selfish and elitist. They also claimed it would create shortages and thus deprive the public of blood.

"We answered all of those points," Dr. Feldschuh says. "Frankly, if someone can't be a donor to anyone else, they'd be adding to the supply because by storing their own, they wouldn't need someone else's blood. Those who can donate can still donate to others. To me, it's something that would appear to be common sense. People should have the right to store their own blood, and it's not very expensive."

Public records show that government regulators were none too thrilled with the Idant autologous blood bank. Published sources and insiders indicate that what followed was a series of inspections, claimed violations, and license suspensions that inactivated the company's blood and semen banks for several years. At one point, a city health inspector was discovered on the blood bank's premises after hours, trying to drill holes into the blood storage freezers to ruin the contents. Idant was reimbursed for the costs and the inspector was permitted to resign from his job. Did he act on his own, or was he doing what he was told? No one would ever know. But when the chaos died down years later and the lawsuits and problems were gone, Dr. Feldschuh and his board of directors vowed to continue operating Idant's blood bank.

Dr. Feldschuh believes that if enough people used autologous blood banking, it would eventually become self-supporting and be part of the overall blood system.

"Think of it as reserves," he says. "In an emergency, autologous blood stores could be freed up for general use and people could re-donate to themselves. It's good all around. We will always need a donor system. But unless the current system focuses more on testing, people should have the choice to store their own blood. It's their right."

References

1. Available at: http://www.fda.gov/opacom/factsheets/justthefacts/15blood.html. Accessed July 31, 2006.

2. Available at: http://www.ombwatch.org/article/articleview/2387/1/280. Accessed July 31, 2006.

3. H.R. Rep. No. 104–746 (1996).

Fish Oil Now Available by Prescription!

by William Faloon

FOR DECADES, THE PHARMACEUTICAL INDUSTRY HAS SOUGHT to limit competition by trying to get the FDA to regulate high-potency supplements as drugs. It was only because of intense consumer backlash that Congress passed legislation that protected the free sale of most supplements in the United States.

The introduction of an overpriced prescription fish oil drug provides absolute proof that every letter to Congress was well worth sending. Americans were perceptive enough to not let the drug industry (and federal government) trample our liberties under the guise of "protecting" us against "unproven" products.

PRESCRIPTION FISH OIL

The scientific evidence documenting the effects of fish oil in the body is overwhelming.[1-3] One of the substantiated benefits of fish oil supplementation is lowering elevated triglycerides in the blood.[4-6]

An enterprising company used the scientific findings about fish oil and conducted a study on humans with extremely high triglycerides (over 500 mg/dL).[7] As would be expected, compared to placebo, the triglyceride levels of the patients who received the fish oil were reduced by 51.6%. This company then applied to the FDA to have its fish oil approved as a new drug. The FDA granted the approval based on the company-sponsored clinical study showing that fish oil does exactly what it had previously been shown to do—that is, lower triglyceride levels.

With prescription drug status, this company is now free to make specific health claims about fish oil and aggressively sell it through cardiologists. If this company's marketing efforts are successful, it stands to earn an enormous amount of money from unwitting patients who do not realize that they can obtain fish oil supplements for a fraction of the price of this prescription fish oil drug.

WHY WOULD YOU EVER BUY YOUR FISH OIL BY PRESCRIPTION?

This new prescription fish oil product, containing 180 one thousand-milligram capsules per bottle, costs a whopping $236.89! That is about nine times more expensive than what this amount of fish oil sells for in a health food store.

The company selling this prescription fish oil drug knew that some consumers might question why they should pay such a high price. In their marketing materials, the company tries to differentiate their fish oil drug from what is available in health food stores by stating the following:

> The US Food and Drug Administration (FDA) has not approved nonprescription, dietary supplement omega-3s for the treatment of any specific disease or medical

condition, like very high triglyceride levels. Dietary supplement omega-3, or so-called fish oil, is not a substitute for prescription (fish oil) because they are not bioequivalent.[8]

Those who feel more comfortable using FDA-approved products can choose to pay the outlandish price of $236.89 for each bottle of this prescription-only fish oil drug. Even people with health insurance may find that their co-pay for this fish oil drug is still higher than what they could freely pay for fish oil supplements at a health food store. That is to say nothing of how much health insurance premiums could increase if too many patients are deceived into using this overpriced fish oil drug.

GREATER CONCENTRATION OF EPA/DHA IN PRESCRIPTION FISH OIL

This expensive fish oil drug does provide more EPA and DHA in each capsule than do most fish oil products sold by supplement companies. What this means is that five or six ordinary fish oil capsules might be needed to get the same amount of EPA/DHA contained in four capsules of this prescription-only version. But on a cost-per-milligram basis, the price for the prescription fish oil is still much higher than the non-prescription supplement.

WHAT OTHER NEW PRESCRIPTION FISH OIL DRUGS MIGHT THE FDA APPROVE?

Fish oil has been shown to prevent or alleviate a wide variety of ailments, including depression,[9–19] osteoporosis,[20–23] arthritis,[24–28] stroke,[29–31] heart attack,[32–44] Alzheimer's disease,[45–54] and some forms of cancer.[55–61]

Might there be future prescription fish oil products approved by the FDA as antidepressant drugs, as bone-protecting prescription drugs, as anti-arthritis prescription drugs, and even as cancer-preventive prescription drugs?

If so, some drug companies stand to make a lot of money. Elderly patients who are unaware of lower-cost fish oil supplements might have to do without some basic necessities in order to afford their fish oil prescriptions. This is unfortunate, as these high-priced fish oil drugs provide the same omega-3 fatty acids that health-conscious Americans have been supplementing with for the past 35 years.

References

1. Guesnet P, Alessandri JM, Vancassel S, Zamaria N. Analysis of the 2nd symposium "Anomalies of fatty acids, ageing and degenerating pathologies." *Reprod Nutr Dev*. 2004 May–Jun;44(3):263–71.

2. Horrocks LA, Yeo YK. Health benefits of docosahexaenoic acid (DHA). *Pharmacol Res*. 1999 Sep;40(3):21 1–25.

3. Roland I, De Leval X, Evrard B, Pirotte B, Dogne JM, Delattre L. Modulation of the arachidonic cascade with omega3 fatty acids or analogues: potential therapeutic benefits. *Mini Rev Med Chem*. 2004 Aug;4(6):659–68.

4. Available at: http://www.ahrq.gov/news/press/pr2004/omega3pr.htm. Accessed June 29, 2006.

5. Bruckner G. Microcirculation, vitamin E and omega 3 fatty acids: an overview. *Adv Exp Med Biol*. 1997; 415:195–208.

6. Mori TA, Vandongen R, Beilin LJ, Burke V, Morris J, Ritchie J. Effects of varying dietary fat, fish, and fish oils on blood lipids in a randomized controlled trial in men at risk of heart disease. *Am J Clin Nutr*. 1994 May;59(5):1060–8.

7. Harris WS, Ginsberg HN, Arunakul N, et al. Safety and efficacy of Omacor in severe hypertriglyceridemia. *J Cardiovasc Risk*. 1997 Oct-Dec;4(5–6):385–91.

8. Available at: http://www.omacorrx.com/About_OMACOR/What_to_Expect_on_OMACOR.html. Accessed June 29, 2006.

9. Visioli F, Galli C. Oleuropein protects low density lipoprotein from oxidation. *Life Sci*. 1994;55(24):1965–71.

10. Tiemeier H, Van Tuijl HR, Hofman A, Kiliaan AJ, Breteler MM. Plasma fatty acid composition and depression are associated in the elderly: the Rotterdam Study. *Am J Clin Nutr.* 2003 Jul;78(1):40–6.

11. Su KP, Huang SY, Chiu CC, Shen WW. Omega-3 fatty acids in major depressive disorder. A preliminary double-blind, placebo-controlled trial . *Eur Neuropsychopharmacol.* 2003 Aug;13(4):267–71.

12. Nemets B, Stahl Z, Belmaker RH. Addition of omega-3 fatty acid to maintenance medication treatment for recurrent unipolar depressive disorder. *Am J Psychiatry.* 2002 Mar;159(3):477–9.

13. Peet M, Horrobin DF. A dose-ranging study of the effects of ethyl-eicosapentaenoate in patients with ongoing depression despite apparently adequate treatment with standard drugs. *Arch Gen Psychiatry.* 2002 Oct;59(10):913–9.

14. Edwards R, Peet M, Shay J, Horrobin D. Omega-3 polyun-saturated fatty acid levels in the diet and in red blood cell membranes of depressed patients. *J Affect Discord.* 1998 Mar;48(2–3):149–55.

15. Peet M, Murphy B, Shay J, Horrobin D. Depletion of omega-3 fatty acid levels in red blood cell membranes of depressive patients. *Biol Psychiatry.* 1998 Mar 1;43(5):315–9.

16. Maes M, Christophe A, Delanghe J, Altamura C, Neels H, Melt-zer HY. Lowered omega-3 polyunsaturated fatty acids in serum phospholipids and cholesteryl esters of depressed patients. *Psychiatry Res.* 1999 Mar 22;85(3):275–91.

17. Stoll AL, Severus WE, Freeman MP, et al. Omega-3 fatty acids in bipolar disorder: a preliminary double-blind, placebocontolled trial. *Arch Gen Psychiatry.* 1999 May;56(5):407–12.

18. Hibbeln JR. Fish consumption and major depression. *Lancet.* 1998 Apr 18;351(9110):1213.

19. Maes M, Smith R, Christophe A, et al. Fatty acid composition in major depression: decreased omega 3 fractions in choles-teryl esters and increased C20: 4 omega 6/C20:5 omega 3 ratio in cholesteryl esters and phospholipids. *J Affect Disord.* 1996; 38:35–46.

20. Kruger MC, Coetzer H, de Winter R, Gericke G, van Papendorp DH. Calcium, gamma-linolenic acid (GLA) and eicosapentaenoic acid (EPA) supplementation in senile osteoporosis. *Aging (Milano).* 1998 Oct;10(5):385–94.

21. van Papendorp DH, Coetzer H, Kruger MC. Biochemical profile of osteoporotic patients on essential fatty acid supplementation. *Nutr Res.* 1995; 1 5(3):325–34.

22. Bhattacharya A, Rahman M, Banu J, et al. Inhibition of osteoporosis in autoimmune disease prone MRL/Mpj-Fas(lpr) mice by N-3 fatty acids. *J Am Coll Nutr.* 2005 Jun; 24(3):200–9.

23. Kesavalu L, Vasudevan B, Raghu B, et al. Omega-3 fatty acid effect on alveolar bone loss in rats. *J Dent Res.* 2006 Jul;85 (7):648–52.

24. Berbert AA, Kondo CR, Almendra CL, Matsuo T, Dichi I. Supplementation of fish oil and olive oil in patients with rheumatoid arthritis. *Nutrition.* 2005 Feb;21 (2): 131–6.

25. de la Puerta R, Martinez-Dominguez E, Ruiz-Gutierrez V. Effect of minor components of virgin olive oil on topical antiinflammatory assays. *Z Naturforsch* [C]. 2000 Sep-Oct;55(9–10):814–9.

26. Alexander JW. Immunonutrition: the role of omega-3 fatty acids. *Nutr.* 1998 Jul-Aug;14(7–8):627–33.

27. Ariza-Ariza R, Mestanza-Peralta M, Cardiel MH. Omega-3 fatty acid in rheumatoid arthritis: an overview. *Semin Arthritis Rheum.* 1998 Jun;27(6):366–70.

28. Kremer JM, Lawrence DA, Petrillow GF, et al. Effects of high-dose fish oil on rheumatoid arthritis after stopping non-steroidal antiinflammatory drugs. *Arthritis Rheum.* 1995 Aug;38(8):1107–14.

29. Serhan CN. Novel eicosanoid and docosanoid mediators: resolvins, docosatrienes, and neuroprotectins. *Curr Opin Clin Nutr Metab Care.* 2005 Mar;8(2):1 15–21.

30. Li H, Ruan XZ, Powis SH, et al. EPA and DHA reduce LPS-induced inflammation responses in HK-2 cells: evidence for a PPAR-gamma-dependent mechanism. *Kidney Int.* 2005 Mar;67(3):867–74.

31. Iso H, Rexrode KM, Stampfer MJ, et al. Intake of fish and omega-3 fatty acids and risk of stroke in women. *JAMA.* 2001 Jan 1 7;285(3):304–1 2.

32. Thorngren M, Gustafson A. Effects of 11-week increases in dietary eicosapentaenoic acid on bleeding time, lipids, and platelet aggregation. *Lancet.* 1981 Nov 28;2(8257):1 190–3.

33. Hjerkinn EM, Seljeflot I, Ellingsen I, et al. Influence of long-term intervention with dietary counseling, long-chain n-3 fatty acid supplements, or both on circulating markers of endothelial activation in men with long-standing hyperlipidemia. *Am J Clin Nutr.* 2005 Mar;81 (3):583–9.

34. Trichopoulou A, Bania C, Trichopoulou D. Mediterranean diet and survival among patients with coronary heart disease in Greece. *Arch Intern Med.* 2005 Apr 25;165(8):929–35.

35. Mori TA, Beilin LJ. Omega-3 fatty acids and inflammation. *Curr Atheroscler Rep.* 2004 Nov;6(6):461–7.

36. Calder PC. n-3 fatty acids and cardiovascular disease: evidence explained and mechanisms explored. *Clin Sci* (Lond). 2004 Jul; 107(1): 1–11.

37. Yam D, Bott-Kanner G, Genin I, Shinitzky M, Klainman E. The effect of omega-3 fatty acids on risk factors for cardiovascular diseases. *Harefuah.* 2001 Dec;140(12):1 156–8, 1230.

38. Connor WE. n-3 Fatty acids from fish and fish oil: panacea or nostrum? *Am J Clin Nutr.* 2001 Oct;74(4):415–6.

39. Dewailly E, Blanchet C, Lemieux S et al. n-3 Fatty Acids and cardiovascular disease risk factors among the Inuit of Nunavik. *Am J Clin Nutr.* 2001 Oct;74(4):464–73.

40. Marchioli1 R. Dietary supplementation with n-3 polyunsaturated fatty acids and vitamin E after myocardial infarction: results of the GISSI-Prevenzione trial. *Lancet.* 1999 Aug 7;354(9177):447–55.

41. von Schacky C, Angerer P, Kothny W, Theisen K, Mudra H. The effect of dietary omega-3 fatty acids on coronary atherosclerosis. A randomized, double-blind, placebo-controlled trial. *Ann Intern Med.* 1999 Apr 6;130(7):554–62.

42. Singh RB, Niaz MA, Sharma JP, Kumar R, Rastogi V, Moshiri M. Randomized, double-blind, placebo-controlled trial of fish oil and mustard oil in patients with suspected acute myocardial infarction: the Indian experiment of infarct survival-4. *Cardiovasc Drugs Ther*. 1997 Jul;1 1(3):485–91.

43. Das UN. Essential fatty acid metabolism in patients with essential hypertension, diabetes mellitus and coronary heart disease. *Prostaglandins Leukot Essent Fatty Acids*. 1995 Jun;52(6):387–91.

44. Garcia-Closas R, Serra-Majem L, Segura R. Fish consumption, omega-3 fatty acids and the Mediterranean diet. *Eur J Clin Nutr*. 1993 Sep;47 Suppl 1:S85–90.

45. Lukiw WJ, Cui JG, Marcheselli VL, et al. A role for docosahexaenoic acid-derived neuroprotectin D1 in neural cell survival and Alzheimer's disease. *J Clin Invest*. 2005 Oct;1 15(10):2774–83.

46. Bourre JM. Omega-3 fatty acids in psychiatry. *Med Sci* (Paris). 2005 Feb;21(2):216–21.

47. Bourre JM. Dietary omega-3 fatty acids and psychiatry: mood, behaviour, stress, depression, dementia and aging. *J Nutr Health Aging*. 2005 9(1):31–8.

48. Bourre JM. [The role of nutritional factors on the structure and function of the brain: an update on dietary requirements]. *Rev Neurol* (Paris). 2004 Sep;160(8–9):767–92.

49. Favreliere S, Perault MC, Huguet F, et al. DHA-enriched phospholipid diets modulate age-related alterations in rat hippocampus. *Neurobiol Aging*. 2003 Mar-Apr;24(2):233–43.

50. Martin DS, Lonergan PE, Boland B, et al. Apoptotic changes in the aged brain are triggered by interleukin-1 beta-induced activation of p38 and reversed by treatment with eicosapentaenoic acid. *J Biol Chem*. 2002 Sep 13;277(37):34239–46.

51. Youdim KA, Martin A, Joseph JA. Essential fatty acids and the brain: possible health implications. *Int J Dev Neurosci*. 2000 Jul-Aug; 1 8(4–5):383–99.

52. Conquer JA, Tierney MC, Zecevic J, Bettger WJ, Fisher RH. Fatty acid analysis of blood plasma of patients with Alzheimer's disease, other types of dementia, and cognitive impairment. *Lipids*. 2000 Dec;35(12):1305–12.

53. Morris MC, Evans DA, Bienias JL, et al. Consumption of fish and n-3 fatty acids and risk of incident Alzheimer's disease. *Arch Neurol*. 2003 Jul;60(7):940-6.

54. Kyle DJ, Schaefer E, Patton G, Beiser A. Low serum docosahexaenoic acid is a significant risk factor for Alzheimer's dementia. *Lipids*. 1999;34 Suppl:S245.

55. Hardman WE. n-3 fatty acids and cancer therapy. *J Nutr*. 2004 Dec;134(12 Suppl):3427S-430S.

56. Burns CP, Halabi S, Clamon GH, et al. Phase I clinical study of fish oil fatty acid capsules for patients with cancer cachexia: cancer and leukemia group B study 9473. *Clin Cancer Res*. 1999 Dec; 5(12):3942-7.

57. Tsuda H, Iwahori Y, Asamoto M, et al. Demonstration of organotropic effects of chemopreventive agents in multiorgan carcinogenesis models. *IARC Sci Publ*. 1996 (139):143-50.

58. Lai PB, Ross JA, Fearon KC, Anderson JD, Carter DC. Cell cycle arrest and induction of apoptosis in pancreatic cancer cells exposed to eicosapentaenoic acid in vitro. *Br J Cancer*. 1996 Nov;74(9):1375-83.

59. Gonzalez MJ. Fish oil, lipid peroxidation and mammary tumor growth. *J Am Coll Nutr*. 1995 Aug;14(4):325-35.

60. Zhu ZR, Agren J, Mannisto S, et al. Fatty acid composition of breast adipose tissue in breast cancer patients and patients with benign breast disease. *Nutr Cancer*. 1995;24(2):151-60.

61. O'Connor TP, Roebuck BD, Peterson F, Campbell TC. Effect of dietary intake of fish oil and fish protein on the development of L-azaserine-induced preneoplastic lesions in the rat pancreas. *J Natl Cancer Inst*. 1985 Nov;75(5):959-62.

Popular Misconceptions About Skin Cancer Prevention

by Steven V. Joyal, MD

P EOPLE APPLY SUNSCREEN TO PROTECT AGAINST SUNBURN, skin aging, and skin cancer. Because of the way sunscreen products are labeled by FDA mandate, consumers are often confused about which ingredients they need to achieve optimal protection against the sun's damaging and deadly rays.

Fortunately, scientific data have emerged indicating that health-conscious individuals can achieve broad-spectrum protection against the increasing onslaught of ultraviolet light penetrating our atmosphere.

Like clockwork, the sound bites occur on television news programs at the start of the summer season: "To prevent skin cancer and premature aging of the skin, apply sunscreen before going out in the sun."

Well known to scientists, physicians, and the average person alike, sun exposure is the main environmental risk factor for skin cancer,[1] and sunburn is a well-established risk factor for skin cancer.[2]

Sun exposure in the form of ultraviolet light not only accelerates skin aging, but can also result in debilitating disfigurement from skin cancer. Some types of skin cancer can even lead to premature death. Furthermore, we are in the midst of a veritable epidemic of skin cancer. The incidence of basal and squamous cell carcinoma is increasing, as is the occurrence of deadly malignant melanoma, a dangerous form of skin cancer that develops in the pigment-producing cells of the skin, known as melanocytes.

Conventional wisdom indicates that, in addition to avoiding sun exposure, sunscreen is your best bet for preventing skin cancer. However, the sun protection factor (SPF) rating system used by the FDA to regulate sunscreen products has an inherent flaw that renders its ratings dangerously inaccurate. This may create a false and potentially disastrous sense of security in sunscreen users.

FLAWS IN THE SPF RATING SYSTEM

Basal cell and squamous cell skin cancers are caused primarily by a particular spectrum of sunlight called ultraviolet B, or UV-B. It is UV-B radiation that also causes sunburn. The FDA's SPF rating system rates sunscreen for protection against UV-B light, but not against ultraviolet A (UV-A) light. UV-A, the longer-wavelength ultraviolet light, penetrates deeper than UV-B through the outer portion of the skin. This is very important, because UV-A damage is largely responsible for premature aging of the skin. Moreover, UV-A light exposes the melanocytes, which are the pigment-producing cells in the skin, to damage that can potentially result in malignant melanoma, the deadliest form of skin cancer.

MELANOMA MORTALITY

The American Cancer Society estimates that the mortality rate from melanoma has increased 50% since 1973. Nearly 8,000 Americans die of the disease every year.[3]

FDA FAILS TO WARN PUBLIC OF UV-A DANGERS

The FDA appears to recognize the limitations of its SPF rating system for sunscreen, yet has done nothing of substance to remedy the problem!

Back in 2000, the FDA discussed some of these issues in its consumer magazine, in which it described the inadequacy of UV-A rating as an "unresolved technical dilemma."[4]

Six years later and counting, the FDA's "unresolved technical dilemma" remains unresolved, while the population remains at risk. Is it any surprise that skin cancer has reached epidemic proportions?

References

1. Solar and ultraviolet radiation (IARC). Monographs on the evaluation of the carcinogenic risk of chemicals to humans. *IARC*. 1992;55.

2. Naylor MF, Farmer KC. The case for sunscreens. A review of their use in preventing actinic damage and neoplasia. *Arch Dermatol*. 1997 Sep; 133(9): 1146–54.

3. Available at: www.cancer.org/docroot/CRI/content? CRI_2_4_1X-What_are_the_key_ statistics_for_melanoma_50. asp? sitearea. Accessed March 27, 2006.

4. Available at: www.fda.gov/FDAC/features/2000/400_sun.html. Accessed March 27, 2006.

FDA Threatens to Raid Cherry Orchards

by William Faloon

A S AMERICANS STRUGGLE TO EAT A HEALTHIER DIET, THE FDA has taken draconian steps to suppress information about foods that reduce disease risk.

While various agencies of the federal government encourage us to eat more fruits and vegetables, the FDA has issued an edict that precludes cherry companies from posting scientific data on their websites. This censorship of published peer-reviewed studies denies consumers access to information that could be used to make wiser food choices.

Tobacco products kill 450,000 Americans each year.[1] Few people understand, however, that poor dietary habits are responsible for more deaths than tobacco. Considering the plethora of toxic foods advertised on television, it is easy to understand why so many consumers eat themselves to death. Just imagine if all you ate is what you saw advertised in the mass media.

The government stopped protecting the tobacco companies long ago, but the FDA continues to take actions that steer Americans away from certain fruits and vegetables that have proven disease-preventive effects.

FDA INTIMIDATES CHERRY GROWERS

There is not much profit in selling fresh fruits and vegetables. Growers of such foods cannot afford to advertise their produce in a meaningful way. Fortunately, the advent of the Internet has allowed cherry growers to enlighten the public about scientific studies showing that nutrients contained in cherries have significant health benefits.[2-15] Until recently, consumers could learn of the health benefits of cherries just by logging on to a cherry company's website. Some individuals might be impressed enough with this data to actually buy cherries at the grocery store instead of trans fat-laden snacks being advertised every second in the mass media.

On October 17, 2005, the FDA banned information about cherries' health benefits from appearing on websites.[16,17] The FDA sent warning letters to 29 companies that market cherry products. In these letters, the FDA ordered the companies to stop publicizing scientific data about cherries.[18] According to the FDA, when cherry companies disseminate this information, the cherries become unapproved drugs subject to seizure. The FDA warns that if those involved in cherry trafficking continue to inform consumers about these scientific studies, criminal prosecutions will ensue.[17]

WHY AMERICANS DON'T EAT MORE FRUIT

The processed food industry has earned enormous profits by loading cheap and dangerous foods with sugar, salt, preservatives, trans fats, saturated fats, and other unhealthy byproducts. Processed foods taste good to most people and are quite inexpensive compared to fresh produce. In order to convince the public to switch from toxic foods that damage the arterial wall, mutate DNA, and induce age-related disease, those who sell fresh fruits need to inform the public about the benefits scientists have discovered about plant foods.[19–37]

Fresh fruit can be expensive and it spoils relatively quickly. Many consumers have developed a taste addiction to processed foods, and find it challenging to switch to a healthier diet that costs more and is not as pleasing to the palate.

By censoring scientific information about cherries, the FDA is in effect shutting down an opportunity for more Americans to learn about the remarkable health benefits that have been discovered about this fruit.

DO CHERRIES PREVENT CANCER?

In a warning letter to Friske Orchards of Ellsworth, MI, the FDA recites the following information contained on this orchard's website:[38] "Tart cherries may reduce the risk of colon cancer because of the anthocyanins and cyanidin contained in the cherry."

The FDA goes on to say in its warning letter:

> These claims cause your product to be a drug as defined in section 201(g). . . . Because this product is not generally recognized as safe and effective when used as labeled, it is also defined as a new drug in section 201(p). . . . Under section 505 of the Act (21 USC 355), a new drug may not be legally marketed in the United States without an approved New Drug Application. . . .

Interestingly, the FDA is not denying the veracity of this information. Instead, it insists that a new drug application has to be approved before the public can be informed about the scientific data supporting cherries. The FDA also asserts, without any basis, that cherries "have not been recognized as safe and effective when used as labeled."[38] According to the FDA's interpretation of the law, cherry growers are engaged in criminal conduct by relaying findings that have been published in peer-reviewed scientific journals. Whether you or other Americans develop cancer does not appear to be a consideration of an agency whose written mission statement includes the following:

> The FDA is responsible for advancing the public health by helping to speed innovations that make medicines and foods more effective, safer, and more affordable; and helping the public get the accurate, science-based information they need to use medicines and foods to improve their health.[39]

As Life Extension documented many years ago, the FDA does the opposite of what it pretends to do. Instead of "helping the public get the accurate, science-based information they need to use foods to improve their health," the FDA has gone to extreme lengths to deny American citizens the right to learn about scientific studies substantiating the health benefits discovered about cherries (and other fruits).

A MEDICAL ATROCITY!

In November 2004, Dr. David Graham, associate director for science at the FDA's Office of Drug Safety, testified before Congress that Vioxx® had caused 88,000 to 139,000 excess cases of heart attack and stroke.[40] Dr. Graham severely criticized his own employer (the FDA) for intentionally covering up information about the lethal side effects of Vioxx®.

As you will read in this month's issue, the FDA is greatly concerned that cherry companies are disseminating scientific data showing that cherries are more effective than FDA-approved drugs in alleviating arthritis inflammation and pain.

The FDA is willing to throw cherry growers in jail for suggesting that their fruit may safely alleviate arthritis discomfort, yet the irrefutable facts are that the FDA intentionally concealed the dangers of Vioxx® for years, thereby causing the needless death of tens of thousands of Americans. Who are the real criminals here?

The FDA says it is responsible for "protecting the public health" by assuring the safety of drugs. It does not take much brainpower to see that the FDA's purported mission is nothing more than a hoax to protect the economic interests of the pharmaceutical giants.

It would appear that the FDA is concerned that if too many arthritis sufferers discover that eating cherries could alleviate inflammation and pain, the multibillion-dollar market for anti-inflammatory drugs would be detrimentally affected. Pharmaceutical industry profits have been spared for the moment by the flagrant acts perpetrated against cherry companies by the FDA.

CONGRESS RECOGNIZES PROBLEMS WITH FDA

As this nation faces a worsening healthcare crisis that threatens to bankrupt corporations, aging adults, and the government itself, members of Congress are becoming incensed that the FDA is suppressing proven methods to prevent and treat disease.

On November 10, 2005, a bill was introduced in the United States House of Representatives that would prohibit the FDA from denying consumers access to truthful health information. The name of this bill is the Health Freedom Protection Act (H.R. 4282).[41]

The original sponsors of this bill introduced it by exposing the FDA's inappropriate censorship of life-saving scientific information. Here is an excerpt from this historic speech:

> Because of the FDA's censorship of truthful health claims, millions of Americans may suffer with diseases and other healthcare problems they may have avoided by using dietary supplements. For example, the FDA prohibited consumers from learning how folic acid reduces the risk of neural tube defects for four years after the Centers for Disease Control and Prevention recommended every woman of childbearing age take

folic acid supplements to reduce neural tube defects. This FDA action contributed to an estimated 10,000 cases of preventable neural tube defects!

The FDA also continues to prohibit consumers from learning about the scientific evidence that glucosamine and chondroitin sulfate are effective in the treatment of osteoarthritis; that omega-3 fatty acids may reduce the risk of sudden death heart attack; and that calcium may reduce the risk of bone fractures.

The Health Freedom Protection Act will force the FDA to at last comply with the commands of Congress, the First Amendment, and the American people by codifying the First Amendment standards adopted by the federal courts. Specifically, the Health Freedom Protection Act stops the FDA from censoring truthful claims about the curative, mitigative, or preventative effects of dietary supplements, and adopts the federal court's suggested use of disclaimers as an alternative to censorship. The Health Freedom Protection Act also stops the FDA from prohibiting the distribution of scientific articles and publications regarding the role of nutrients in protecting against disease.[42]

CITIZENS REVOLT AGAINST BUREAUCRATIC CORRUPTION

When Life Extension stated in 1989 that the law had to be changed to allow scientific information about foods and supplements to be freely disseminated, everyone told us that it was impossible to beat the entrenched FDA on Capitol Hill. As we went on national television and radio shows in the early 1990s to expose the incompetence and fraud perpetrated against the public by the FDA, a growing number of health-conscious individuals began to realize the magnitude of the problem.

In October 1994, by a nearly unanimous margin, Congress enacted the Dietary Supplement Health and Education Act (DSHEA), which allowed the public to learn about some of the health benefits attributed to certain nutrients.[43]

Despite significant losses in the federal courts regarding how DSHEA should be interpreted, the FDA is continuing to dedicate substantial resources to suppressing scientific information about how certain foods may prevent and treat disease. The FDA's arrogance is appalling in light of the record number of prescription drugs that have been withdrawn because too many users are dying from side effects. In the case of cherries, many of the scientific studies the FDA is concerned about relate to this fruit's anti-arthritic effect.[4-6,44,45]

The FDA's flagrant disregard for the First Amendment and DSHEA is one reason why the Health Freedom Protection Act was introduced. Members of Congress and the American public are fed up with the abuse of power perpetrated by an agency whose track record shows a reckless disregard for human life.

DRUG COMPANIES CONTROL FDA

The FDA has come under fire by the media and Congress for its failure to protect consumers against dangerous drugs. Life Extension has long contended that large drug companies exert tremendous influence over the FDA. The result is that toxic drugs remain on the market while the sale of dietary supplements (and now even cherries) is impeded by FDA.

One reason doctors prescribe dangerous drugs is that pharmaceutical companies persuade the FDA to omit information concerning side effects from the drug's label. An egregious example of the incestuous control that drug companies exert over the FDA came to light with the Vioxx® scandal.

Based on evidence showing increased heart attack rates in Vioxx® users, the FDA suggested putting a cardiovascular warning on the label. Merck, the maker of Vioxx®, vehemently objected. On November 8, 2001, when talks with the FDA were not going to Merck's liking, the head of Merck's research department sent an email to his top scientists stating:

> Twice in my life I have had to say to the FDA, "That label is unacceptable, we will not under any circumstances accept it." . . . I assure you I will NOT sign off on any label that has a cardiac warning for Vioxx®.[46]

Vioxx® was withdrawn from the market on September 30, 2004, after a clinical trial showed the risk of heart attack and stroke doubled for patients taking Vioxx® for more than 18 months.[47–49] The FDA knew about the cardiovascular risks of Vioxx® years before it was withdrawn, but succumbed to drug company pressure to omit this information from the drug's warning box. It did appear many months later on the label's "precautions box," which is normally too voluminous for anyone to read.

The statement by the Merck official that he would "not under any circumstances accept" a cardiovascular warning on Vioxx® provides a startling glimpse into how much control drug companies have over the FDA. Consumers are relegated to ingest toxic drugs while the FDA takes extraordinary measures to censor information showing the anti-arthritis efficacy of cherries.

References

1. Available at: http://www.cdc.gov/tobacco/factsheets/Tobacco_Related_Mortality_factsheet.htm. Accessed December 12, 2005.

2. Kang SY, Seeram NP, Nair MG, Bourquin LD. Tart cherry anthocyanins inhibit tumor development in Apc(Min) mice and reduce proliferation of human colon cancer cells. *Cancer Lett.* 2003 May 8;194(1):13–9.

3. Pratico D, Tillmann C, Zhang ZB, Li H, FitzGerald GA. Acceleration of atherogenesis by COX-1-dependent prostanoid formation

in low density lipoprotein receptor knockout mice. *Proc Natl Acad Sci USA*. 2001 Mar 13;98(6):3358–63.

4. Tall JM, Seeram NP, Zhao C, et al. Tart cherry anthocyanins suppress inflammation-induced pain behavior in rat. *Behav Brain Res*. 2004 Aug 12;153(1):181–8.

5. Wang H, Nair MG, Strasburg GM, et al. Cyclooxygenase active bioflavonoids from Balaton tart cherry and their structure activity relationships. *Phytomedicine*. 2000 Mar;7(1):15–9.

6. Seeram NP, Momin RA, Nair MG, Bourquin LD. Cyclooxygenase inhibitory and antioxidant cyanidin glycosides in cherries and berries. *Phytomedicine*. 2001 Sep;8(5):362–9.

7. Wang H, Nair MG, Strasburg GM, et al. Antioxidant and antiinflammatory activities of anthocyanins and their aglycon, cyanidin, from tart cherries. *J Nat Prod*. 1999 Feb;62(2):294–6.

8. Kolayli S, Kucuk M, Duran C, Candan F, Dincer B. Chemical and antioxidant properties of Laurocerasus officinalis Roem. (cherry laurel) fruit grown in the Black Sea region. *J Agric Food Chem*. 2003 Dec 3;51(25):7489–94.

9. Wakabayashi H, Fukushima H, Yamada T, et al. Inhibition of LPS-stimulated NO production in mouse macrophage-like cells by Barbados cherry, a fruit of Malpighia emarginata DC. *Anti-Cancer Res*. 2003 Jul;23(4):3237–41.

10. Nagamine I, Akiyama T, Kainuma M, et al. Effect of acerola cherry extract on cell proliferation and activation of ras signal pathway at the promotion stage of lung tumorigenesis in mice. *J Nutr Sci Vitaminol* (Tokyo). 2002 Feb;48(1):69–72.

11. Jacob RA, Spinozzi GM, Simon VA, et al. Consumption of cherries lowers plasma urate in healthy women. *J Nutr*. 2003 Jun;133(6):1826–9.

12. Rimm EB, Katan MB, Ascherio A, Stampfer MJ, Willett WC. Relation between intake of flavonoids and risk for coronary heart disease in male health professionals. *Ann Intern Med*. 1996 Sep 1;125(5):384–9.

13. Burkhardt S, Tan DX, Manchester LC, Hardeland R, Reiter RJ. Detection and quantification of the antioxidant melatonin in

Montmorency and Balaton tart cherries (Prunus cerasus). *J Agric Food Chem*. 2001 Oct;49(10):4898–902.

14. Available at: http://pubs.acs.org/pressrelease/jafc/release3. html. Accessed December 15, 2005.

15. Available at: http://www.wholehealthmd.com/print/ view/1,1560,SU_10015,00.html. Accessed December 15, 2005.

16. Available at: http://www.wjla.com/news/stories/1005/272655. html. Accessed December 15, 2005.

17. Available at: http://www.fda.gov/bbs/topics/news/2005/ new01246.html. Accessed December 15, 2005.

18. Available at: http://www.cfsan.fda.gov/~dms/chrylist.html. Accessed December 15, 2005.

19. Available at: http://aspartametruth.com/ blaylock/interaction. html. Accessed December 15, 2005.

20. Available at: http://www.inmotionmagazine.com/ geff4.html. Accessed December 15, 2005.

21. Sasso FC, Carbonara O, Nasti R, et al. Glucose metabolism and coronary heart disease in patients with normal glucose tolerance. *JAMA*. 2004 Apr 21;291(15):1857–63.

22. Reiser S. Effect of dietary sugars on metabolic risk factors associated with heart disease. *Nutr Health*. 1985;3(4):203–16.

23. Pamplona R, Bellmunt MJ, Portero M, Prat J. Mechanisms of glycation in atherogenesis. *Med Hypotheses*. 1993 Mar;40 (3):174–81.

24. Reyes FG, Valim MF, Vercesi AE. Effect of organic synthetic food colours on mitochondrial respiration. *Food Addit Contam*. 1996 Jan;13(1):5–11.

25. Jagerstad M, Skog K. Genotoxicity of heat-processed foods. *Mutat Res*. 2005 Jul 1;574(1–2):156–72.

26. Sasaki YF, Kawaguchi S, Kamaya A, et al. The comet assay with 8 mouse organs: results with 39 currently used food additives. *Mutat Res*. 2002 Aug 26;519(1–2): 103–19.

27. Tsuda S, Murakami M, Matsusaka N, et al. DNA damage induced by red food dyes orally administered to pregnant and male mice. *Toxicol Sci*. 2001 May;61(1):92–9.

28. Ashida H, Hashimoto T, Tsuji S, Kanazawa K, Danno G. Synergistic effects of food colors on the toxicity of 3-amino-1,4¬dimethyl-5H-pyrido[4,3-b]indole (Trp-P-1) in primary cultured rat hepatocytes. *J Nutr Sci Vitaminol* (Tokyo). 2000 Jun;46(3):130–6.

29. Tjaderhane L, Larmas M. A high sucrose diet decreases the mechanical strength of bones in growing rats. *J Nutr*. 1998 Oct;128(10):1807–10.

30. Veromann S, Sunter A, Tasa G, et al. Dietary sugar and salt represent real risk factors for cataract development. *Ophthalmologica*. 2003 Jul;217(4):302–7.

31. Michaud DS, Liu S, Giovannucci E, et al. Dietary sugar, glycemic load, and pancreatic cancer risk in a prospective study. *J Natl Cancer Inst*. 2002 Sep 4;94(17):1293–300.

32. Molteni R, Barnard RJ, Ying Z, Roberts CK, Gomez-Pinilla F. A high-fat, refined sugar diet reduces hippocampal brain-derived neurotrophic factor, neuronal plasticity, and learning. *Neuroscience*. 2002;112(4):803–14.

33. Blacklock NJ. Sucrose and idiopathic renal stone. *Nutr Health*. 1987;5(1–2):9–17.

34. Moerman CJ, Bueno de Mesquita HB, Runia S. Dietary sugar intake in the aetiology of biliary tract cancer. *Int J Epidemiol*. 1993 Apr;22(2):207–14.

35. Kruis W, Forstmaier G, Scheurlen C, Stellaard F. Effect of diets low and high in refined sugars on gut transit, bile acid metabolism, and bacterial fermentation. *Gut*. 1991 Apr;32(4):367–71.

36. Yudkin J, Eisa O. Dietary sucrose and oestradiol concentration in young men. *Ann Nutr Metab*. 1988;32(2):53–5.

37. De Stefani E, Deneo-Pellegrini H, Mendilaharsu M, Ronco A, Carzoglio JC. Dietary sugar and lung cancer: a case-control study in Uruguay. *Nutr Cancer*. 1998;31(2):132–7.

38. Available at: http://www.fda.gov/foi/warning_letters/g5531d.htm. Accessed December 15, 2005.

39. Available at: http://www.fda.gov/opacom/morechoices/mission.html. Accessed December 15, 2005.

40. Available at: http://www.finance.senate.gov/ sitepages/ hearing111804.htm. Accessed December 15, 2005.

41. Available at: http://thomas.loc.gov/. Accessed December 15, 2005.

42. Available at: http://www.house.gov/ paul/congrec/congrec2005/ cr111005.htm. Accessed December 15, 2005.

43. Available at: http://www.fda.gov/opacom/laws/dshea.html. Accessed December 15, 2005.

44. Available at: http://www.arthritis.org/resources/ arthritistoday/2002_archives/2002_09_10_OnCall.asp. Accessed December 15, 2005.

45. Blando F, Gerardi C, Nicoletti I. Sour cherry (Prunus cerasus L) anthocyanins as ingredients for functional foods. *J Biomed Biotechnol*. 2004;2004(5):253–8.

46. Martinez B. Novartis fights eczema drug's cancer warning. *Wall Street Journal*. April 8, 2005.

47. Bresalier RS, Sandler RS, Quan H, et al. Cardiovascular events associated with rofecoxib in a colorectal adenoma chemoprevention trial. *N Engl J Med*. 2005 Mar 17;352(11):1092–102.

48. Topol EJ. Failing the public healthrofecoxib, Merck, and the FDA. *N Engl J Med*. 2004 Oct 21;351(17):1707–9.

49. Martinez B. Merck documents shed light on Vioxx® legal battles. *Wall Street Journal*. February 7, 2005

2005

Inside the FDA's Brain

by William Faloon

THE FDA HAS RELEASED A DETAILED REPORT THAT STATES, "it is highly unlikely that green tea reduces the risk of prostate cancer."[1]

The FDA made it clear that it evaluates lots of evidence when deciding whether to allow a health claim. Most of this evidence, however, is eliminated from further review because it does not meet the agency's standards.

While there are numerous published studies on green tea and prostate cancer, the FDA determined that only two met its standards. The first study cited by the agency showed that drinking three cups of green tea a day reduced prostate cancer risk by 73%.[2] The second study did not provide statistically significant data, but showed that drinking two to 10 cups of green tea daily reduced prostate cancer risk by 33%.[3] According to the FDA, "both studies received high methodological quality ratings."

Based on these two human studies, the FDA will allow the following health claim for green tea beverages:

> One weak and limited study does not show that drink-
> ing green tea reduces the risk of prostate cancer, but
> another weak and limited study suggests that drinking
> green tea may reduce this risk. Based on these studies,
> FDA concludes that it is highly unlikely that green tea
> reduces the risk of prostate cancer.[1]

WHY FDA CALLS THESE "WEAK" STUDIES

The FDA's gold standard is tightly controlled studies that consist of an active component and a placebo arm. The two green
tea studies chosen by the FDA evaluated the effects of historical consumption of green tea beverages on prostate cancer risk.

The studies showed that the greater the consumption of green
tea, the lower the prostate cancer risk. This does not, however,
impress the FDA as much as a carefully designed study where
half of the men would drink three to 10 cups of green tea a day
while the other half drank a placebo beverage.

While the FDA admits that the study showing a 73% reduction in prostate cancer risk is significant, the agency believes
the study that showed a non-statistically significant 33% risk
reduction cancelled out the better study. According to the FDA,
"replication of scientific findings is important in order to substantiate results."[4,5]

THE OMITTED STUDY

While the FDA claims to have extensively reviewed the scientific
literature to find the truth about green tea and prostate cancer,
one important study was overlooked.

In a tightly controlled clinical setting, men with pre-malignant
prostate disease were given either 600 mg a day of green tea extract
or a placebo. Compared to those who received the placebo, men

with this pre-malignant condition who received the green tea extract were 90% less likely to develop prostate cancer.[6]

While the FDA may argue that green tea supplements differ from green tea beverages, the fact is that this placebo-controlled study existed, but was omitted from the FDA's report. The FDA's report concluded:

> Based on FDA's review of the strength of the total body of publicly available scientific evidence for a claim about green tea and reduced risk of prostate cancer, FDA ranks this evidence as the lowest level for a qualified health claim. For the reasons given above, FDA concludes that it is highly unlikely that green tea reduces the risk of prostate cancer.[4]

THE FDA PRESS RELEASE

The FDA issued a press release to alert the world that green tea has little or no value in preventing cancer. The news media picked up on the FDA's negative findings about green tea and echoed the agency's claims that green tea does not prevent cancer.

Newspapers and television stations reported that consumers were wasting their money by drinking green tea. None of these media sources bothered to check the National Library of Medicine's database to find over 600 studies relating to green tea and cancer. Even a cursory review of these studies reveals a very different story than what was contained in the FDA's press release.

The National Library of Medicine is part of the US Department of Health and Human Services, the same parent agency as the FDA!

CONSUMERS NEED TO KNOW THE FACTS

The United States faces a worsening healthcare crisis as aging baby boomers financially exhaust the nation's medical systems.

The FDA is empowered to regulate almost every aspect of our healthcare, yet this federal agency continues to behave in a manner that promotes illness. An unbiased review of the published scientific literature reveals health properties attributed to green tea, but the FDA has restricted what Americans are allowed to read on the labels of green tea beverages.

If the data about green tea and prostate cancer risk turn out to be only partially accurate, the lives of millions of men could be saved and billions of dollars shaved off future healthcare expenditures. Yet the law still allows the FDA to censor truthful information about foods and dietary supplements.

WE CAN CHANGE THE LAW

On May 12, 2005, a bill was introduced in the US House of Representatives that would give consumers access to truthful, non-misleading health information. This bill—the Consumers' Access to Health Information Act (H.R. 2352)[7]—seeks to amend the Food, Drug and Cosmetic Act to ensure that:

- Accurate health claims are not suppressed;
- Consumers are given truthful and complete information about the curative, mitigation, treatment, and prevention effects of foods and dietary supplements on disease or health-related conditions;
- The FDA honors the intent of the Congress not to censor accurate health claims.

This is one of the most critical pieces of legislation to ever come before Congress. Passage of the Consumers' Access to Health Information Act would enable the American public to learn how to prevent many of the degenerative diseases of aging. This bill could help avert the healthcare crisis that is threatening to bankrupt Medicare, corporations, and aging adults.

References

1. FDA issues information for consumers about claims for green tea and certain cancers [press release]. Washington, DC: US Food and Drug Administration; June 30, 2005.

2. Jian L, Xie LP, Lee AH, Binns CW. Protective effect of green tea against prostate cancer: a case-control study in southeast *China*. *Int J Cancer*. 2004 Jan 1;108(1):130–5.

3. Sonoda T, Nagata Y, Mori M et al. A case-control study of diet and prostate cancer in Japan: possible protective effect of traditional Japanese diet. *Cancer Sci*. 2004 Mar;95(3):238–42.

4. Available at: http://www.cfsan.fda.gov/~dms/qhc-gtea.html. Accessed August 19, 2005.

5. Wilson EB Jr. Replication of scientific findings is important for evaluating the strength of scientific evidence. In: *An Introduction to Scientific Research*. Mineola, NY: Dover Publications;1990:46–48.

6. Available at: http://www.aacr.org/Default.aspx?p=1066&d=432. Accessed August 19, 2005.

7. Available at: http://thomas.loc.gov/cgi-bin/query/z?c109:H.R.2352.IH. Accessed August 19, 2005.

Drug Makers Abuse FDA Approval Process

by Linda M. Smith, RN

MOST DRUG COMPANIES BENEFITING FROM THE FDA'S "accelerated approval" process—a means of expediting approval of drugs intended for patients with life-threatening illness—have not conducted legally required post-marketing studies on their products, according to Rep. Edward J. Markey (D-MA).[1]

Created in 1992, the FDA's accelerated approval process uses preliminary data indicating drug safety and efficacy to help bring drugs to the marketplace more quickly. This process greatly reduces the typical 10-to-15-year time period required to conceive, develop, and thoroughly test new drugs in animals and humans. In return for the enormous marketing advantages realized by drug makers, it was agreed that rigorous studies validating the preliminary data would continue in accordance with normal approval procedures.

Released on June 1, 2005, Rep. Markey's report, *Conspiracy of Silence: How the FDA Allows Drug Companies to Abuse the Accelerated Approval Process*, reveals that at least 17 drug companies have not completed the FDA-required post-marketing studies. Of the 91 post-marketing studies promised since 1992, only 49 have been completed. Of the 42 pending studies, half have not even been initiated, though some of the approved drugs have been on the market for years; three are in progress but behind schedule; and only 18 are currently meeting scheduled milestones.

Although the FDA has the authority to withdraw drugs from the market in the absence of supporting data, it has not done so in any cases. The need for post-approval studies is well illustrated by AstraZeneca's Iressa®, approved in May 2003 to treat non-small cell lung cancer. While preliminary data suggested that Iressa® would benefit 10% of patients, the FDA's review of the mandated follow-up studies by AstraZeneca concluded that Iressa® provided no survival benefit and that patients taking it should discuss treatment alternatives with their physicians.

The FDA must enforce its requirements for post-marketing studies by drug makers in order to protect public safety.

Reference

1. Available at: http://www.house.gov/markey/Issues/iss_health_pr050601.pdf. Accessed June 15, 2005.

FDA Fails to Protect Domestic Drug Supply

by William Faloon

I F YOU TAKE THE INFORMATION ON THE FDA'S WEBSITE AT FACE value, you would be convinced that the FDA has guaranteed the safety of our drug supply—as long as you do not import any prescription drugs from outside the United States.

According to the FDA's website, medications not approved for sale in the US may not have been manufactured under this nation's rigid quality assurance procedures that ensure a safe, effective product. These imported drugs may not have been evaluated for safety and effectiveness in the US, and thus might be addictive or even contain dangerous substances. Moreover, according to the FDA's website, some imported medications— even those bearing the name of a US-approved product—may be counterfeit versions that are unsafe or even completely inef- fective. The FDA suggests that you need not worry about these dangers if you buy drugs from domestic pharmacies.[1]

Joe McCallion, a consumer safety officer in the FDA's Office of Regulatory Affairs, sums it up this way: "If you buy drugs that come from outside the US, the FDA doesn't know what you're getting, which means safety can't be assured."[1]

On the other hand, the FDA website notes that drugs sold in the US must be made in accordance with good manufacturing practices, and all products must have proper labeling that conforms to FDA requirements. As part of the FDA's "high" standards, drugs can be manufactured only at plants registered with the agency, and manufacturers are subject to ongoing FDA inspections. Along with these legal requirements, US pharmacists and wholesalers must be licensed or authorized in the states where they operate.[1] These safeguards in the process of getting drugs onto US pharmacy shelves ensure that the products you buy are safe and effective.

It is a great argument, designed to assure us that the FDA has things well under control. If only it were true.

THE REAL STORY

In fact, the drugs you buy pass through a network of wholesalers operating under lax state supervision and virtually no FDA supervision. You probably assume the drug manufacturers ship their products directly to pharmacies, maintaining strict control all along the way. Not so. Big pharmaceutical companies use middlemen that buy, sell, sort, repackage, and distribute 98% of the nation's medicine. These middlemen, numbering about 6,500 in all, range from publicly traded giants with pristine warehouses to small, obscure, backroom operators. While the three largest companies control 90% of this market, below them are some 15 regional wholesalers, and below them are scores of smaller secondary wholesalers.

All of these middlemen, regardless of size, aim to buy medicine as cheaply as possible and resell it for a profit, a system of arbitrage made possible by widely varying drug prices. Drug companies offer an array of targeted discounts that result in their selling the exact same drug for any number of prices.

These varying prices often spark frenetic trading among the wholesalers. The "Big Three" distributors have trading divisions that scout the secondary wholesale market for discounted medicine, and they have been known to boast how much they saved by purchasing heavily discounted medicine from obscure wholesalers. The secondary wholesalers contend that this aggressive trading helps reduce drug prices for mom-and-pop pharmacies and local hospitals that lack the buying power of the big chains.

However, the bargains also drive a parallel and illegal process called diversion, in which some middlemen resort to fraud or misrepresentation to obtain discounted medicine. Corrupt wholesalers often solicit "closed-door" pharmacies (those that supposedly buy only for themselves) and others that qualify for discounts to buy more medicine than they need and sell the rest out the back door for kickbacks. In 2000, the National Association of Boards of Pharmacy estimated that up to four-fifths of the closed-door pharmacies that received discounted medicine illegally resold at least a portion of it to outside buyers.

STOLEN DRUGS

In her book, *Dangerous Doses: How Counterfeiters Are Contaminating America's Drug Supply*, investigative medical reporter Katherine Eban details the results of a two-year exploration of America's secret ring of drug counterfeiters, following the trail of medicine as it winds its way from a seemingly minor break-in to a sprawling national network of drug polluters. She follows the progress of a team of Florida criminal investigators as they uncover sickening examples of stolen medicine that is resold as the genuine article without any of the safeguards we assume exist for prescription drugs.[2]

While the FDA has an Office of Criminal Investigations, the agency does not aggressively pursue these matters. The wholesalers profiled in Dangerous Doses use this confusion to their advantage. They have state licenses, lawyers, accountants, and all the trappings of legitimacy. Their goal is to buy low, sell high, and make money. But they have little incentive to maintain drugs in pristine condition.[2]

Three years ago in Florida, it was laughably easy to become a pharmaceutical wholesaler. All you needed was a refrigerator, an air conditioner, an alarm to secure your products, $200 for a security bond, and $700 for a license. No experience or particular knowledge was required. You had to certify that you had no criminal record, but the state's pharmaceutical bureau did not actually check for a criminal background. Through this loophole slipped all sorts of unsavory characters: former cocaine dealers looking for good money with less chance of jail time, real estate hucksters, and others. Once established, a pharmaceutical wholesaler had little reason to worry about FDA inspections. State authorities alone regulated your business. And each inspector had some 300 companies to look after.[2]

With this regulatory framework, Florida's pharmaceutical wholesale companies proliferated like rabbits, far beyond any need for them. By 2002, Florida had licensed 1,399 wholesalers, one for every three pharmacies in the state. The vast majority of these companies were based out of state, though some actually were Florida operations. The wholesalers set up "corporate headquarters" by rerouting their calls and faxes to make it appear that they had offices everywhere.[2]

Not surprisingly, criminal elements were drawn to this regulatory vacuum like moths to a flame. The state investigation began when a two-bit burglar stole cancer medicine from an unlocked refrigerator at Jackson Memorial Hospital in Miami. Caught in the act, he cooperated with police in return for leniency, agreeing to carry a hidden microphone while he sold his stolen goods. The woman who bought the drug, a licensed wholesaler, threw it in the hot trunk of her car while she did errands, destroying the potency of this delicate medicine without any obvious indication of damage. According to the investigators, this adulteration happens frequently, with the end-user of the drug being the hapless victim. Arrested later that day, she also agreed to cooperate, and in time the state investigators worked their way to the kingpins of the trade, who were making millions from this illicit activity.[2]

RECYCLED DRUGS

One of these men was Michael Carlow, who pocketed $2.5 million in a single eight-month period. Duffel bags delivered to his house were filled with pill bottles, medicine vials, and bags of blood derivatives, all culled from different sources and some still bearing the labels of the patients to whom they had been dispensed.[2]

His conspirators maintained the flow of discounted inventory by buying anti-cancer and anti-AIDS drugs from patients treated at health clinics in Miami's slums. Some of those infected with HIV/AIDS were crack addicts who preferred getting high to getting well. Carlow's associates waited for them outside the clinics and swayed them to sell their Medicaid-supplied medicine (including growth hormone that retails for more than $1,000) for a few $20 bills.[2]

Carlow sold the medicine through his licensed wholesale businesses, using a variety of aliases to make them appear to be independently owned. The buyers of his goods would sometimes meet Carlow or an assistant at a gas station to exchange medicine for checks or cash. At Carlow's office, the state investigators found nail polish remover, lighter fluid, and paint remover cluttering the worktables and desks. The employees apparently used these products to remove patient dispensing labels and any other evidence of a product's origin. However, Carlow did not stop at selling to small, obscure companies. He developed a lucrative relationship with one of the Big Three distributors. In 2000, Carlow sold almost $2 million in contaminated or even counterfeit products to National Specialty Services, a Big Three division that at the time was the nation's largest supplier of blood products, cancer drugs, and other specialty pharmaceuticals to hospitals.[2]

STOLEN BLOOD

Carlow was not the only kingpin to be trapped in the state investigators' dragnet. In January 2002, thieves stole 344 vials of specialty blood products from a refrigerator in the warehouse of BioMed Plus, one of the nation's largest wholesale distributors of these drugs. These products, worth $335,000 wholesale, were destined for patients with compromised immune systems, hemophilia, and other rare disorders. Incredibly, the owner of BioMed Plus received a call a few days later from a wholesaler who offered to let him buy back a list of products identical to his list of stolen goods for a discounted price of $229,241. This medicine is rare and is almost never traded freely, so BioMed's owner knew the goods were his. He cooperated with investigators to retrieve the stolen drugs, but had to destroy the medicine because he could not guarantee that it had been properly stored during the heist.[2]

COUNTERFEIT DRUGS

The state investigators also discovered a filthy Miami warehouse filled with $15 million worth of counterfeit, diverted, and illegally re-imported medicine, as well as pill-making machines and 2 million tablets of counterfeit Lipitor®.

By the end of 2004, the state investigators had arrested 55 suspects—more than 30 of them on racketeering charges—and seized $33 million in bad medicine and almost $3 million in cash. Sixteen suspects agreed to cooperate, most pleading guilty to an array of charges. As a result of these state and local investigations, the Florida Legislature tightened its regulation of wholesalers, reducing their numbers by 50% (still one for every six pharmacies). Statewide Medicaid costs plunged for certain categories of drugs that had been overprescribed, billed to Medicaid, diverted to clinics, and prescribed again.[2]

Throughout the entire investigation, the FDA did nothing to help track down and bring these criminals to justice.

FDA FAILS TO PROTECT CONSUMERS

This story provides yet another example of how the FDA places the profits of drug companies and wholesalers above the health of the American consumer. The FDA has the authority to go after the counterfeiters and prosecute them aggressively. However, doing so would expose the current lack of safety to the glare of publicity, showing that the agency is not doing its job despite its power to do so. Far better to cast negative aspersions on the safety of imported drugs and allege that the supposed dangers are so great that we must construct a protective wall around our borders, within which pharmaceutical companies can charge a king's ransom for drugs available at a fraction of the price overseas.

When the author of Dangerous Doses called the public relations director of a major drug company to inform him that numerous lots of his company's lifesaving drug had been relabeled to appear 20 times their actual strength and that a licensed distributor was suspected of trafficking in counterfeit versions of that same medicine, his response was, "I'd hate to have you short the stock [try to profit from a decline in the share price] because of these local and contained incidents."[2] This outrageous response professes not anger at the possible contamination and threat to public health, but concern about a possible financial loss if word of the counterfeiting problem were to get out. Obviously, this executive's fear about the value of his stock options trumped any concern that people could suffer and perhaps die because of incidents that are by no means "local and contained."

It is bad enough that Americans have to pay an arm and a leg in the US for drugs that can be purchased for less money in Canada and Europe. Now, due to the investigative reporting in Dangerous Doses and the diligent efforts of Florida investigators, we are finding that drugs we purchase in the US may actually be more dangerous than those the FDA says we should not obtain from abroad.

The FDA pretends to protect consumers against contaminated drugs, but the sordid facts do not support this self-serving assertion. FDA complicity has enabled criminals to get potentially dangerous drugs into our local pharmacies.

References

1. Available at: http://www.fda.gov/fdac/features/2002/502_import.html. Accessed May 18, 2005.
2. Eban K. *Dangerous Doses: How Counterfeiters Are Contaminating America's Drug Supply*. Orlando, FL: Harcourt, Inc; 2005.

APRIL 2005

Inside the Vioxx® Debacle

by Jon VanZile

In an exclusive Life Extension *interview, the FDA's Dr. David Graham explains why he blew the whistle on his own employer, why Vioxx® will not be the last FDA-sanctioned drug scandal, and why only Congress can reform the FDA.*

O N A CRISP NOVEMBER DAY IN 2004, DR. DAVID GRAHAM, a senior FDA scientist, asked members of the US Senate Finance Committee to imagine the unimaginable. "What would you do if two to four aircraft had crashed, killing all aboard, every week for the past five years?" he asked. "What would you want to know? And what would you do about it?"

Of course, airline safety was not Dr. Graham's concern that day. He was referring to the biggest prescription drug scandal in history: the approval and continued use of the pain drug Vioxx®. And he was talking about the campaign of harassment and intimidation waged against him by senior FDA officials when he tried to alert the public to the dangers associated with Vioxx®.

Before it was removed from the market in late 2004, Vioxx®
had been implicated in about 160,000 cases of heart attack and
stroke in the US between 1999 and 2004—the equivalent of
100,000 unnecessary deaths.[1]

A CATASTROPHE IN THE MAKING

Produced by Merck & Company, Vioxx® belongs to a class of selective nonsteroidal anti-inflammatory drugs, or NSAIDs, called
COX-2 inhibitors. These drugs work by reducing an enzyme called
cyclooxygenase-2 (COX-2) that is responsible for converting arachidonic acid into prostaglandin E2 (PGE2). A hormone-like substance,
PGE2 has been linked to inflammatory diseases, including arthritis.

When Vioxx® gained FDA approval in 1999, it was hailed, along
with Pfizer's pain drug Celebrex®, as a miracle drug for people
suffering from chronic arthritis. Merck marketed Vioxx® as an
effective painkiller that did not cause the gastrointestinal side
effects of other common pain drugs such as aspirin or ibuprofen.

Even before Vioxx® was approved, however, there were clear
warnings that it was linked to heart attack and stroke. Nevertheless, the drug hit the market in a flurry of consumer advertising
and favorable media coverage. Between 1999 and 2004, more
than 20 million Americans took Vioxx®.[2]

But the evidence against Vioxx continued to accumulate.
Finally, in September 2004, a study was released linking chronic
Vioxx® use to increased rates of heart attack and stroke. Merck
halted the study early when researchers uncovered the cardiovascular risk associated with Vioxx®.

The public outcry was immediate and enormous. In the days
following the announcement, Merck's shares tumbled and the
Vioxx® story was front-page news across the country. On September 30, Merck voluntarily withdrew Vioxx® from the market.
The company today faces hundreds of lawsuits over Vioxx® and
about $2 billion a year in lost revenue.

But the fallout over Vioxx® did not stop with Merck. Attention soon turned to the FDA. As the public's alleged watchdog agency, the FDA is responsible for ensuring that dangerous drugs like Vioxx® do not make it to the market. Yet somehow, Vioxx® had slipped through the system. Worse yet, there were indications that the FDA had actively tried to protect Vioxx® despite evidence that it was dangerous.

Even before the drug was approved, an internal Merck study had found a sevenfold increase in heart attack risk associated with low-dose Vioxx®. A year later, another internal Merck study linked high-dose Vioxx® to heart attack and stroke. The company tried to explain away the results, but its argument was unconvincing. Not long afterward, the nonprofit public interest organization Public Citizen recommended that people stop taking Vioxx®.

Given its role as a protector of the public, the FDA should have taken action based on this information alone. Indeed, in 2000, after the second Merck study, a mild warning was added to the Vioxx® label concerning the dangers of high-dose Vioxx®. But the agency implemented no ban, and sales of high-dose Vioxx® were not affected.

FINDINGS PROVOKE FDA INTIMIDATION

Worried about the mounting evidence against the drug, Dr. Graham, associate director for the Office of Drug Safety and a 20-year FDA veteran, launched a study of Vioxx® in 2001. His team included researchers from California-based Kaiser Permanente and the Vanderbilt University School of Medicine in Nashville, TN. They analyzed data from 1.4 million people in California who had taken Vioxx® between 1999 and 2004.

They worked for three years, compiling data. Finally, in early August 2004, almost two months before Vioxx® was removed from the market, Dr. Graham completed the study. The results were explosive—his team found that high-dose Vioxx® increased heart attack risk 3.7-fold, while low-dose Vioxx® increased the risk 1.5-fold.

Dr. Graham prepared his findings for presentation at the International Conference on Pharmacoepidemiology in Bordeaux, France. He concluded that high-dose Vioxx® should not be prescribed or used by patients. As part of normal FDA procedure, he submitted this conclusion for internal review by the FDA. His superiors did not react favorably.

> "These conclusions triggered an explosive response from the Office of New Drugs," Dr. Graham told the Senate committee, referring to the FDA office responsible for granting new drug approvals. "The response from senior management in my office, the Office of Drug Safety, was equally stressful."

Instead of acting to protect the public, FDA officials at the highest levels lashed out at Dr. Graham. He was intimidated, pressured to change his conclusions, and forced to delay publication of his study. One senior FDA official even wrote to the editorial board of the prestigious *British Medical Journal The Lancet*—which had accepted the study for publication in September 2004—raising questions about the integrity of Dr. Graham's research. As a result, *The Lancet* delayed publication of the study for more than three months.

Internal emails show that FDA officials even wanted Dr. Graham to send his results to Merck before the study's release.

After being repeatedly attacked by senior staff members at the FDA, Dr. Graham finally responded in an email to Dr. Paul Seligman, director of the Office of Pharmacoepidemiology and Statistical Sciences, stating, "I've gone about as far as I can without compromising my deeply held conclusions about these safety questions."

Nevertheless, they had gotten to him. When Dr. Graham presented his findings in France, he had altered his conclusion about high-dose Vioxx®. The FDA later used this as evidence that Dr.

Graham had questioned his own research. Agency spokespeople announced that Dr. Graham had "voluntarily" changed his conclusions.

According to Dr. Graham, however, the real story was somewhat different. "There's voluntary and there's voluntary," he explained in an exclusive interview with *Life Extension*. "If someone puts a gun to your head and says, 'Sign over your house,' and you sign over your house, that's technically voluntary."

Dr. Graham said he changed his conclusions because the information was so important that it overshadowed his own convictions.

"They weren't going to allow me to go to France with my conclusion the way it was," he said. "I decided it was more important to get this information out into the scientific community than to make my conclusion what I really believed. The FDA can maintain it was voluntary, but the fact is, if it was voluntary, the conclusions would have remained."

By attacking Dr. Graham, the FDA was doing everything within its power to withhold this damaging information from the public for as long as possible. Even after Vioxx® was withdrawn, the FDA was slow to act. On November 2, 2004—the day of the US presidential election—the FDA quietly posted Dr. Graham's study on the Internet. By then, Vioxx® had already been off the market for more than a month.

THE TOLL: 100,000 NEEDLESS DEATHS

In Dr. Graham's view, the FDA is to blame for as many as 100,000 needless deaths due to Vioxx®. Although Merck was responsible for defending its drug in light of the mounting evidence against it, the FDA's job is to guarantee that prescription drugs approved for sale in the US meet the highest safety standards. By any standard, the FDA failed that responsibility.

"The FDA has let the American people down, and sadly, betrayed a public trust," Dr. Graham told members of the Senate Finance

Committee. "We are talking about a catastrophe that I strongly believe could have, should have been, largely avoided. But it wasn't, and over 100,000 Americans have paid dearly for this failure."

As of this writing, Dr. Graham is still employed at the FDA, as associate director of the Office of Drug Safety. However, he told *Life Extension* that his life has been "surreal" since the Vioxx® scandal broke. His superiors have ostracized him, and every day he has to face the same people who tried to destroy him professionally for simply telling the truth about Vioxx®.

"It's very difficult," he said. "I periodically have to sit down with supervisors who I knew in November were lying to Congress about me, lying to *The Lancet* about me, and who tried to prevent my getting protection as a government whistleblower. They were doing hateful things, and now they pretend nothing happened."

But Dr. Graham is also quick to note that this kind of treatment comes only from FDA senior management.

"At the staff level, I'm very respected and supported," Dr. Graham said. "If anything, esteem for me has increased because they realize I told the truth. They know the reality of what we're dealing with."

The reality is that the FDA has been hopelessly corrupted. The agency's problems are wide-ranging and fundamental. It will probably require action by Congress to wean the FDA off its reliance on pharmaceutical industry money and to change the defensive institutional mindset of an agency that cannot admit to its own mistakes.

Dr. Graham hopes that his testimony and experience will be the first steps in reforming the FDA—and there are some hopeful signs. Following Dr. Graham's testimony, Senate Finance Committee Chairman Charles Grassley (R–IA) issued a blistering statement:

> Americans rely on scientists at the FDA as front-line defenders to ensure the safety of prescription drugs. . . . A giant pharmaceutical company, which

announced a voluntary global recall in September, said studies showed the use of its multibillion-dollar Vioxx® could put cardiovascular health at risk. And now it appears the FDA did nothing about mounting evidence that suggested this risk. . . . My bottom line is this: The FDA must remember its mission. To put the public health and safety first and foremost. The American people must be the FDA's first and only concern.

Other signs, however, are less promising. At various times since the Vioxx® scandal broke, FDA officials have "categorically denied" Dr. Graham's charges or, alternatively, tried to argue that because all prescription drugs pose some degree of risk, the agency was not lax in its oversight of Vioxx®. The road ahead to true FDA reform appears to be long and difficult.

VIOXX®: TIP OF THE ICEBERG?

The situation might not be so bad if Vioxx® were an isolated case. But it is not. In recent years, other FDA scientists have come forward with their own stories. Unfortunately, the treatment they received was no better than the intimidation directed at Dr. Graham.

"I wasn't surprised at the FDA's reaction because the tradition at the FDA has been to react negatively to new information that illustrates how the FDA's policies are inadequate or wrong," Dr. Graham said. "When you illustrate that the FDA's policies are harmful, the reaction is negative and immediate."

In fact, Dr. Graham was the second FDA scientist to appear before the Senate Finance Committee in late 2004. The first was Dr. Andrew Mosholder, an FDA epidemiologist who testified last fall that FDA superiors had asked him to soften recommendations concerning antidepressants.

In 2004, Dr. Mosholder conducted a meta-analysis of 22 studies on the use of antidepressants in children. His research showed that children who took antidepressants, such as Prozac® and Zoloft®, were twice as likely to become suicidal as children who took a placebo.

Once again, however, senior FDA officials intervened before Dr. Mosholder could make his results public. Dr. Mosholder was told to alter his research findings in material that was submitted to Congress, and was threatened with disciplinary action by the FDA's Office of Internal Affairs if he went to the media. On another occasion, he was barred from testifying at a public hearing on antidepressants and children.

And once again, there had been warning signs. According to the Senate investigation, the link between antidepressants and children had been studied since 1996, yet no drug label changes were made and no drugs were taken off the market.

"There is something terribly rotten at the FDA," Rep. Peter Deutsch (D-FL) told the *Los Angeles Times* after Mosholder's testimony. "No agency charged with protecting the public health should have behaved with such indifference."[3]

The only thing unusual about these cases is that they became public, according to Dr. Graham. In fact, without urgent reform at the FDA, it seems almost inevitable that another Vioxx®-sized disaster will occur. Dr. Graham himself has identified several other drugs that demand immediate action:

- Meridia®, used for weight loss, has been associated with high blood pressure and stroke.
- Crestor®, used to lower cholesterol, has been associated with renal failure and other serious side effects.
- Accutane®, used to treat acne, has been linked to birth defects, and Dr. Graham believes its sale should be restricted immediately.
- Serevent®, used to treat asthma, can actually aggravate and cause death due to asthma.

Dr. Graham, along with other consumer groups such as Public Citizen, are calling on the FDA to scrutinize other COX-2 inhibitors, such as Bextra® and Celebrex®. In late January 2005, Public Citizen filed a petition with the FDA, demanding that it remove Bextra® and Celebrex® from the market.

"The Food & Drug Administration should immediately ban the sale of Celebrex® and Bextra®, which put millions of people, many of them elderly, at risk of heart attack," said Dr. Sidney Wolfe, director of Public Citizen's Health Research Group. "These drugs are not only more expensive and more dangerous than older, safer pain relievers, they are no better at protecting the gastrointestinal tract."

Even the FDA's own scientists lack faith in the agency's ability to protect the American people. December 2004 saw the release of a previously unpublished FDA internal management review, in which 846 FDA scientists were asked to complete an extensive survey. About half answered. The study found that:

■ Two thirds of FDA scientists lack confidence that the agency "adequately monitors the safety of prescription drugs once they are on the market."

■ More than a third (36%) were not at all or only somewhat confident that "final decisions adequately assess the safety of a drug."

■ Nearly 20% said they "have been pressured to approve or recommend approval [for a drug] despite reservations about the safety, efficacy, or quality of the drug."

With findings like these, it is no wonder the FDA tried to prevent the survey from ever seeing the light of day. In fact, it might never have been made public if not for the efforts of two public interest groups, Public Employees for Environmental Responsibility (PEER) and the Union of Concerned Scientists (UCS).

"Many concerns had been raised about the manipulation of science within the [Bush] administration," said Suzanne Shaw,

UCS director of communications. "There had also been concerns raised at the FDA. In thinking about how to design a tool to get more data, we heard about the survey. But when we tried to see the actual results, we were told we couldn't see the report."

Eventually, it took a request under the Freedom of Information of Act to pry the report loose from the FDA.

SERVING DRUG COMPANIES, NOT THE PUBLIC

Dr. Graham is certain that without urgent reform, Vioxx® is only the beginning of the disasters that will flow from FDA incompetence and arrogance. Congress must act, because the FDA's problems are so fundamental that nothing except reform forced on the agency from the outside can work.

The basic problem, according to Dr. Graham, is that the FDA does not serve the American public, but instead serves the pharmaceutical industry.

Under FDA regulations, pharmaceutical companies submit new drugs to the FDA's Office of New Drugs. These companies are always racing against time because their drugs are protected by a patent for only 17 years, which includes the time it takes to get the drug approved in the first place.

To speed drug approval, the FDA charges fees to pharmaceutical companies during the approval process. The fees help "expedite" the complicated but required evaluation of human and animal studies. This means that the FDA accepts money from the very industry it is supposed to regulate.

"You want to be evidence based, but the FDA would rather suspend its judgment so it can better serve its clients: industry," said Dr. Graham.

This process results in a biased flow of information, dictated almost entirely by pharmaceutical companies. During the approval process and afterward, the drug makers are not required to release studies that reflect poorly on their drugs.

The real trouble begins, however, once a drug is approved. No matter how extensive the pre-approval process, there is no substitute for experience. In the case of Vioxx®, the drug was approved based on studies involving 5,000 subjects. That may seem like a lot, but it is a tiny fraction compared to the millions who eventually used Vioxx®. Sometimes researchers do not and cannot learn about a dangerous drug until they study the side effects across whole populations of people.

Given the way the FDA is structured, however, that almost never happens. Dr. Graham launched a study on Vioxx® after its approval, and that is the exception rather than the norm. In most cases, once drugs are approved, no further steps are taken to ensure their safety. In fact, the FDA culture actively discourages scientists from pursuing safety concerns in approved drugs, according to Dr. Graham. And that goes for the manufacturer as well.

"There's no incentive for the company to do post-marketing studies," said Dr. Graham. "They've already been given a free pass on safety. It's all downside for the company, and the FDA has no incentive to do post-marketing studies because it only cares about getting new drugs on the market. The FDA's main client is industry."

As Dr. Graham's story demonstrates, once questions are raised, the Office of New Drugs is willing to say or do virtually anything—including pressuring its senior scientists to alter their conclusions, and even trying to destroy their careers and reputations—to protect drug company interests.

As long as the FDA remains beholden to the pharmaceutical companies, financially and otherwise, it will be unable to protect the American public. Considering the FDA's recent history, there is no reason to believe the agency can reform itself. The only real hope is that Congress will act to dismantle and rebuild the FDA from the ground up.

"Right now, it's the FDA's fault, but if it happens again, Congress will be partly responsible," said Dr. Graham. "I'm an idealist. I hope people can rise above their political philosophy and unite to create a system of drug safety. If they don't unite, another disaster will come, and it might be a family member of someone in Congress. Then they will become believers. The men and women in Congress need to understand that these are people's lives."

References

1. Topol EJ. Failing the public health—rofecoxib, Merck, and the FDA. *N Engl J Med.* 2004 Oct 21;351(17):1707–9.

2. Martinez B. Merck documents shed light on Vioxx® legal battles. *Wall Street Journal.* February 7, 2005.

3. FDA fails to act on information on link between antidepressants, suicide risk in children, say lawmakers. *Medical News Today.* September 27, 2004.

2004

Pharmacies Sue FDA Over Compounding Limits

by Stephen Laifer

A COALITION OF PHARMACIES FROM TEXAS, ARIZONA, ALAbama, Wisconsin, California, and Colorado filed suit against the Food and Drug Administration in September, claiming that the agency is illegally enforcing an arbitrary regulation that is out of its jurisdiction. The suit accuses the FDA of conducting unlawful inspections, illegal interventions, and intimidation of law-abiding pharmacies.

At issue is the centuries-old practice of compounding medications from bulk ingredients. In this process, a pharmacist combines, mixes, or alters the administration of ingredients to prepare a medication, prescribed by a physician or veterinarian, that is tailored to an individual patient's needs. Compounding protection laws were enacted in 1962 to ensure the best healthcare for patients and pets.

The FDA has no legal authority over pharmacies, whether or not they prepare compound preparations. Last year, however, the FDA issued a compliance policy guideline that made the use of bulk ingredients in the preparation of medications illegal. The agency has since waged an aggressive inspection campaign to enforce the guideline.

Ten compounding pharmacies have petitioned a US District Court in Texas to be able to continue filling prescriptions from doctors and veterinarians using pure "bulk ingredients" that are manufactured in facilities that are registered, inspected, and approved by the FDA.

"If the FDA is successful, this would deprive veterinarians and physicians of critical treatment options that relieve the suffering of their patients and improve their health," said Steven F. Hotze, MD, president of Premier Pharmacy in Katy, TX.

Compounded drugs typically offer superior treatment options because they are tailored to the individual patient. Moreover, restrictions on compounded medications prevent many prescription drugs from being offered at more affordable prices. The FDA's illegal actions work to the benefit of large pharmaceutical companies, which continually lobby the agency in efforts to stifle competition and keep prices high.

FDA Permits New Fish Oil Health Claim

by William Faloon

I T WAS LONG AGO ESTABLISHED THAT CONSUMPTION OF COLD-water fish reduces the risk of heart attack.[1] In fact, just two to three servings of fish a week may protect against many diseases, including arthritis, stroke, certain cancers, and a host of inflammation-related disorders.[2-9]

When scientists sought to discover which components of fish are responsible for preventing heart attacks, they found that the oil plays a critical role. Coldwater fish oil is high in omega-3 fatty acids that function in multiple ways to reduce cardiovascular disease risk.[10]

Based on the published scientific evidence about fish oil, a lawsuit was filed against the FDA in 1994 by Durk Pearson and Sandy Shaw, seeking to force the agency to allow the following health claim on fish oil supplement labels: "Consumption of omega-3 fatty acids may reduce the risk of coronary heart disease." The FDA rejected this one-sentence claim and a multiyear litigation battle ensued.

In their lawsuit, Durk and Sandy pointed out that consumers would benefit by learning of the value of fish oil in protecting against heart disease. They also argued that the FDA lacked the constitutional authority to ban this truthful health claim.

The FDA contended that this health claim was not adequately backed by scientific studies and that the agency had the legal authority to ban these kinds of health claims.

Seven years of extensive litigation ensued as the FDA asserted that it had the sole authority to dictate what Americans could read on the label of fish oil supplements. After an onslaught of irrefutable scientific evidence was presented, including articles published in the most prestigious scientific journals in the world, the FDA capitulated and said it would permit the following claim:

> Consumption of omega-3 fatty acids may reduce the risk of coronary heart disease. FDA evaluated the data and determined that although there is scientific evidence supporting the claim, the evidence is not conclusive.

LIFE EXTENSION CHALLENGES FDA ON FISH OIL HEALTH CLAIM

The FDA's compromise health claim that the evidence was "not conclusive" did not satisfy the Life Extension Foundation. The scientific literature provided overwhelming validation that consuming coldwater fish or fish oils dramatically lowers heart attack risk.

To substantiate this position, a massive document enumerating the scientific studies backing the benefits of omega-3 fatty acids was filed, along with legal arguments supporting the constitutional right to disseminate this truthful information.

The Life Extension Foundation Buyers Club, Inc., and Wellness Lifestyles, Inc., filed a health claim petition against the FDA on June 23, 2003. The petition urged the FDA to reconsider its permitted health claim for omega-3 fatty acids and coronary heart disease risk, and to allow the following revised claim: "Consumption of omega-3 fatty acids may reduce the risk of coronary heart disease."

Also included in the petition was a calculation of how many American lives were needlessly being lost because of the FDA's restriction of this simple health claim. Epidemiological data were presented showing that if all Americans regularly took fish oil supplements or ate about two coldwater fish meals a week, it would prevent about 150,000 deaths a year. Life Extension further argued that during the seven years it took to litigate this case against the FDA, Americans suffered over 1 million preventable sudden-death heart attacks.

THE POLITICAL BATTLE OVER WHAT AMERICANS EAT

Junk food is big business in the United States. Processed food companies have historically used their political clout to persuade the federal government to defend the safety of dangerous food products. The cost of treating diseases caused by poor diet has become so staggering, however, that the government is recommending that Americans eat healthier.

For nearly two decades, the FDA protected the economic interests of companies selling high-fat and high-cholesterol foods by making it illegal to promote a healthy diet as a way of preventing heart disease. Heart attack rates were three times higher in the 1950s than in the 1990s. The FDA's censorship of healthy dietary information caused tens of millions of Americans to unnecessarily succumb to cardiovascular and other diseases.

FDA CAPITULATES TO SCIENTIFIC REALITY

On September 8, 2004, the FDA announced that it would allow an expanded health claim on products containing the omega-3 fatty acids eiscosopentaenoic acid (EPA) and docosahexaenoic acid (DHA).

According to Acting FDA Commissioner Dr. Lester M. Crawford, "Coronary heart disease is a significant health problem that causes 500,000 deaths annually in the United States. This new qualified health claim for omega-3 fatty acids should help consumers as they work to improve their health by identifying foods that contain these important compounds (EPA and DHA)."

The FDA now permits the following statement to be printed on the label of fish oil supplements: "Supportive but not conclusive research shows that consumption of EPA and DHA omega-3 fatty acids may reduce the risk of coronary heart disease."

The FDA went on to recommend that consumers not exceed more than 3 grams per day of EPA and DHA omega-3 fatty acids, with no more than 2 grams per day derived from a dietary supplement. Life Extension argues that many scientific studies show that higher amounts of EPA and DHA are often needed to obtain optimal benefits, such as reduction of triglycerides and prevention of restenosis (re-occlusion of a blocked artery).[11]

This battle over what can be stated about fish oil began back in 1994. While the FDA's announcement of a broader health claim represents a significant legal victory, Life Extension is still not satisfied with the FDA's latest health claim on fish oil supplements. We reiterate our position that evidence from peer-reviewed scientific publications supporting the benefit of EPA and DHA supplements in reducing heart attack risk is conclusive and not merely "supportive" as the FDA contends.

Attorney Jonathan Emord put hundreds of hours of productive work into this case over the past ten years. Jonathan filed the initial lawsuit against the FDA on behalf of Durk Pearson and Sandy

Shaw that resulted in a precedent-setting legal victory against FDA censorship. Jonathan then prepared the petition on behalf of Life Extension and Wellness Lifestyles that resulted in the FDA allowing this new expanded health claim to be made about the protective effect of fish oils against cardiovascular disease.

References

1. FTC Press Release, November 29, 2000. "FTC Reaches Record Price-fixing Settlement to Settle Charges of Price-fixing in Generic Drug Market."

2. Price quoted by Hollywood Discount Pharmacy in Hollywood, Florida on Jan 15, 2002.

3. Associated Press, October 4, 2001. "Drugmaker to pay $875 million fine."

4. Robert Pear (*New York Times* News Service). "Health spending jumps 6.9%—Main factors: hospitals and drug costs, managed care resistance, *The Herald*, Tuesday, January 8, 2002.

5. Faloon William, "Dying from Deficiency," *Life Extension* magazine, October 2001.

6. *National Vital Statistics Reports*, Vol. 48, No.11.

7. *Wall Street Journal*, December 24, 2001, pp-A3, "Schering Fines Could Total $500 Million."

8. http://www.cnn.com/HEALTH/9804/14/drug.reaction/Chicago CNN. "Study: Drug reactions kill an estimated 100,000 a year," April 14, 1998.

9. David Willman, "The Rise and Fall of the Killer Drug Rezulin," *Life Extension* magazine, September 2000.

10. http://news.ft.com/ft/gx.cgi/ftc?pagename=View&c=Article&cid=FT3HZ3AFMWC &live=true&tagid=IX LHT5GTICC&subheading=heal By David Firn in London, "More deaths linked to Bayer's Lipobay," January 18, 2002. 19:44. Last Updated: January 18 2002 19:48

11. Calder PC. n-3 fatty acids and cardiovascular disease: evidence explained and mechanisms explored. *Clin Sci* (Lond). 2004 Jul; 107(1): 1–11.

FDA Approves Deadly Drugs, Delays Lifesaving Therapies

by William Faloon

HAT IF A DIETARY SUPPLEMENT WAS SHOWN TO KILL
100 Americans and cause 56,000 emergency room visits each year?[1] Without a doubt, the supplement would
be banned immediately and those who knowingly marketed such
a lethal product would be subject to severe criminal penalties.

On January 22, 2004, the FDA confirmed that acetaminophen
is extremely dangerous.[2] Acetaminophen is sold under the brand
name Tylenol® and is contained in 600 other drug products. The
toxicity of acetaminophen was clear more than 12 years ago, and
Life Extension harshly criticized the FDA for not mandating that
the label of acetaminophen products warn those with liver or
kidney problems to avoid the drug.

In 2002, an FDA scientific advisory committee urged that warnings be put on the labels of acetaminophen drugs.[3,4] Despite overwhelming documentation confirming acetaminophen's toxicity,[5–28] the FDA said no to its own scientific advisors. Instead, the agency has budgeted a mere $20,000[29,30] to develop material that it hopes will be run in major magazines and distributed by pharmacy chains for free! This is the bureaucratic equivalent of doing nothing.

The agency spends tens of millions of dollars a year attacking companies selling natural health products that have harmed no one. Yet the FDA is making virtually no effort to prevent the 100 deaths and 56,000 emergency room visits that the agency itself admits are caused by acetaminophen drugs every year![31]

ACETAMINOPHEN RISKS UNDERSTATED

Back in 1992, research showed that many more people are dying because of acetaminophen than the number indicated by the official statistics. While the FDA was preoccupied with acetaminophen-induced liver failure, it overlooked studies showing that regular users of acetaminophen may be doubling their risk of kidney cancer.[11,13,32]

What does that translate to in actual numbers of victims? Each year, almost 12,000 Americans die of kidney cancer.[33] The incidence of kidney cancer in the US has risen 126% since the 1950s,[34] a jump that may be tied to the growing use of drugs containing phenacetin or acetaminophen.

Phenacetin is a painkiller that was banned because it causes severe kidney toxicity.[35–40] Acetaminophen is the major metabolite of phenacetin, which means that some of the destructive properties exhibited by phenacetin could have been caused by its breakdown to acetaminophen in the body. So while phenacetin was withdrawn because too many people's kidneys were shutting down, the FDA had no problem letting the major metabolite of phenacetin (acetaminophen) be freely marketed without any consumer warning whatsoever.

If acetaminophen is responsible for even a small percentage of the overall kidney cancer cases, this drug may have already killed tens of thousands of Americans—and the FDA has done nothing to stop this carnage!

Because acetaminophen generates damaging free radicals throughout the body, it may very well increase the risk of many age-related diseases. In fact, scientists can consistently induce cataracts in the eyes of laboratory animals by giving them acetaminophen. They consider acetaminophen a "cataratogenic agent." Interestingly, if antioxidants are provided to the animals, the cataract-inducing effects of acetaminophen are often completely neutralized.[41-46]

The antioxidant N-acetylcysteine helps neutralize destructive free radicals. When a person acutely overdoses on acetaminophen, the standard medical therapy is to administer N-acetylcysteine over a period of weeks. Unfortunately, the FDA bans the combination of an over-the-counter drug (acetaminophen) with a dietary supplement (N-acetylcysteine), so it is "illegal" to make a safe acetaminophen drug.

Despite the overwhelming evidence that acetaminophen use should be strictly limited, the FDA capitulates to pharmaceutical companies that earn billions of dollars a year selling this lethal class of analgesic drug.

By failing to mandate a warning on the label of acetaminophen products, the FDA once again demonstrates its propensity for protecting the pharmaceutical industry's economic interests at the expense of the American public's health.

FDA DENIES ALZHEIMER'S DRUG FOR 14 YEARS

At any given time, 4 million Americans suffer the devastating consequences of Alzheimer's disease.[47] Alzheimer's has no cure, and all victims suffer a progressive neurodegenerative process that results in total disability and death.

In 1990, a drug used in Germany was found to slow the progression of the disease.[48] The drug's generic name is memantine, and Life Extension has long recommended it to family members of Alzheimer's victims.[49]

Memantine does not offer miraculous benefits. The studies show that some patients experience improvements in memory and cognitive skills.[50] For the vast majority, however, memantine merely slows the pace of deterioration, enabling patients to perform certain functions a little longer than would otherwise be possible.[51,52] For example, the drug enabled some patients to go to the bathroom independently for an additional six months, a benefit caregivers called very important.[53]

The July 2001 issue of *Life Extension* featured an in-depth report on the clinical value of memantine in treating a wide range of disorders, including Parkinson's disease, glaucoma, and diabetic neuropathy.[54] It was highly critical of the FDA's attempts to deny Alzheimer's patients residing in the US access to this safe and partially effective medication.

Starting this year, Americans can now purchase memantine sold under the brand name Namenda® at American pharmacies. One reason memantine is available now is the intense pressure put on the FDA by family members of Alzheimer's victims who had to order the drug from Europe and risk FDA seizure.

Americans had to wait 14 years to gain legal access to a drug proven to work in Europe. In 1991, the FDA was sued for denying access to the drug tacrine for Alzheimer's patients. Tacrine's mechanism of action inhibits the acetylcholinesterase enzyme, thus making more of the neurotransmitter acetylcholine available to brain cells. Six months after the lawsuit was dropped, the FDA approved tacrine.[55] And few years later still, the FDA approved a safer drug called Aricept® that shares some of tacrine's same mechanisms of action but is less toxic.[56]

Memantine works by a different mechanism than tacrine or Aricept®. Memantine blocks a reaction known as "excitotoxicity," a pathological process in which too much glutamate is released in the brain, severely damaging the neurons. Those seeking to protect their healthy neurons against the damaging effects of excitotoxicity use dietary supplements such as methylcobalamin and vinpocetine. That it took litigation, harsh media criticism, and a citizens' uprising to motivate the FDA to approve these Alzheimer's drugs is a testament to the agency's inability to differentiate between safe, effective medications that should be approved and lethal drugs that should be removed.[57]

WHO WILL PROTECT US FROM THE FDA?

The FDA pretends to protect Americans from dangerous and ineffective products, yet even a cursory review of the agency's track record reveals the opposite to be true. Dangerous and ineffective drugs are approved, while novel lifesaving therapies and natural approaches to disease prevention are brutally suppressed.[58-69]

The FDA's failure to mandate a warning on the label of acetaminophen products is just one example of its failure to protect consumers against lethal drug side effects. The agency's inexcusable delay in approving drugs to alleviate the miseries of Alzheimer's disease reveals its lack of compassion for human beings who have lost the cognitive ability to take care of themselves.

Since 1980, the Life Extension Foundation has recommended drugs that the FDA has not yet approved.[70-73] In many cases, what we recommended was eventually approved, which means that our scientific analysis—as opposed to the FDA's politically motivated decision-making process—was medically correct.

Regrettably, some non-patentable therapies will never receive FDA approval because of the high cost of navigating the agency's bureaucratic labyrinth. When it comes to disease prevention, the FDA has made extraordinary efforts to censor information about proper diet and supplements that would provide guidance to consumers who want to adopt healthier lifestyles.[74]

References

1. Available at: http://www.kvue.com/shared content/ nationworld/nation/0 1 2204cccanat painkillers.40e6c22 1. html. Accessed February 27, 2004.

2. Available at: http://www.fda.gov/bbs/topics/ NEWS/2004/ NEW01 008.htm. Accessed February 27, 2004.

3. Available at: http://www.fda.gov/ohrms/ dockets/ac/02/ agenda/3882A_Draft.doc. Accessed February 27, 2004.

4. Available at: http://www.fdanews.com/ 1_1 /dailynews/ 7334–1 .html. Accessed February 27, 2004.

5. Anand BS, Romero JJ, Sanduja SK, Lichtenberger LM. Phospholipid association reduces the gastric mucosal toxicity of aspirin in human subjects. *Am J Gastroenterol.* 1999 Jul; 94(7):1818–22.

6. Blakely P, McDonald BR. Acute renal failure due to acetaminophen ingestion: a case report and review of the literature. *J Am Soc Nephrol.* 1995 Jul;6(1):48–53.

7. Bonkovsky HL, Kane RE, Jones DP, Galinsky RE, Banner B. Acute hepatic and renal toxicity from low doses of acetaminophen in the absence of alcohol abuse or malnutrition: evidence for increased suscep tibility to drug toxicity due to cardiopul monary and renal insufficiency. *Hepatology.* 1994 May;19(5):1 141–8.

8. Clemmesen JO, Ott P, Dalhoff KP, Astrup LB, Tage-Jensen U, Poulsen HE.Recommendations for treatment of paracetamol poisoning. *Ugeskr Laegr.* 1996 Nov 25; 158(48):6892–5.

9. Conti M, Malandrino S, Magistretti MJ. Protective activity of silipide on liver damage in rodents. *Jpn J Pharmacol.* 1992 Dec;60 (4):31 5–21.

10. DeLeve LD, Kaplowitz N. Glutathione metabolism and its role in hepatotoxicity.*Pharmacol Ther.* 1991 Dec;52(3):287–305.

11. Derby LE, Jick H. Acetaminophen and renal and bladder cancer. *Epidemiology.* 1996 Jul;7(4):358–62.

12. Dunjic BS, Axelson J, Ar'Rajab A, Larsson K, Bengmark S. Gastroprotective capability of exogenous phosphatidylcholine in experi mentally induced chronic gastric ulcers in rats. *Scand J Gastroenterol.* 1993 Jan;28(1):89–94.

13. Gago-Dominguez M., Yuan JM, Castelao JE, Ross RK, Yu MC. Regular use of anal gesics is a risk factor for renal cell carcino ma. *Br J Cancer.* 1999 Oct;81(3):542–8.

14. Graudins A, Aaron CK, Linden CH. Overdose of extended-release acetamino phen. *N Engl J Med.* 1995 Jul 20;333(3):196.

15. Jaeschke H, Werner C, Wendel A. Disposition and hepatoprotection by phosphatidyl choline liposomes in mouse liver. *Chem Biol Interact.* 1987;64(1–2):127–37.

16. Jones AL. Mechanism of action and value of N-acetylcysteine in the treatmentof early and late acetaminophen poisoning: a critical review. *J Toxicol Clin Toxicol.* 1998;36(4):277–85.

17. Kaye JA, Myers MW, Jick H. Acetaminophen and the risk of renal and bladder cancer in the general practice research database. *Epidemiology.* 2001 Nov; 1 2(6):690–4.

18. Kind B, Krahenbuhl S, Wyss PA, Meier-Abt PJ. Clinical-toxicological case (1). Dosage of N-acetylcysteine in acute paracetamol poisoning. *Schweiz Rundsch Med Prax.* 1996 Aug 2; 85(31–32):935–8.

19. Lieber CS. Role of oxidative stress and antioxidant therapy in alcoholic andnon-alcoholic liver diseases. *Adv Pharmacol.* 1 997;38:601-28.

20. Lieber CS. Alcohol: its metabolism and interaction with nutrients. *Annu Rev Nutr.* 2000;20:395–430.

21. McLaughlin JK, Blot WJ, Mehl ES, Fraumeni JF Jr. Relation of analgesic use to renal cancer: population-based findings. *Natl Cancer Inst Monogr.* 1985 Dec;69:217–22.

22. Mitchell T, Needham A. Over-the-counter drug is treatment for Alzheimer's. *Life Extension*. November 2000:50–5.

23. Price LM, Poklis A, Johnson DE. Fatal acetaminophen poisoning with evidence ofsubendocardial necrosis of the heart. *J Forensic Sci*. 1991 May;36(3):930–5.

24. Richie JP Jr, Lang CA, Chen TS. Acetaminophen-induced depletion of glutathione and cysteine in the aging mouse kidney. *Biochem Pharmacol*. 1992 Jul 7;44(1):129–35.

25. Siegers CP, Moller-Hartmann W. Cholestyramine as an antidote against paracetamol-induced hepato-and nephro-toxicity in the rat. *Toxicol Lett*. 1989 May;47(2):179–84.

26. Uhlig S, Wendel A. Glutathione enhancement in various mouse organs and protection by glutathione isopropyl ester against liver injury. *Biochem Pharmacol*. 1990 Jun 15;39(12):1877–81.

27. Werner C, Wendel A. Hepatic uptake and antihepatotoxic properties of vitamin E and liposomes in the mouse. *Chem Biol Interact*. 1990;75(1):83–92.

28. Zhao J, Agarwal R. Tissue distribution of silibinin, the major active constituent of silymarin, in mice and its association with enhancement of phase II enzymes: implications in cancer chemoprevention. *Carcinogenesis*. 1999 Nov;20(1 1):2101–8.

29. Available at: http://www.fda.gov/cder/drug/ analgesics/ letter.htm. Accessed February 27, 2004.

30. Available at: http://www.fda.gov/cder/drug/ analgesics/ SciencePaper. htm. Accessed February 27, 2004.

31. Available at: http://www.fda.gov/ohrms/ dockets/ac/02/ transcripts/3882T1 .htm. Accessed February 27, 2004.

32. Kaye JA, Myers MW, Jick H. Acetaminophen and the risk of renal and bladder cancer in the general practice research database. *Epidemiology*. 2001 Nov; 1 2(6):690–4.

33. Available at: http://www.kidney-cancer-symptoms.com. Accessed February 27, 2004.

34. Available at: http://www.kidney-cancer symptoms.com. Accessed February 27, 2004.

35. Piper JM, Tonascia J, Matanoski GM. Heavy phenacetin use and bladder cancer in women aged 20 to 49 years. *N Engl J Med.* 1985 Aug 1;313(5):292–5.

36. Linet MS, Chow WH, McLaughlin JK, et al. Analgesics and cancers of the renal pelvis and ureter. *Int J Cancer.* 1995 Jul 4;62 (1):15–8.

37. McCredie M, Stewart JH, Day NE. Different roles for phenacetin and paracetamol in cancer of the kidney and renal pelvis. *Int J Cancer.* 1993 Jan 21 ;53(2):245–9.

38. Brunner FP, Selwood NH. End-stage renal failure due to analgesic nephropathy, its changing pattern and cardiovascular mortality. EDTA-ERA Registry Committee. *Nephrol Dial Transplant.* 1994;9(10):1371–6.

39. Stewart JH, Hobbs JB, McCredie MR. Morphologic evidence that analgesic-induced kidney pathology contributes to the progression of tumors of the renal pelvis. *Cancer.* 1999 Oct 15;86(8):1576–82.

40. Dubach UC, Rosner B, Pfister E. Epidemiologic study of abuse of analgesics containing phenacetin. Renal morbidity and mortality (1968–1979). *N Engl J Med.* 1983 Feb 17;308(7):357–62.

41. Rathbun WB, Killen CE, Holleschau AM, Nagasawa HT. Maintenance of hepatic glutathione homeostasis and prevention of acetaminophen-induced cataract in mice by L-cysteine prodrugs. *Biochem Pharmacol.* 1996 May 3;51(9):1111–6.

42. Rathbun WB, Holleschau AM, Cohen JF, Nagasawa HT. Prevention of acetaminophen and naphthalene-induced cataract and glutathione loss by CySSME. *Invest Ophthalmol Vis Sci.* 1996 Apr;37(5):923–9.

43. Nagasawa HT, Shoeman DW, Cohen JF, Rathbun WB. Protection against acetaminophen-induced hepatotoxicity by L-CySSME and its N-acetyl and ethyl ester derivatives. *J Biochem Toxicol.* 1996;1 1(6):289–95.

44. Zhao C, Shichi H. Prevention of acetaminophen-induced cataract by a combination of diallyl disulfide and N-acetylcysteine. *J Ocul Pharmacol Ther.* 1998 Aug;14(4):345–55.

45. Qian W, Shichi H. Cataract formation by a semiquinone metabolite of acetaminophen in mice: possible involvement of Ca(2+) and calpain activation. *Exp Eye Res*. 2000 Dec;71(6):567–74.

46. Qian W, Shichi H. Acetaminophen produces cataract in DBA2 mice by Ah receptor-independent induction of CYP1A2. *J Ocul Pharmacol Ther*. 2000 Aug;16(4):337–44.

47. Available at: http://www.alz.org/AboutAD/ Statistics.asp. Accessed February 27, 2004.

48. Ditzler K. Efficacy and tolerability of memantine in patients with dementia syndrome. A double-blind, placebo controlled trial. *Arzneimittelforschung*. 1991 Aug;41(8):773–80.

49. Available at: http://www.lef.org/magazine/ mag2001/july2001_ awsi.html. Accessed February 27, 2004.

50. Ambrozi L, Danielczyk W. Treatment of impaired cerebral function in psychogeriatric patients with memantine—results of a phase II double-blind study. *Pharmacopsychiatry*. 1988 May;2 1(3): 144–6.

51. Wilcock G, Mobius HJ, Stoffler A; MMM 500 group. A double-blind, placebo-controlled multicentre study of memantine in mild to moderate vascular dementia (MMM500). *Int Clin Psychopharmacol*. 2002 Nov;17(6):297–305.

52. Ferris SH. Evaluation of memantine for the treatment of Alzheimer's disease. *Expert Opin Pharmacother*. 2003 Dec;4 (1 2):2305–1 3.

53. Tariot PN, Farlow MR, Grossberg GT, et al. Memantine treatment in patients with moderate to severe Alzheimer's disease already receiving donepezil: a randomized controlled trial. *JAMA*. 2004 Jan 21;291(3):317–24.

54. Available at: http://www.lef.org/magazine/ mag2001/july2001_ report_brain_01 .html. Accessed February 27, 2004.

55. Available at: http://www.fda.gov/cder/ogd/ RLD/rld_labeling_ approved_June_2001 .html. Accessed February 27, 2004.

56. Available at: http://www.fda.gov/cder/foi/ appletter/2001/20690s16ltr.pdf. Accessed February 27, 2004.

57. Available at: http://www.pbs.org/wgbh/ pages/frontline/ shows/prescription/. Accessed February 27, 2004.

58. Available at: http://www.commondreams.org/ pressreleases/ Dec98/120298c.htm. Accessed February 27, 2004.

59. Available at: http: //www.cato.org/dailys/1-29-97.html. Accessed February 27, 2004.

60. Available at: http://www.pbs.org/wgbh/ pages/frontline/ shows/prescription/hazard/. Accessed February 27, 2004.

61. Available at: http://www.lef.org/magazine/ mag2001/ june2001_report_fda.html. Accessed February 27, 2004.

62. Available at: http://www.lef.org/magazine/ mag2000/sep2000_ report_rezulin.html. Accessed February 27, 2004.

63. Available at: http://www.life-enhancement.com/ article_template.asp?ID=206. Accessed February 27, 2004.

64. Available at: http://www.lef.org/magazine/ mag2002/jul2002_ awsi_01 .html. Accessed February 27, 2004.

65. Available at: http://www.lef.org/magazine/ mag2003/ mar2003_cover_effects_02.html. Accessed February 27, 2004.

66. Available at: http://www.lef.org/magazine/ mag2000/dec2000_ awsi.html. Accessed February 27, 2004.

67. Available at: http://www.newmediaexplorer.org/ chris/2003/07/22/access_to_medical_treatment_act_amta. htm. Accessed February 27, 2004.

68. Available at: http://www.newmediaexplorer.org/chris/control_ tactics.htm. Accessed February 27, 2004.

69. Available at: http://www.lef.org/magazine/mag2001/ sep2001 _awsi.html. Accessed February 27, 2004.

70. Available at: http://www.lef.org/magazine/ mag2001/ july2001_awsi.html. Accessed February 27, 2004.

71. Available at: http://www.lef.org/featured-articles/track2.html. Accessed February 27, 2004.

72. Available at: http://www.lef.org/magazine/ mag2001/ feb2001_awsi.html. Accessed February 27, 2004.

73. Available at: http://www.lef.org/magazine/mag99/ may99-cover.html. Accessed February 27, 2004.

74. Available at: http://tobaccodocuments.org/pm/ 2046936740-6743.html. Accessed February 27, 2004.

Dangerous Medicine

by William Faloon

HE FDA CLAIMS THAT THE DRUGS IT APPROVES ARE "SAFE."
This charade is rapidly collapsing. PBS television's investigative series *Frontline* has aired a shocking exposé of dangerous prescription drugs and the FDA's complicity in allowing this outrage to occur.[1]

The *Frontline* producers initially investigated drugs that had been withdrawn from the market. After filming began, current and former FDA employees started coming forward to give a powerful critique of what really goes on inside the agency. As the story evolved, rather than making a documentary about drug safety, *Frontline* ended up shifting its focus to the FDA itself.

A major emphasis of the documentary was the FDA's reliance on drug companies' research of their own products to determine safety. As *Frontline* found out, the FDA does not conduct clinical trials, because the agency is not in the business of conducting medical research. The FDA instead reviews the results submitted by pharmaceutical companies. This means that the basis for FDA approval of a new drug is often "safety data" provided by the very company that makes the drug!

Frontline exposed this questionable drug approval sham to the world in a one-hour broadcast aired November 17, 2003. It was FDA drug reviewers who made the most appalling disclosures. These current and former FDA employees revealed incidences in which drug dangers were clearly present but were ignored or covered up by higher-level FDA officials. Only after many injuries and deaths were these drugs withdrawn or relabeled. A survey of all FDA employees showed a significant number felt they were pressured by others in the agency to give favorable reviews to dangerous and ineffective drugs.

The most absurd part of this saga is the FDA's historical record of attempting to restrict consumers' access to dietary supplements. The FDA deceitfully implies that supplements have hidden dangers. Yet the data supporting the safety and efficacy of nutrients usually come from independent sources, as opposed to the company-sponsored studies the FDA relies on to certify drug safety.

Frontline showed that in too many cases, the safety data supplied by drug companies are flawed and altered, with the result being an alarming number of injuries and deaths from prescription drug toxicities. Deaths from adverse drug reactions have become so commonplace that they rarely make the news.

For the past 18 years, *Life Extension* has harshly criticized this corrupt system of drug approval. What Life Extension lacked was the "inside" data gathered by *Frontline* that show specifically how the FDA conspires with the drug industry to approve dangerous drugs. Even more disturbing are instances in which the FDA allows toxic drugs to remain on the market even after injuries and deaths are reported. If the FDA had even a vestige of credibility remaining about its role of "protecting" the public against dangerous drugs, this *Frontline* documentary tore it to shreds. The emperor (the FDA) clearly has no clothes (credibility).

DRUGS OFTEN DO NOT WORK

In a stunning admission, a senior executive with Britain's largest pharmaceutical company has stated that most prescription medicines do not work on half the patients who take them.

Dr. Allen Roses is worldwide vice-president of genetics at GlaxoSmithKline. He is a world-class pioneer in the branch of medicine that studies the relationship between our genes and our response to individual drugs. On December 8, 2003, a British newspaper quoted Dr. Roses telling a scientific conference in London: "The vast majority of drugs only work in 30 or 50% of the people."[2]

Dr. Roses predicted that in a few years, scientists would be able to give patients a simple genetics test that would predict which medicines would work for them. Drug companies could use the information to tailor new drugs aimed at the 50% of people not helped.

It is an open secret within the pharmaceutical industry that most of its products are ineffective in most patients, but this is the first time that such a senior drug boss has gone public. Dr. Roses' admission corroborates what FDA reviewers told *Frontline*—not only are many dangerous drugs wrongfully approved, but they often are only minimally effective!

GOVERNMENT-PROTECTED MEDICINE IS DANGEROUS MEDICINE

The word regulate can be defined as "to control or direct according to rule, principle, or law."[3]

In the US, all aspects of medical care are heavily "regulated" by the government. The end result is that healthcare is expensive, complicated, dangerous, and often ineffective.

The only way out of this bureaucratic abyss is serious free-market reform. This will not happen as long as the public thinks it needs government "protection." The producers of *Frontline* exposed the fact that the FDA does not protect Americans against unsafe drugs. Soon after the *Frontline* program aired, the most popular news program in the US contacted Life Extension seeking information about problems with prescription drugs. It appears that the mainstream media may finally be targeting the FDA.

References

1. Dangerous prescription [transcript]. "*Frontline*." PBS television. November 17, 2003.

2. Glaxo chief: our drugs do not work on most patients. *The Independent*. December 8, 2003.

3. Available at: http://www.dictionary.com/. Accessed December 31, 2003.

Dr. Julian Whitaker Files a Petition Against the FDA

by William Faloon

JULIAN WHITAKER, MD, FILED A PETITION AGAINST THE FDA that meticulously documented the many lethal effects that would occur if patients prescribed statin drugs were not supplemented with 100–200 mg a day of coenzyme Q10. The objective of this petition was to force the FDA to mandate on the package insert that patients taking statin drugs should also take coenzyme Q10.

DR. WHITAKER'S PROPOSED WARNING FOR STATIN DRUGS

Dr. Whitaker petitioned the FDA to mandate that the following warning be included in the package inserts of all statin drugs, with a big black box warning surrounding the text:

Warning: HMG CoA reductase inhibitors (statin drugs)
block the endogenous biosynthesis of an essential cofac-
tor, coenzyme Q10, required for energy production. A
deficiency of coenzyme Q10 is associated with impairment of myocardial function, with liver dysfunction
and with myopathies (including cardiomyopathy and
congestive heart failure). All patients taking HMG CoA
reductase inhibitors should therefore be advised to take
100 to 200 mg per day of supplemental coenzyme Q10.[35]

Dr. Whitaker's petitions state that statins deplete coenzyme
Q10 stores in the body and increase congestive heart failure and
cardiomyopathy risk. They call on the FDA commissioner to take
immediate action to safeguard the millions of statin drug users.

Dr. Whitaker's petition explains that statin drug use may be
inducing adverse effects in as many as 575,000 people worldwide.
The petitions go on to state that statin drugs work by blocking
production of cholesterol and coenzyme Q10 in the same pathway, and that consumption of 100–200 mg per day of coenzyme
Q10 can reverse depletion induced by statins.

Dr. Whitaker asserts that most patients and doctors do not
realize that statin drugs block the production of coenzyme Q10.
Dr. Whitaker went on to describe how coenzyme Q10 has been
found to be essential for cellular energy production as well as for
the functioning of the heart muscle. According to Dr. Whitaker:

Statin drugs have proven in clinical trials to deplete
coenzyme Q10, the 'sparkplugs' of the human body.
Patients who take statin drugs without coenzyme Q10,
particularly those with a history of heart disease, are
especially prone to developing complications that can
have fatal consequences.[35]

FDA FAILS TO PROTECT STATIN USERS

Dr. Whitaker's meticulously documented petition was filed on May 24, 2002. For the past 20 months, however, the FDA has ignored it. The result is that millions of statin drug users are needlessly being subjected to lethal side effects.

The failure of the FDA to amend the drug package insert to recommend that statin users supplement with coenzyme Q10 is a medical travesty. Since the underlying science is irrefutable, this is a blatant example of large drug companies influencing the FDA into not taking actions that would save lives.

Drug companies may not want this label change as it could reduce sales of their statin drugs. After all, if doctors told patients that statin drugs could cause heart muscle degeneration, many cardiac patients would refuse to take this class of drug. There is also an economic issue. Those covered by health insurance often have their prescription drugs subsidized, while government programs provide low-income people with free drugs. If these patients were told they had to buy coenzyme Q10 supplements if they are prescribed a statin drug, many would not be willing or able to bear this extra cost.

On the flip side, more statin drugs could be sold if there were fewer side effects encountered, such as muscle pain, fatigue, liver toxicity, heart failure, etc. A lot of statin drug prescriptions are not refilled because of side effects, so drug companies may be shortchanging themselves in the long run by not recommending coenzyme Q10 supplementation.

The fact that the FDA does not mandate this warning on the package insert of statin drugs demonstrates the political nature of the agency's decisions. The FDA pretends to be a consumer protection agency, but its actions clearly show that its primary function is to protect the economic interests of the drug industry. Statin drugs cause potentially lethal coenzyme Q10 deficiencies in millions of Americans, but drug company profits are obviously more important to the FDA than saving Americans' lives.

FORMER FDA COMMISSIONER MAKES SURPRISING ADMISSION

Jere Goyan, MD was FDA commissioner from 1979 to 1981. During that era, the FDA exerted totalitarian authority over what Americans were allowed to read about dietary supplements and drugs. According to the FDA at that time, any advertising claim that even implied that a supplement provided a health benefit automatically turned that supplement into an illegal "unapproved new drug."

Dr. Goyan was FDA commissioner when the Life Extension Foundation published its first newsletter in 1980. Even though Life Extension was not selling products, we were cautioned to avoid any relationship with a supplement maker, as that could draw us into a "criminal conspiracy" if we were to publish information about a particular supplement's health benefits.

How times have changed! A consumer uprising resulted in Congress passing several bills that limited the FDA's censorship powers. Federal courts have ruled against the FDA's suppression of health claims based on First Amendment grounds. Back in 1980, the legal consensus was that the First Amendment did not apply to the FDA.

In response to growing reports that drug companies are engaged in all kinds of nefarious behavior that result in consumers being prescribed dangerous drugs, Dr. Goyan was quoted in the *Detroit Free Press* on November 5, 2003 as stating: "We as patients have got to raise the questions ourselves and take care of our own selves."[2]

Considering the FDA's historically rigid position that American consumers are too stupid to make their own healthcare choices and therefore need the FDA to "protect" them, this statement by a former FDA commissioner that people have to "take care of their own selves" is a revolutionary admission. Too bad so many innocent people had to die because the FDA denied them access to the findings from scientific journals about the disease-prevention benefits of dietary supplements. Consumers back then had a hard time "taking care of their own selves" when the FDA uniformly censored all health claims.

FDA SOUGHT TO BAN COQ10

What is truly ironic is that from 1985 to 1994, the FDA made a concerted effort to completely outlaw coenzyme Q10. One of the FDA's arguments was that because coenzyme Q10 is sold as a prescription drug in Japan, it should not be freely available to Americans as a dietary supplement.

The FDA tried to embargo imports of coenzyme Q10 from Japan and launched criminal investigations against those who promoted it in the United States.

Life Extension's CoQ10 supplements were seized twice (and won back both times in legal actions). The FDA's excuse for the first seizure was that the cardiovascular health claims made by Life Extension turned the coenzyme Q10 into an illegal "drug." During the second seizure, the FDA claimed that coenzyme Q10 was so "dangerous" that it posed an "imminent threat" to the health of the American public. These allegations were of course baseless, and fortunately federal judges eventually saw through the FDA's charade.

The sad facts were that statin drugs (approved by the FDA) were killing Americans by causing lethal coenzyme Q10 deficiencies. Instead of addressing the statin drug issue, the FDA sought to ban CoQ10—the best antidote for statin drug toxicity.

The FDA continues to proclaim that it "protects" the health of Americans by denying "unproven" therapies. The FDA's statements about "protecting" consumers' health may go down in history as one of the greatest medical hoaxes of all time.

References

1. Dangerous prescription [transcript]. *Frontline*. PBS television. November 17, 2003.

2. Huang HY, Appel LJ. Supplementation of diets with alpha-tocopherol reduces serum concentrations of gamma-and delta-tocopherol in humans. *J Nutr*. 2003 Oct;133(10):3137–40.

2003

Patient Advocates Sue FDA Over Drug Access

by William Faloon

I T TAKES THE FOOD AND DRUG ADMINISTRATION AN AVERAGE of nearly seven years to approve promising new anti-cancer drugs. For most terminally ill patients, that's not nearly fast enough. Now patient advocates are taking the FDA to court in an effort to force the agency to streamline its approval process.

In late July, the Washington Legal Foundation sued the FDA and the Department of Health and Human Services in US District Court on behalf of the Abigail Alliance for Better Access to Developmental Drugs, a Virginia-based advocacy group for terminally ill patients. The lawsuit contends that the FDA's tortuous drug-approval process effectively denies terminally ill cancer patients access to experimental anti-cancer drugs, thereby violating their constitutional rights.

Alliance founder Frank Burroughs named the group after his daughter Abigail, who two years ago succumbed to cancer at age 21 after trying unsuccessfully to obtain access to two experimental anti-cancer drugs. The group's lawsuit also details the struggles faced by other Alliance patients who were urged by their physicians to try experimental drugs after traditional therapies failed. None of the Alliance patients was able to get into the very limited group who participated in the drug companies' clinical trials.

The lawsuit calls on the FDA to give special initial approval to experimental drugs that show effectiveness and to permit their sale and distribution to patients with no other approved treatment options. The FDA was withholding comment pending review of the lawsuit.

FDA's Lethal Impediment

by William Faloon

THE FDA STIFLES THE DISCOVERY AND AVAILABILITY OF LIFE-
saving therapies by making the cost of getting them
approved prohibitively expensive. The FDA is a major
obstacle that prevents scientific findings from being translated
into therapies to stave off age-related disease.

Compared to the advancement of other technologies over the
past 40 years, medicine has progressed the slowest as far as finding solutions for lethal diseases. Those in the medical establishment may debate this assertion, but the undeniable fact is that
for most types of cancer and neurological diseases, there have
been few substantive improvements in survival, let alone a cure.

Most of you remember attending funerals in the 1960s to 1970s
of those who perished from cancer. You might have been certain
that a cure for cancer would have been found by year 2000. In
fact, the propaganda being released by the cancer establishment

at that time was that doctors were on the verge of eradicating most cancers. (This misguided optimism was primarily based on the premise that chemotherapy was the solution.)

When it comes to therapies designed to slow or reverse aging, the FDA still does not officially recognize aging as a disease process. That means when a company tries to gain approval to market an anti-aging therapy, it first has to overcome the hurdle of educating the FDA that aging is indeed a lethal disease. The new therapy then has to show sufficient efficacy to warrant approval. To date, no one has succeeded in convincing the FDA to approve an anti-aging drug.

In today's world of ever-expanding technological achievement, the fact that medicine remains bogged down in a regulatory quagmire is a disgrace. More than 6,000 Americans die every single day, yet most of these deaths could be prevented if it were not for the strangulation of innovation caused by the FDA, State regulatory agencies, HMOs and apathetic physicians.

DOES GERON HAVE AN EFFECTIVE CANCER VACCINE?

Geron Corporation was originally established to develop anti-aging drugs. Their research, however, led them to discover a potentially effective cancer treatment. On March 18, 2003, Geron released the results of a study that an experimental cancer vaccine might be effective against all types of cancer. This bold announcement was based on a study published in the journal *Cancer Gene Therapy* (March 2003).

Geron's vaccine works in a relatively simple manner. It programs powerful dendritic immune cells to attack cells that express high levels of an enzyme called telomerase. It just so happens that 85% of human tumor cells overly express telomerase[1] whereas normal healthy adult cells express very low and/ or transient telomerase levels. Using telomerase as the target for dendritic cells, Geron's vaccine was shown to provoke a massive attack against prostate and kidney cancer cells as well as breast, melanoma and bladder cancer.

Most cancer cells require high levels of telomerase to prevent them from undergoing a healthy cellular removal process called apoptosis (programmed cell death). The concept of attacking cells high in telomerase makes cancer cells particularly vulnerable, because if they try to hide from this vaccine by making less telomerase, then they will die via normal apoptosis.

There are 558,000 people in the United States who will die of cancer over the next 12 months. Most of them know they are likely to die. We believe these cancer-stricken individuals should have the right to access any potentially effective therapy under the guidelines of an objective yet humanistic formal scientific protocol. While there is no assurance that Geron's new vaccine will cure cancer, the FDA should not withhold this and other potential cancer therapies.

The cancer establishment maintains that only carefully controlled studies can establish safety and efficacy. This sounds reasonable. The reality, however, is that the FDA's current clinical trial requirement has produced flawed data that enabled bad drugs to be approved while potentially effective drugs are denied.[2]

It takes so long for a new drug to make it through the FDA approval process, that if Geron's new drug is effective, most cancer patients reading this column today will perish long before the vaccine ever became available. A real world example of this occurred with an anti-cancer agent for childhood leukemia called Vumon®. This drug was first studied in 1972, but only attained FDA approval in 1992.

A Phase I study of Geron's telomerase vaccine is currently underway in patients with prostate cancer at Duke University in North Carolina. There are two fundamental problems with Phase I studies. First of all, they usually mandate that cancer patients fail all "proven" therapies first.

As has been repeatedly shown in published scientific studies, most so-called "proven" cancer therapies do not cure the disease. Since Phase I studies only test for safety, extremely small doses of the anti-cancer agent are used. This dooms virtually all the terminal cancer patients who participate in Phase I trials to certain death, but it does supply the FDA with the safety data it mandates. In other words, as long as the patient dies of their cancer and not the new drug, it is now permissible to move on from Phase I to Phase II studies where a potentially effective dose of the anti-cancer drug can be given.

HOW THE FDA PERPETUATES THE CANCER EPIDEMIC

It is clear that the bureaucratic process is incredibly long for the approval of anticancer and other therapies used in the treatment of life-threatening diseases. To add insult to injury, the very same approval process has geographic boundaries that create inhumane and unacceptable delays for approval of a critical drug in one country that may be a few miles away from a country where the drug is already studied, reviewed and accepted.

For example, it took years for Taxotere, one of the most impressive anti-cancer agents used to treat breast and prostate cancer, to finally gain FDA approval in the United States. This occurred despite hundreds of studies supporting its efficacy published in the European literature that were not acceptable to the FDA.

Ironically, now that Taxotere has gained FDA approval for the treatment of metastatic prostate cancer in the USA, countries such as Germany do not permit its use in the treatment of prostate cancer because no published papers on this subject have emanated from Germany. This becomes even more incredulous when one realizes that the pioneering research on Taxotere emanated from Germany's next-door neighbor France. The approval agencies such as the FDA here and its counterparts abroad are allowing bureaucratic ego, and perhaps economics, to interfere with the saving of life. Think about this! American and German physicians and scientists are engaged in a battle against a common enemy (cancer) while the respective regulatory agencies (those that approve the use of a drug) of each country use national borders to say "yes" or "no" to a life-saving drug or therapy. This is a violation of human rights within so-called civilized societies. People from all over the world should unite in protest to such atrocity.

Not only do FDA policies delay life-saving drugs from being approved, but they often keep effective medications off the market forever! If a small company like Geron were to run out of money before they could conclude the expensive clinical trials, their vaccine research program could come to a grinding halt.

Contrast this with a libertarian policy of giving dying cancer patients the choice to try Geron's new vaccine immediately. Under this system, it could be possible to determine whether the vaccine worked within months, as opposed to the multiyear period currently mandated by the FDA. If it worked, then millions of cancer patients lives would be saved. If the vaccine failed, then these terminally ill cancer patients will have died, as they would have anyway.

The FDA does have a "compassionate use" exemption that allows cancer patients access to experimental therapies. The problem is that the FDA mandates that these cancer patients first fail so-called "proven" therapies. When cancer cells are exposed to "proven" therapies like radiation or chemotherapy, they mutate in a way that causes them to become super-resistant to future therapies. The patient's healthy cells (including dendritic cells of the immune system) are often seriously impaired when exposed to these "proven" therapies, thus making therapies like Geron's telomerase vaccine less likely to be effective.

PROMISING OVARIAN CANCER DRUG

Ovarian cancer kills more than 14,000 women each year. What makes this type of cancer so insidious is that there are few early warning signs, meaning the disease is usually well advanced when diagnosed.

In May 2003, an announcement was made about a drug called phenoxodiol that induced cell death in 100% of ovarian cancer cells, including those cells resistant to chemotherapy drugs such as Taxol® and carboplatin. The tests were conducted on human cell lines at Yale University School of Medicine.

Phenoxodiol was discovered when scientists were studying the anti-cancer properties of isoflavonoid plant extracts. They used data collected from this research to synthesize phenoxodiol. This drug works by altering a signal pathway in cancerous cells that prevent them from undergoing apoptosis (programmed cell death). These findings indicate that the drug could be successful at treating other cancer types as well. The study was published in the May 1, 2003, issue of *Oncogene*.

FDA-mandated Phase I studies involve giving advanced cancer patients low doses of a new drug to verify safety. The dose is usually so small that the drug has no chance of curing end-stage cancer victims. In the case of phenoxodiol, five Phase I human trials have been completed with few if any side effects. Preliminary results of a trial conducted at the Cleveland Clinic found that more than half of the 10 patients tested on the experimental drug showed some response. Each of these patients had different types of advanced cancer that did not respond to chemotherapy.

It is very difficult to kill cancer cells once they have become resistant to chemotherapy. That is because the cancer cells not killed by chemo develop multisurvival mechanisms that make them extremely difficult to eradicate. What has surprised researchers at Yale was that phenoxodiol killed all ovarian cancer cells (in the laboratory setting), regardless of their immunity to chemo agents.

A phase II trial using phenoxodiol is under way at Yale for women with chemo-resistant ovarian cancer. In this Phase II study, a therapeutic dose of the drug is given with the hope of improving survival or achieving a complete response. The researchers also tested phenoxodiol in mice and found that when dosed at 20 mg/kg every day for six days there was a three-fold reduction in tumor mass compared to a control group. No side effects were noted.

Phenoxodiol functions via several unique mechanisms to induce cancer cells to undergo programmed cell death (apoptosis). Normal cells undergo apoptosis in a controlled manner so they can be replaced with healthier functioning cells. Cancer cells, on the other hand, have gene mutations that prevent them from self-destructing. The ultimate goal of a cancer therapy is to induce malignant cells to undergo apoptosis, instead of indefinitely proliferating out of control.

Under today's antiquated system, a new drug cannot be marketed until it has been thoroughly investigated in clinical trials. These trials can take many years to complete. The results of these numerous trials are then submitted in a new drug application to the FDA. The FDA sends these results to a committee for review. The committee may ask for more studies, reject the application or recommend the drug be approved. The FDA then takes the committee's report and decides whether to approve the drug as safe and effective. This can happen quickly, or it can become bogged down in the FDA's regulatory quagmire. Until the FDA reaches its final verdict, no marketing can take place. It can take 10 or more years after a promising cancer drug has been discovered before the FDA is even in a position to approve it. One reason for this long delay is that after the drug has been discovered, money has to be raised to fund the clinical studies and negotiations with the FDA have to be completed to get approval for the study design itself.

Every month, more than 1,000 women succumb to ovarian cancer. Phenoxodiol was discovered in April 2002. If this drug turns out to be even partially effective, the delay in getting it into cancer victims' hands would have caused thousands of needless deaths.

SAVING CANCER PATIENTS' LIVES

Large amounts of monies have been spent on *Cancer Research*, yet the findings from this research are not being incorporated into clinical oncology practice.

In May 2003, the FDA released news of an initiative to speed the identification and development of new cancer drugs. It appears that the FDA is in the beginning stages of a long overdue reform of Byzantine bureaucracy in order to properly fulfill its public service mission. We have printed the news release in its entirety below. As you will read, what the FDA proposes is not nearly enough. The FDA, in essence, is trying to put out a forest fire with a garden hose.

NCI and FDA Announce Joint Program to Streamline Cancer Drug Development

Under an agreement between the Food and Drug Administration (FDA) and the National Cancer Institute (NCI), which is part of the National Institutes of Health (NIH), the two agencies will share knowledge and resources to facilitate the development of new cancer drugs and speed their delivery to patients.

FDA Commissioner Mark McClellan, MD, PhD, and NCI Director Andrew von Eschenbach, MD, said today that they will establish a multipart Interagency Agreement to enhance the efficiency of clinical research and the scientific evaluation of new cancer medications. The planned agreement, to be announced formally at this week's meeting of the American Society of Clinical Oncology in Chicago, will enhance existing programs and add new joint programs to the existing close cooperative relationship between NCI and FDA, both of which are part of the Department of Health and Human Services (HHS).

"This new collaboration between two key HHS agencies means that federal researchers and regulators will be working together more effectively than ever before," said HHS Secretary Tommy Thompson. "The result will be a more unified, integrated, and efficient approach to the technology development and approval process at a critical time for a disease that affects too many lives," Secretary Thompson said.

The agreement offers potential benefits for the more than one million Americans who are diagnosed with cancer each year.

"The FDA is committed to finding better ways to get safe and effective treatments to patients with life-threatening diseases as quickly as possible," said McClellan. "At a time when the opportunities to reduce the burden of cancer are greater than ever, sharing tools and resources with our colleagues at the National Cancer Institute will help us fulfill that mission," he said.

"The effort between NCI and FDA in cancer therapies is a prototype that should inform and eventually be applied across all areas of research," said NIH Director Elias A. Zerhouni, MD "Dr. McClellan and I are committed to NIH and FDA working closely to find innovative ways to more rapidly make the fruits of our discoveries available to the public."

"The collaboration will help the two agencies take full advantage of their combined knowledge base at a time when many new kinds of anti-cancer agents are in the pipeline," said von Eschenbach. "Molecularly targeted drugs and other novel agents offer great promise, but they also present new challenges that require more collaboration between those involved in their discovery and development," he said.

References

1. Wang Z, Ramin SA, Tsai C, et al. Telomerase activity in prostate sextant needle cores from radical prostatectomy specimens. *Urol Oncol* 6:57–62, 2001.

2. A Life-Saving Drug Discovered In the United States Over 20 Years Ago Is Saving Lives Around the World . . . But Not Yet Here. *Life Extension* magazine, July 2001, p. 54–62.

JUNE 2003

The FDA's Safety Charade

by William Faloon

THE FDA CLAIMS TO BE A CONSUMER PROTECTION AGENCY, yet it continues to permit the sale of a drug (Tambocor®) that is proven to cause twice as many heart attacks than if patients take nothing at all.

On the flip side, the FDA argues against allowing any drug to come in from Canada because this is "exposing the public to significant potential risks." Here is a news bulletin obtained from the FDA's website on March 31, 2003:

FDA Supports Oklahoma Action
Against Pharmacy Obtaining Canadian Drugs

FDA is supporting Oklahoma's petition for an injunction seeking to stop RxDepot from violating state law by obtaining unapproved drugs from Canada for customers in the United States. FDA says the company is

exposing the public to significant potential risks associated with unregulated imported prescription medicines. FDA is concerned that the company has made
misleading assurances about the safety of the drugs.

The FDA admitted to ABC News in 1995 that drug company lobbying caused Tambocor® and similar drugs to be approved before
adequate safety data could be compiled. Drug company lobbying
again is motivating the FDA to pretend that prescription drugs
imported from Canada are "dangerous," when the FDA knows
these are the identical medications sold in American pharmacies. The FDA's actions substantiate that the agency is a puppet
of the drug industry.

Americans are being defrauded out of their money because
the FDA won't let lower cost imports to freely enter the United
States. Thousands of Americans are losing their lives each year
because the FDA allows the sale of drugs that have been proven
to kill. This is not consumer protection.

Supplement Benefit Claims Finally Allowed by the FDA

by William Faloon

O N FEBRUARY 21, 2003, THE FDA AUTHORIZED THE USE of two claims regarding the benefit of the dietary supplement selenium against cancer.* The FDA had to relent in the face of substantial scientific evidence concerning these nutrient-disease effects. The language allowed on the label will now state:

> Selenium may reduce the risk of certain cancers. Some scientific evidence suggests that consumption of selenium may reduce the risk of certain forms of cancer.

---

* The "qualified health claims," as the FDA calls them, which they allowed for selenium were reduced in 2009. This reduction, along with other FDA denials of qualified health claims, has led to further litigation.

However, FDA has determined that this evidence is limited and not conclusive.

Selenium may produce anticarcinogenic effects in the body. Some scientific evidence suggests that consumption of selenium may produce anticarcinogenic effects in the body. However, FDA has determined that this evidence is limited and not conclusive.

Back in 1983, the Life Extension Foundation made a similar claim about selenium based on its own research. Unfortunately, at the time, the FDA determined that Life Extension Foundation was out to harm rather than help people. As a result Life Extension had to endure the illegal seizure by the US government of their selenium products which resulted in a lengthy and costly legal battle. Now years later, the government has reluctantly realized that it can no longer limit or control information that benefits the health and wellbeing of the American public.

Days after the FDA allowed the above selenium claim, it also approved an important claim concerning the benefit of phosphatidylserine with regard to cognitive dysfunction and dementia. On February 24, 2003, the FDA agreed to allow the following statements to be placed on the labels of dietary supplements containing phosphatidylserine:

Phosphatidylserine (PS) may reduce the risk of cognitive dysfunction in the elderly. Very limited and preliminary scientific research suggests that PS may reduce the risk of cognitive dysfunction in the elderly. FDA concludes that there is little scientific evidence supporting this claim.

Phosphatidylserine (PS) may reduce the risk of dementia in the elderly. Very limited and preliminary scientific research suggests that PS may reduce the risk of dementia in the elderly. FDA concludes that there is little scientific evidence supporting this claim.

The Life Extension Foundation originally introduced phosphatidylserine and its brain-function benefits to the American public in 1988. Despite the clear-cut applications for the elderly, the FDA interceded and fought to keep this supplement off the market. On two occasions, the FDA seized Life Extension's phosphatidylserine (PS), and on both occasions Life Extension was able to win the detained product back. The FDA then made a concerted effort to incarcerate Life Extension's founders for promoting and selling a phosphatidylserine supplement. Through persistence and costly legal battles, Life Extension eventually prevailed and those who needed it the most, were able to use phosphatidylserine to alleviate one of the more devastating effects of aging. These two recent victories are an outgrowth of the legal battles that Life Extension has been fighting for the past 18 years. The right to take supplements to protect and enhance one's own health has been hard won.

A New Day at FDA?

After years of battling in the courts, the FDA may finally be forced to comply with the law . . . *again*

OVER FIVE HUNDRED YEARS BEFORE THE DRAFTING OF THE United States Constitution, medieval barons in England fed up with regal abuse created their own set of laws known as the Magna Carta. Latin for "Great Charter," the Magna Carta was a series of written promises designed to force any king—in this case John—to govern the land according to the customs of law and not by whim.

Although originally unwilling to yield any of his royal power, after months of violent battle—and being literally at the point of a sword—the reluctant King John finally agreed to the demands of his barons and signed the document.

Centuries later, the FDA—this time at the point of a legal sword—finally acquiesced to judicial pressure and protests by health activists and created the "Better Health Information for Consumers" initiative, a policy that allows for greater latitude when disseminating information about health foods and nutritional supplements.

In this article, we examine the latest First Amendment victory won in the courts and the FDA's recent capitulation on the issue of dietary supplement health claims.

The Food and Drug Administration (FDA) has consistently fought the use of any statement describing how a nutritional supplement can promote health. Over the past several years, a series of historic court cases has systematically required the FDA to revamp its restrictive policies and allow manufacturers to make health benefit claims for nutritional supplements and foods. The FDA, however, has not always chosen to comply fully with the rulings of the court.

Each of these court cases focused on just a few simple sentences of information that the FDA deemed dangerous and illegal. The result of this litigation and the FDA's partial compliance are finally becoming visible in the marketplace as supplement labels and foods begin to carry expanded information concerning their potential health benefits. For example, bottles of vitamin E may now claim that the supplement helps boost the immune system as well as maintain red blood cells and cardiac muscles. Prior to these court cases, the FDA prohibited such statements. While these rulings support the health industry, the clear winner is the American public, who can now make more informed choices concerning the maintenance of its own health.

WINNING OUT OVER CENSORSHIP

Recently, there have been two new significant developments in the quest to limit the FDA's censorship of health claims. The first was the announcement by the FDA on December 18, 2002, of a broad new initiative, "Better Health Information for Consumers," aimed at making available more information about the health benefits of dietary supplements and foods for the prevention of disease. This new policy represents a 180-degree turn from the traditional FDA stance that no nutrient-disease claims should be allowed for foods or supplements unless they are proven to a "near conclusive degree."

The second development occurred on December 23, 2002, when the FDA lost yet another court case (Whitaker vs. Thompson) concerning its continued suppression of a health claim. What the FDA objected to was the simple statement, "Consumption of antioxidant vitamins may reduce the risk of certain kinds of cancers." This legal action was brought by Dr. Julian M. Whitaker, along with Durk Pearson, Sandy Shaw and Pure Encapsulations, Inc., among others.

REMEMBERING THOSE WHO PERISHED NEEDLESSLY

A great philosopher once stated, "Those who forget the past are condemned to relive it." the Life Extension Foundation is dedicated to reminding the public about the past atrocities committed against the health of the American public by the FDA. We must never forget the tens of millions of innocent Americans who perished while the FDA did everything in its power to suppress information about the importance of disease prevention. These pointless deaths continue as potentially lifesaving medications remain bogged down in the FDA's bureaucratic approval quagmire.

Judge Gladys Kessler of the United States District Court for the District of Columbia ruled that these censoring actions by the FDA were a violation of the Constitution's free speech clause. This is the second time that the FDA was brought into court over this exact statement of antioxidant benefit. The first time was in the 1999 case of Pearson vs. Shalala (commonly referred to as Pearson I) in which the judge ordered the FDA to allow the antioxidant claim with the disclaimer, "These statements have not been evaluated by the Food and Drug Administration." Despite the court's decision, the FDA refused to comply. According to Jonathan W. Emord, the attorney for the plaintiffs in all of these cases, "these victories have resulted in a First Amendment revolution at the FDA. The agency must now expand health information that will enable the public to reduce the risk of disease and live longer."

Judging by the December 18 announcement, the FDA seems to have finally gotten the message. In the past, whenever the court ruled against FDA censorship, the agency strategically took one-step forward and two steps back. The result was that the FDA only partially complied with the Judge's order and additional legal motions had to be filed to bring the FDA in line.

PREVIOUS FIRST AMENDMENT VICTORIES

As a background to the recent victory of Whitaker vs. Thompson, it is essential to look at its two predecessors, Pearson I and Pearson II.

The complaint against the FDA in Pearson I was that the agency refused to allow the following four health claims:

- Consumption of antioxidant vitamins may reduce the risk of certain kinds of cancer. (This was again taken up in Whitaker vs. Thompson.)
- Consumption of fiber may reduce the risk of colorectal cancer.
- Consumption of omega-3 fatty acids may reduce the risk of coronary heart disease.
- 800 mcg of folic acid in a dietary supplement is more effective in reducing the risk of neural tube defects than a lower amount in foods in common form.

The plaintiffs (Durk Pearson, Sandy Shaw, Julian Whitaker, et al.) fought to have the FDA's health claim ban deemed unconstitutional. The court ruled that suppression of these statements was a violation of the First Amendment and ordered the FDA to allow these four claims to enter the marketplace. In reviewing the case, the court found the standard by which the FDA measured the efficacy of a health claim to be purely subjective. It is interesting to note that the FDA was not banning actual products, but only specific claims that spoke to the application of these nutritional products.

For the next two years, the FDA failed to comply with the court's original decision in Pearson I. As a result, attorney Emord and his clients went back to court to seek enforcement of Pearson I as well as relief from the FDA's continued speech suppression.

Their new case in 2001, titled Pearson II, focused on the FDA's refusal to allow the original claim that folic acid supplements were effective in reducing neural tube defects. The court stated, "The scientific consensus, even as acknowledged by the FDA, confirms that taking folic acid substantially reduces a woman's risk of giving birth to an infant with a neural tube defect. The public interest is well served by permitting information about the ability of folic acid to reduce the risk of neural tube defects to reach as wide a public audience as possible." Again, the court ruled in Pearson et al's favor on the same folic acid statement. The FDA was again ordered to comply. In effect, the court had stripped the FDA of any power to ban health claims of nutritional supplements unless the FDA had solid evidence that the claims actually mislead.

What was especially egregious about the FDA's failure to immediately respond to the court's first decision was the potential harm it was causing to unborn children. Folic acid is a safe and low-cost nutrient to prevent neural tube defects. Yet the FDA would not move from its position of refusing to allow such an important statement into the marketplace. This is a perfect example of how public health can be harmed by excessive regulation. Thankfully, despite the FDA's attempt at suppression of this information, the mass media picked up on the story and the public quickly learned about the benefits of folic acid supplements for pregnant women. Doctors now routinely encourage their patients during pregnancy to follow a regimen that includes folic acid in order to prevent unnecessary birth defects.

FDA RESPONDS TO COURT LOSSES

All of this repeated litigation finally began to have an impact on the FDA's policy makers. On December 18, 2002 FDA Commissioner Dr. Mark McClellan, in conjunction with the White House, announced the agency's "Better Health Information for Consumers." This initiative is the FDA's attempt to comply with the requirements of both Pearson I and Pearson II. According to a statement by the FDA, it "anticipates that this policy will facilitate the provision to consumers of additional, scientifically supported health information" and that "the dissemination of current scientific information concerning the health benefits of conventional foods and dietary supplements should be encouraged to enable consumers to make informed dietary choices yielding potentially significant health benefits."

Before this announcement the FDA permitted limited health claims only for certain dietary supplements but not for conventional foods—even though there is much more scientific data available to support the health benefits of foods. Now average consumers will become aware of the specific health benefits of, say, eating broccoli or salmon. According to FDA documents, the consumer health information initiative is focused on three main areas:

- Helping consumers obtain accurate, up-to-date and scientifically-based information about conventional food and dietary supplements.
- Allowing only those health claims for conventional foods and dietary supplements that have been pre-approved by FDA and meet the weight of scientific evidence.

■ Enforcing against false or misleading claims about dietary supplements.

The FDA now states "consumers are more likely to respond to health messages in food labeling if the messages are specific with respect to the health benefits associated with particular substances in the food." The FDA goes on to say that consumers' incorporating "beneficial foods into their diets improves public health." Providing the public with such enhanced nutritional information will hopefully contribute to the decline of such current health epidemics as diabetes, heart disease and cancer.

In "Better Health Information for Consumers," the FDA makes it clear that it is finally responding to the enormous growth of nutritional awareness by the American consumer. A recently released FDA document, the Dietary Supplement Enforcement Report, states that over 158 million consumers use dietary supplements for "ensuring good health" and "preventing various illnesses." It certainly appears the FDA has realized a vast number of Americans are taking responsibility for enhancing their own health by utilizing supplements with or without FDA approval.

Dr. McClellan sums up the initiative by stating, "Our mission at the FDA is to improve health outcomes for the nation, and some of the best opportunities for improving health involve informed choices by consumers." Hopefully, this statement signals the beginning of a new and enlightened position for the FDA.

The impact of the court decisions and the FDA's new initiative are likely to be profound and far-reaching:

■ Americans will have access to much more information regarding the therapeutic benefits of supplements and various food products. This will enable them to make proactive choices in managing their health. Ideally, a better-informed public will become a healthier public focusing on prevention rather than pharmaceutical cures.

- Manufacturers will now be encouraged to research and develop targeted nutriceuticals aimed at specific conditions. In the near future we might see manufacturers making the same therapeutic claims for nutritional products as for standard pharmaceuticals—but without the side effects. The FDA's initiative will remove the barriers for innovation in the expanding nutriceutical field.
- Doctors will be more likely to suggest nutritional protocols along with traditional pharmaceuticals to their patients.

BATTLE TO PROTECT FREE SPEECH CONTINUES

While these recent developments are encouraging, much remains to be done and the battle against the FDA and its restrictive policy toward nutrient claims continues. A Federal Court recently denied manufacturers the right to state on the label the benefits of saw palmetto in reducing the symptoms of mild benign prostatic hypertrophy. As it has repeatedly done in the past, the FDA refused to review the claim, stating in this case that it was "a treatment claim and, hence was not covered under the provisions for health claims." This decision will be appealed. According to attorney Jonathan Emord, he is "not finished with the FDA until it allows health claims for foods and dietary supplements that can be used to treat diseases, not just help prevent them." The battle continues.

DON'T BELIEVE THE FDA'S PROPAGANDA

The FDA was forced to launch its "Better Health Information for Consumers" policy and pretends now that they are in favor of allowing consumers to learn about the benefits of dietary supplements.

The reality is that health activists, Congress, and Federal Judges forced the FDA to capitulate on this critical First Amendment issue. It took decades of protests by American consumers, passage of the Dietary Supplement Health and Education Act (DSHEA) in 1994, and countless losses in the Courts to compel the FDA to pull this public relations stunt (the "Better Health Information for Consumers" initiative) that makes it appear as if they are the good guys. The facts are that Congress passed laws denying the FDA's power to suppress truthful health information and Federal Courts have mandated that the FDA adhere to the law.

The FDA is in an embarrassing situation; they have been cornered into a position that they cannot constitutionally get out of, i.e. Congress has grown increasingly hostile to new regulatory proposals and judges are ruling against them on First Amendment issues. Instead of admitting defeat, they created the "Better Health Information For Consumers" as a charade to make it appear that the FDA came up with the idea to uncensor health information and let consumers learn some of the proven health benefits of certain foods and supplements.

The sad fact is that tens of millions of Americans needlessly died during most of the past century, as the FDA prohibited manufacturers of dietary supplements from disseminating information about peer-reviewed published scientific studies. The FDA went further by actively discouraging Americans from using dietary supplements and conducting nationwide seizure actions against companies who dared to make health claims.

Patriotic Americans who have participated in this successful health-freedom battle should feel proud to have helped defend the United States Constitution against one its most abusive domestic enemies, the FDA.

References

Emord & Associates, "FDA Implements Pearson Decision; Expands to Foods," 2002 Dec 18.

Emord & Associates, Whitaker vs. Thompson; 2002 Dec 26.

Emord, Jonathan. Interview, 2003, Jan 8.

Faloon, William, "What's Wrong With the FDA?" *Life Extension*, 2001 May:26–29.

US Food and Drug Administration, Dietary Supplement Enforcement Report; 2002 Dec 18:1.

US Food and Drug Administration, *FDA News*, "FDA Announces Initiative to Provide Better Health Information for Consumers," 2002 Dec 18: 1.

US Food and Drug Administration, Guidance for Industry, "Qualified Health Claims in the Labeling of Conventional Foods and Dietary Supplements," 2002 Dec 18: 2.

Pearson, Durk; Shaw, Sandy, *FDA Folds: The First Amendment Wins After Eight Years of Battle*; 2002:7.

Medications Side Effects

by Jay S. Cohen, MD

P RESCRIPTION DRUGS HELP MILLIONS OF PEOPLE. STILL, MOST people don't like taking drugs, although many of us ultimately need to. So how can you get the treatment you need while minimizing the risks?

Mainstream medicine's record on preventing medication side effects is poor. A 1998 article in the *Journal of the American Medical Association (JAMA)* defined the scope of the problem: 106,000 deaths and 2,000,000 severe reactions from medications annually in US hospitals, making side effects the fourth leading cause of death in America.[1] These numbers aren't new. The side effect problem has continued for decades and persists unrecognized by many doctors and authorities.

But patients understand. Patients' first concern about medications is safety. They know intuitively that, as a leading drug reference states, "Any drug, no matter how trivial its therapeutic actions, has the potential to do harm."[2]

How can you maximize safety while getting the treatment you need? There are ways, ways in accordance with scientific principles and proven by medical studies, yet routinely ignored by drug companies, the FDA and doctors.

THE FIRST KEY TO AVOIDING SIDE EFFECTS

Side effects occur because most drugs aren't specific in their actions. We may call a drug an "anti-inflammatory" or "antidepressant," but medications don't just go to the cells involved in these problems. They go to most of the cells of our bodies, which can provoke undesirable effects. Thus, an anti-inflammatory may reduce your joint pain, but it may also cause stomach bleeding, kidney failure or anxiety. An antidepressant can improve mood but can also cause insomnia, nausea, weight gain or diminished sex drive.

Most of these unintended effects—side effects—are dose-related. In the 1998 *JAMA* study cited above, 76.2% of all side effects were dose-related. *Melmon and Morrelli's Clinical Pharmacology* places the number at 75% to 85%.[3] The number may be higher, because many drug interactions are also dose-related. When people take multiple drugs, higher doses cause more adverse interactions than lower doses. Whatever the actual number, the first key to avoiding side effects is this: The best way to avoid side effects is to use the lowest dose that works. Excessive dosing merely increases risks.

THE SECOND KEY: INDIVIDUAL VARIATION

Why do side effects occur in some people but not in others? Because people vary tremendously in their sensitivities to medications.

The American Medical Association states that the difference in people's response to a specific drug can vary "4-to 40-fold."[4] So it isn't surprising that some people need 80 mg of the antidepressant Prozac® or the cholesterol-lowering drug Lipitor®, while others need just 2.5 mg.

INDIVIDUAL VARIATION WITH MEDICATIONS ISN'T THE EXCEPTION; IT'S THE RULE

The basis of individual variation is well known. People differ greatly in how they absorb, metabolize and eliminate drugs. The new science of pharmacogenetics has revealed wide variations in the efficiency of people's liver enzymes in processing drugs. People also differ in the sensitivity of their tissues to medication effects. These factors change with age, and many people become more sensitive as they get older.

Because of the great variability between people, it is essential for drug doses to be tailored to each person's needs. I call this precision prescribing. Doctors already practice this with a few drugs—digoxin, insulin, thyroid drugs—but not with most drugs. Many drugs are prescribed one-size-fits-all or at doses that are identical for young and old, big and small, healthy or taking six other drugs at the same time. The failure to match drug doses to individual needs underlies the high incidence of side effects.

CREATING A SIDE EFFECT EPIDEMIC

Drug companies and the FDA routinely ignore the wide differences in people's drug tolerances and the fact that most side effects are dose-related. Doctors, accepting uncritically drug company dosage guidelines, don't think twice about prescribing the same doses of powerful drugs to young and old, big and small, healthy and frail. They ignore patients with long histories of medication reactions. Cookbook dosing is the rule, and an epidemic of side effects is the result.

Even when studies show that half and quarter doses are effective, the data is ignored and dosing is one-size-fits-all. Even when studies show that women or the elderly respond to lower doses, they get the same higher doses as younger, larger men. Something is very wrong when Shaquille O'Neal, Ally McBeal and Grandma

Moses are getting the exact same doses of potent drugs, yet this is exactly how many drugs are prescribed.

"To think that the same dose will do the same thing to all patients is absurd," says Dr. Raymond Woosley, Vice President of Health Services at the University of Arizona. "Patients need to be titrated, starting with the lowest possible dose that could have the desired effect."[5]

Experts everywhere agree with him (Table 1), but that's not how it's done today. The side effect epidemic isn't caused by a few bad drugs, but by bad dosing methods with many drugs.

DOSAGE PROBLEMS WITH ANTIDEPRESSANTS

Doctors follow the guidelines in the drug company-written *PDR*. The *PDR* still advises 75 mg initially for Elavil® (amitriptyline), yet 10 mg or 25 mg is frequently enough for mild depressions or pain syndromes. Effexor® is recommended at 75 mg, but 37.5 mg or 50 mg often is enough initially. Zoloft® is recommended at 50 mg, but 25 mg works well for many mild depressions. Serzone is recommended at 100 mg twice daily, but 50 mg once or twice daily is usually plenty initially.

Similar strategies apply to Paxil®, Wellbutrin®, Celexa®, Norpramin®, Pamelor®, imipramine, doxepin and just about every other antidepressant. "The sales representatives for most antidepressants are now giving out sample packs starting with half-strength doses," Dr. Anthony Weisenberger, a top psychopharmacologist, recently told me. "They lose so many sales because patients get side effects and quit treatment, the drug companies have finally caught on that the dose makes a big difference."

Why is this happening with drug after drug? One reason is that the standard doses of antidepressants are based on studies of major depression—a severe disorder that requires strong treatment. In contrast, the great majority of office patients with depression have mild disorders. Yet, no distinction is made about

Table 1: Medical Experts Agree that Individual Variation Is Common and Matching Doses to Patients Is Essential

Goth's Medical Pharmacology:
"Many adverse reactions probably arise from failure to tailor the dosage of drugs to widely different individual needs."[1]

Goodman and Gilman's The Pharmacological Basis of Therapeutics:
"Therapists of every type have long recognized that individual patients show wide variability in response to the same drug or treatment method."[2]

Hazards of Medication:
"The ultimate hazard is variability of patient response."[3]

American Medical Association Drug Evaluations:
"Almost all drugs cause reasonably predictable toxic reactions when given in excessive doses."[4]

BMJ (British Medical Journal):
"Many drugs have been introduced at doses that later were found to be too high; and usually years have passed, with unnecessary toxicity, before action was taken."[5]

Pharmacoepidemiology and Drug Safety:
"Optimal drug therapy requires appropriate dosing in order to obtain the desired therapeutic effects at minimum risk."[6]

Variability In Drug Therapy—A Sandoz Workshop:
"Even if we try to forget, we are constantly reminded, by one experience or another, that patients differ in their responses to drugs."[7]

Goth's Medical Pharmacology:
"Biologic variation in drug effect is an important reason to individualize dosage and adjust treatment to the requirements of a given patient."[1]

Paracelsus (1493–1541):
"All substances are poisons; there is none which is not a poison. The right dose differentiates a poison and a remedy."[2]

References for Table 1 at the end of the chapter.

treating mild and severe disorders in the dosage guidelines of most antidepressants, so doctors prescribe the same doses to everyone.

DRUGS FOR ELEVATED CHOLESTEROL AND C-REACTIVE PROTEIN

The statins—Lipitor®, Zocor®, Pravachol®, Mevacor®, Lescol®— were the best-selling group of drugs in America in 2001. There's no doubt that statins help millions by reducing heart attacks, strokes and overall cardiac mortality. But statins harm thousands, perhaps millions more, often unnecessarily.

Duane Graveline's first dose of Lipitor® caused amnesia "so severe that I landed in the emergency room of a hospital near my Vermont home. I didn't remember any of it." Dr. Graveline, a retired family doctor, flight surgeon and astronaut, was perplexed. After all, he wasn't usually sensitive to medications, and he'd taken only 10 mg, the lowest dose recommended and marketed by the manufacturer.

Yet, 10 mg of Lipitor® is very strong, much stronger than many people need. It was much stronger than Dr. Graveline needed, because he needed only 2.5 mg of Lipitor®—75% less medication than he got. Experts advise doctors to select statin doses based on the reduction in LDL-C (the bad, low density lipoprotein-cholesterol) that each person needs.[7] 10 mg of Lipitor® reduces LDL-C 39%, a strong response needed by cardiac patients and people with severely elevated cholesterol.

But most people with high cholesterol have mild-to-moderate elevations and no cardiac history, and they require only 20% to 30% reductions in LDL-C. This can be attained with only 2.5 mg or 5 mg of Lipitor®.[8-11] Dr. Graveline required a 25% reduction in LDL-C and should have been started at 2.5 mg mg. Yet, there's no information about 2.5 or 5 mg of Lipitor® in the package insert or PDR and no pills in these doses, so doctors start everyone at 10 mg, or even 20 mg or 40 mg.

EXCESSIVE STATIN DOSES, UNNECESSARY SIDE EFFECTS

Dr. Graveline received 400% more medication than he needed and got a major dose-related side effect because of it. This is a common story. Cognitive and memory problems, sometimes severe and long lasting, occur far more often with statins than doctors recognize. Muscle pain and abdominal discomfort occur frequently. All of these are dose-related.

Liver disorders occur in 1% of patients taking statins. With statins now recommended for 35 million Americans, that's 350,000 people with liver problems, which include liver toxicity and, rarely, death. Dr. W. C. Roberts, the editor-in-chief of the *American Journal of Cardiology*, states, "With each doubling of the dose, the frequency of liver enzyme elevations also doubles."[12] Liver enzyme elevations signify liver injury. So if you get 10 mg of Lipitor® when you only need 2.5 mg, your risk of liver injury is also quadrupled.

Lipitor® is the best-selling drug in America. In 2001, patients filled more than 57 million prescriptions for Lipitor®, and sales are skyrocketing. Zocor®, the third best-selling drug, presents the same dose problems as Lipitor®. Zocor's® standard starting dose, 20 mg, reduces LDL-C 38%. Many people need only 10 mg or even 5 mg, which reduce LDL-C 30% and 26%, respectively.[6] If the standard doses of such widely advertised, top-selling drugs, are so strong, how can we rely on the standard doses of any drug?

DRUGS FOR HIGH BLOOD PRESSURE

Fifty million Americans have high blood pressure (hypertension), and 90% of us will ultimately develop this potentially deadly disease as we age. Hypertension is a particularly vicious disease, a silent destroyer of blood vessels that causes heart attacks, strokes, kidney disease, peripheral vascular diseases and erectile dysfunctions in men. Much of this is preventable with treatment. Yet half of the people starting treatment for hypertension quit within a year. Most do not last 90 days. Why? Medication side effects.

Experts acknowledge the problem: "Often, the cure is perceived as being worse than the disease, and when this is the case, the patient is unlikely to remain [in] treatment."[13]

People get worn down by side effects such as dizziness, weakness, drowsiness, fatigue, diarrhea, muscle cramps and sexual impairments, and give up. Doctors often dismiss so-called "minor" side effects, but minor reactions drive millions from needed treatment—with dire consequences. There's a better solution.

LOWER DOSES RECOMMENDED BY EXPERTS

Because most side effects with antihypertensive drugs are dose-related, experts recommend starting with the very lowest effective doses. But what are they? Most doctors turn to the *PDR*, but the *PDR*'s doses often aren't the lowest. In an analysis I published in the *Archives of Internal Medicine* in 2001, I found that for 23 of 40 top-selling antihypertensive drugs, the initial doses recommended by the drug companies in the *PDR* were much higher than recommended by the Joint National Committee-the national board of medical experts on hypertension.[14]

For example, the manufacturer's initial dose for Norvasc®, the fifth most prescribed drug in the US in 2001, is 5 mg. The experts recommend 2.5 mg, 50% less medication. The manufacturer of Capoten® (captopril) recommends 50 mg to 75 mg/day initially, 100% to 600% more than the 12.5 mg to 25 mg recommended by experts.

When Tenormin® (atenolol) was introduced in 1976, the one-size-fits-all dose was 100 mg. It wasn't until 1980 that a 50 mg dose was available and until 1989 that 25 mg was produced. The manufacturer still recommends 50 mg initially, 100% higher than the 25 mg recommended by the national board.

Similar over-dosing is seen with top-sellers Zestril®, Prinivil®, Altace®, Inderal® (propanolol), Cardura®, Cozaar®, and many others (Table 2). Is it any wonder why so many people quit treatment?

Some savvy doctors recognize that starting with the lowest dose not only reduces risks, but allows people time to improve their diets, lose weight, start exercising and learn stress reduction or meditation. These methods not only lower blood pressure, but can reduce the amount of medication you need. As one specialist put it, "With blood pressure, it's easy to overshoot the mark. That's why I always start low and give people time to make other changes. Very often, their blood vessels relax over a period of time and you wind up ultimately needing less medication. When I start with standard doses, we spend the rest of our lives combating side effects."

Table 2: Lower Initial Doses of Antihypertensive Drugs		
	PDR	**Proven Lower Dose**
ACE INHIBITORS		
Accupril® (quinapril)	10 mg	5 mg
Altace® (ramipril)	2.5 mg	1.25 mg
Capoten® (captopril)	50–75 mg	25 mg
Prinivil®, Zestril® (lisinopril)	10 mg	5 mg
ANGIOTENSIN RECEPTOR BLOCKERS (ARBS)		
Inderal® (propanolol)	80 mg	40 mg
Kerlone® (betaxolol)	10 mg	5 mg
Levatol® (penbutolol)	20 mg	10 mg
Lopressor® (metoprolol)	100 mg	50 mg
Sectral® (acebutolol)	400 mg	200 mg
Zebeta® (bisoprolol)	5 mg	2.5 mg
Calan®, Isoptin®, Verelan® (verapamil)	120–180 mg	90 mg
Cardizem®, Dilacor® (diltiazem)	180–240 mg	120 mg

EXCEPTIONS

There are some drugs for which the low-dose approach does not apply. For example, antibiotics, antifungal and anticancer drugs should be used at full doses. These drugs are not targeting you, but invaders that can be made stronger if inadequate doses are used.

THE ELDERLY

"The overall incidence of adverse drugs reactions in the elderly is two to three times that found in young adults," states the *New England Journal of Medicine*.[15] Although people over age 60 comprise 19% of the population, they account for 39% of all hospitalizations and 51% of all deaths related to medication reactions.[16]

Seniors metabolize drugs more slowly than younger people, so they are frequently more sensitive to their effects. That's why gerontologists recommend extra caution in treating seniors and starting with low doses (Table 3). Yet, for scores of top-selling drugs, drug company guidelines tell doctors to use the same strong doses for young and old. Even when we know that blood levels of drugs rise much higher in seniors, doctors are told to ignore this fact and prescribe the same doses.

For example, Allegra® blood levels rise 99% higher in seniors versus younger adults. Claritin® rises 50% higher. Blood levels of top-selling antihypertensives Zestril® and Prinivil® rise 100% higher. Blood levels of Prilosec® and Nexium® are higher in the elderly. Yet, the recommended doses of all these drugs are the same for young and old.[6]

The FDA itself states, "There is evidence that older adults tend to be more sensitive to drugs than younger adults, due to their generally slower metabolisms and organ functions. The old adage, 'Start low and go slow,' applies especially to the elderly."[17] Yet the FDA keeps approving drugs at identical doses for young and old. Perhaps this explains why 9% of all hospital admissions for seniors are related to side effects from standard doses of prescription drugs.[18]

Table 3: Lower Medication Doses for Older People

Journal of the American Geriatrics Society, **1999:**

"Choosing the correct dose of a drug therapy is critical when prescribing for older people because adverse effects are often dose-related. The conventional wisdom has been to start low and go slow."[1]

Goth's *Medical Pharmacology*

"In general the best approach is to start with lower doses and to increase dosage slowly and in small increments."[2]

Public Citizen's *Worst Pills, Best Pills II*, 1993:

"If drug therapy is indicated, in most cases it is safer to start with the dose which is lower than the usual adult dose."[3]

***Drug Safety*, 1990:**

"Starting doses can often be reduced in the elderly."[4]

***FDA Consumer Magazine*, 1997**

"There is evidence that older adults tend to be more sensitive to drugs than younger adults, due to their generally slower metabolisms and organ functions. [The] old adage, 'Start low and go slow,' applies especially to the elderly."[5]

***Archives of Internal Medicine*, 1986:**

"The elderly are especially sensitive to both the intended pharmacologic effects of drugs and their undesirable adverse reactions."[6]

***BMJ (British Medical Journal)*, 1997:**

"If drug treatment is necessary, the lowest feasible dose of the drug should be used."[7]

***United States Pharmacopeia, Drug Information*, 1994:**

"Some clinicians recommend that geriatric patients, especially those 70 years of age or older, be given one-half of the usual adult dose initially."[8]

***Australian Family Physician*, 1992:**

"[With the elderly,] the starting dose should be lower than that recommended for younger adults; the maximum tolerated dose may well be lower than for younger individuals." "Select the minimum dose of the safest medication. . . . Start low and go slow."[9]

WOMEN

In summer 2002, two studies caused alarm by revealing increased risks of cancer and heart disease with Premarin® and Prempro®, the top-selling hormone replacement therapies (HRT) for menopausal women.[19, 20] The dose of estrogens in these drugs: 0.625 mg. But we've known for years that lower doses of Premarin® (0.3 mg) and other estrogens are often effective and cause fewer risks.[21-24] Might these doses be safe enough today? Quite possibly, but the studies ignored this obvious question, leaving women in the lurch.

The studies also didn't mention that from 1964 through 1999, the recommended dose of Premarin® for hot flashes was 1.25 mg. How much cancer did this double dose cause? Why was such a strong dose approved in the first place? These questions weren't answered.

A similar pattern was seen with birth control pills. The hormone doses in the first pills were 300% to 1000% higher than in today's pills,[25-28] yet it took decades—and hundreds of women's lives—before high-dose pills were withdrawn and replaced with today's lower doses.

Similar problems are seen with other medications. A study of ibuprofen for menstrual pain showed that 44% of women did just fine with the 200 mg over-the-counter dose, but the researchers still recommended 400 mg for all women.[29] Studies of cholesterol-lowering drugs show that many women respond to lower doses,[30-33] but they are routinely prescribed the same doses as men.

Side effects with antihypertensive drugs occur more often in women,[34, 35] which, according to the *American Journal of the Medical Sciences*, "could be due to the fact that women are treated with antihypertensives using the dosage and schedule established with men, even though it is well known that body size, fat distribution and coronary artery size differ in women and men."[35]

Not all women require lower doses, but many do, especially small women. Why aren't doses developed for them? A 2001 report of the US General Accounting Office found not only that women are underrepresented in the dose studies, but even when dose differences are identified, they usually aren't reflected in the final dosage guidelines.[36] A 2001 report by the National Academy of Sciences recommended additional attention to differences between men and women in diseases and treatments.[37] The panel's report added that medical researchers often view men as the norm while underreporting rather than highlighting sex differences. Commenting on this report, Dr. Woosley added that many drug studies he sees "don't consider sex differences at all."[38]

Is this important? In the US, 55% of women versus 37% of men take a prescription drug daily.[39] And of the 11 drugs withdrawn in recent years, eight (maybe nine) affected women more than men.

ENTRENCHED PROBLEMS WITH THE MEDICAL-PHARMACEUTICAL COMPLEX

"It's long been known that for individual subjects the dosage listed on a drug label is not necessarily the right one," Dr. Carl Peck, the highly respected director of Georgetown's Center of Drug Development Science and a former division director at the FDA, stated in September 2002.[40] This is a chilling, and accurate, comment. Yet, the medical—pharmaceutical complex-drug companies, FDA and mainstream doctors—maintain that our medications are as safe as possible. Clearly, this isn't the case.

PROBLEMS IN DRUG INDUSTRY RESEARCH

Why aren't drug doses designed to fit individuals and to prevent side effects? Don't drug manufacturers care?

They do care. "More and more senior executives are concerned that so many patients are dropping out of therapy prematurely," magazine declared in 2002. "So many are asking, "What can I do to increase patient retention?"[41] Each year, patients driven from treatment by side effects cost the drug industry billions in sales.

Yet, many economic factors keep the system from changing (Table 4). Drug companies are profit-driven entities, so marketing issues weigh very heavily. Manufacturers feel great pressure to keep costs down while hastening new drugs to market. And drug companies aren't held responsible for the huge costs of dose-related side effects to the healthcare system. The result is that marketing issues frequently outweigh medical science in drug company decisions.

Indeed, marketing influences affect science so severely that even the medical journals, which depend on drug company advertising, rebelled against them. In September 2001, Reuters Health reported: "Seeking to curb the growing influence exerted by drug firms over research findings, the world's top medical journals announced steps on how to prevent firms that fund studies from manipulating results to favor their drugs and bury studies that are unfavorable."[42] The editors of *JAMA, Lancet*, the *New England Journal of Medicine*, and ten others declared: "We are concerned that the current environment in which some clinical research is [conducted] may threaten medical objectivity. . . . The use of clinical trials primarily for marketing makes a mockery of clinical investigation."[43] The journals implemented new guidelines to ensure the integrity of clinical studies, but a year later few medical schools had adopted them.[44]

Drug marketing is geared toward doctors' preferences, and doctors like drugs that can be dosed simply and quickly. No time is required to match doses to individual patients if drugs are one-size-fits-all. Expediency sells.

So does pumped-up effectiveness. Strong doses produce higher efficacy numbers, which are essential for introducing a new drug

Table 4: Why Don't Drug Companies Produce Doses That Fit Individuals?	
Cost	Good dose studies cost a little more.
Time	Good dose studies take a little more time, placing a company at a disadvantage versus its less diligent competitors.
Unrepresented Populations	Women and seniors are often underrepresented in dose studies. A 2001 GAO analysis found that 78% of subjects in dose trials are male.
Study Designs	Drug companies prefer to study serious disorders because they are more stable and measurable. Serious disorders usually require potent doses. When marketed, these same doses are often prescribed for milder disorders that don't usually require such potent doses
Less Inventory	Fewer doses cost less to manufacture.
Effective Advertising	Higher doses produce higher efficacy rates, which makes great advertising that influences doctors.
Effective Marketing	Simplicity sells. Doctors like onesize-fits-all drugs because they are easy and quick to use.
Weak FDA Regulations	FDA definitions of "effective and safe" do not ensure that the lowest, safest doses are marketed.
FDA Analysis	Fearing long delays if a drug is denied, drug companies use strong doses to ensure that the efficacy passes FDA analysis.
No Public Pressure	The public isn't aware of the side effect epidemic or that most side effects are dose-related, so it doesn't demand change.
No Accountability	The drug industry isn't required to pay the billions for the extra doctors' visits, prescriptions, ER visits and hospitalizations from dose-related side effects.
Basic Economics	With record profits and weak regulation, the drug industry has little incentive to change.

into a competitive market. Dr. Thomas Bodenheimer of the University of California, San Francisco, reported:

> Drug company studies are often done in younger, healthier populations—providing better rates of effectiveness and fewer adverse reactions—than those who will actually receive the drug.[45]

Dr. Alexander Herxheimer, Professor Emeritus at the Cochrane Center in Britain, concurred in *Lancet*. "For quick market penetration, a drug must be simple to use and effective in the greatest number of people. Drugs are often introduced at a dose that will be effective in around 90% of the target population, because this helps market penetration. The 25% of patients who are most sensitive to the drug get much more than they need."[46] With nearly 100 million Americans taking a prescription drug daily, that's 25 million people.

THE FDA'S ROLE

The FDA has not pushed the drug industry to provide better dose studies or a range of doses to match patients' differences. The FDA's decisions about drug doses have been criticized even from within the FDA itself. Based on his recent study showing that dozens of drugs ultimately require dosage reductions years after approval, FDA officer James Cross stated in September 2002, "We've seen a lot of situations where drugs are approved by the FDA and subsequent important information about their optimal dose is not determined until afterward."[47]

Even if the FDA wanted to push the matter, could it? The pharmaceutical industry has the biggest lobby in Washington and is a top contributor to elected officials. With Congress pressuring the FDA to approve drugs faster and faster over the past decade, and the new commissioner vowing to speed approvals even more, the FDA isn't likely to reject drugs for better dose studies. "Making sure the dosages that are used best serve the patients should be near the top of the agenda for regulators and the prescribing community," Dr. Herxheimer insists. "Right now this item seems to be nowhere on the agenda."[48]

CONSEQUENCES OF A FLAWED SYSTEM

The failure of the system is revealed by disaster after disaster. "Discovery of new dangers of drugs after marketing is common," a 1998 study in *JAMA* declared. "Overall, 51% of approved drugs have serious adverse effects not detected prior to approval."[49]

Another study disclosed that 20% of all new drugs ultimately require a new "black box" warning, indicating serious or fatal reactions. The study noted: "Serious adverse drug reactions commonly emerge after FDA approval. The safety of new agents cannot be known with certainty until a drug has been on the market for many years."[50]

How can long-term side effects be minimized? By using the lowest, safest doses. For example, the jury is still out on the long-term safety of statin drugs, but already serious nerve injuries are being reported. A 2002 study found that "people who had taken statins were 4 to 14 times more likely to develop" peripheral nerve injuries (tingling, numbness, shooting or electrical pain, muscle weakness).[51] These reactions occur in one in 2,000 users of statin drugs per year. With 35 million Americans projected to take statins, that's 17,500 cases of peripheral neuropathies each year. Discontinuation doesn't always bring reversal. Most important, the risk is cumulative: the higher the dose, the greater the risk.

DOCTORS AND THE DRUG INDUSTRY

Some doctors are terrific. Some aren't. But even good doctors often don't have all of the information you'd like in order to make good dose decisions.

Doctors ultimately decide which drugs are successful, so doctors are in a position to demand better drug information, a wider range of drug doses to fit patients and better information about non-drug alternatives. Doctors can play a pivotal role, but so far they haven't demanded anything. Many doctors aren't even aware that a problem exists.

"There is an informational void about pharmaceuticals in the training of most doctors, despite the importance of the prescription in medical care," stated Harvard physician Jerry Avorn. "Most of those who have looked thoughtfully at this process have been appalled at its inadequacy."[52]

The result is that doctor's knowledge of medications is less than ideal, which is directly linked to the high rate of side effects. "Much of the morbidity and mortality currently associated with drug therapy is due to well-recognized adverse effects and reflects our inability as health professionals to implement current knowledge fully," Dr. Alastair Wood, Vice Chancellor of Medical Affairs at Vanderbilt, wrote in 1998.[53]

Specialists are usually more knowledgeable about drugs than general physicians, but many specialists don't even understand the importance of precision prescribing. One heart specialist told me, "Most doctors don't think about dose-response. They think you either get side effects or you don't." Dr. Herxheimer agrees: "Clinicians rarely think critically about the dose-response relations of the drugs they use."[48]

"If a medication doesn't work or causes side effects," a pharmacist told me years ago, "most physicians just switch from one to another, then another, then another, until they either find a drug that works, or they or the patient give up. Very few physicians go to the trouble of adjusting drug dosages to fit their patients. Most don't deviate from the drug companies' recommendations."

According to Dr. Woosley, who develops medical training programs. "Only about fifteen of the medical schools today teach formal courses in clinical pharmacology, which is the discipline that emphasizes individual variability in response to drugs. This small effort will never counter the overwhelming message from the drug industry that one dosage is all that is needed and everyone will respond nicely without side effects."

The result is that most doctors accept drug company information uncritically. They assume that the drug companies and the FDA have chosen doses carefully and that the recommended doses are right for everyone. They accept incomplete side-effect lists in the *PDR* as the final word, even when published studies repeatedly say otherwise.

Most doctors get their drug information from the drug company-written *PDR*, the 80,000 drug representatives dispatched to doctors offices, the drug advertising that fills medical journals, drug company-designed studies and drug company-underwritten conferences. Many doctors don't hesitate to accept $500 stipends and fancy dinners to receive drug company-paid presentations. One concerned doctor wrote to the *New England Journal of Medicine*: "The conflicts are obvious to everyone in the field. Who hasn't sat through a company-sponsored presentation by a well-known colleague without squirming a little at the obvious bias in the discussion?"[54] A doctor visiting from Germany, appalled at the overt willingness of doctors to accept drug company goodies, wrote to *JAMA*, "In the long run this behavior will undermine the respect and trust of physicians and the standing of the entire medical profession."[55]

Dr. Marcia Angell, former editor-in-chief of the *New England Journal of Medicine*, chided doctors, "It is well to remember that the costs of the industry-sponsored trips, meals, gifts, conferences, symposiums and honorariums, consulting fees, and research grants are simply added to the prices of drugs and devices."[56] But many doctors eagerly accept these freebies. As one doctor wrote to me, "Physicians as a group have an amazing capacity to rationalize their own greed."

Some doctors are rightfully concerned, but not near enough. "Many physicians have grown accustomed to industry-subsidized education and now resist paying even modest amounts to attend classes" offered by unbiased medical centers, the *Wall Street Journal* reported recently.[57] Yet if you bring your own ideas about drugs and doses to your doctor, don't expect a warm reception. Many doctors get defensive, even hostile, when patients question their methods. If there's any area that defines doctors, it's their ability to prescribe drugs. They are the experts, and too often they choose to defend their turf rather than expand their minds.

"Doctors don't like to be challenged," a pharmacist wrote to me. "One doctor was prescribing Paxil® well above the highest recommended dosage. When I asked him about it, he said, "Are you a doctor? Who are you to be telling me what to do!"

Indeed, some doctors have difficulty admitting even common side effects listed in the *PDR*. Being defensive doesn't strengthen doctor-patient relationships. More and more, doctors are perceived as pill pushers and as defenders of the medical-pharmaceutical machine instead of their own patients.

This perception is enhanced when drug companies can so easily convince doctors to prescribe new drugs even when older, better-known drugs are equally effective. For years, the FDA has warned doctors against using new drugs unless a patient has a specific need. Dr. Janet Woodcock, Director of the FDA Center for Drug Evaluation and Research, has stated, "The sad truth is that, even after all the clinical development that occurs with every drug and even after drugs have been approved for a time, we only have a crude idea of what they do in people."[58] With the FDA approving drugs faster than ever, the American public is frequently the world's first population to try out new drugs.

Yet, doctors repeatedly make new drugs bestsellers within months. Drug reps fill doctors' cabinets with "free" samples, knowing that if patients do well on them, they won't want to switch. Drug advertising seizes upon any difference, no matter how trivial, to sway doctors to prescribe expensive new drugs with no track records, and doctors readily oblige. You'd think that after recent disasters with Baycol®, Rezulin®, Lotronex®, Duract®, Redux® and Fen-Phen®, doctors would learn, but they keep prescribing new drugs like Clarinex®, Nexium® and Bextra® at greater risk and cost. These repeated problems compelled Drs. Marcia Angell and Arnold Relman, another former editor of the *New England Journal of Medicine,* to warn, "Few Americans appreciate the full scope and consequences of the pharmaceutical industry's hold on our healthcare system."[59]

One healthcare observer wrote: "The root cause is the physician, his lack of knowledge or intellectual curiosity. The pharmaceutical companies are trying to make a buck anyway they can, and it is up to the physician to have the fortitude to resist." He has a point. Doctors can't have it both ways. They can't be objective advisors to patients while being so reliant on drug company data and accepting of drug company influences.

Such reliance explains why people today make more visits to alternative practitioners than mainstream doctors. It explains why mainstream doctors remain largely unaware of proven-effective alternatives like omega-3 oils for reducing inflammation and sudden cardiac death, policosanol and inositol hexanicotinate for reducing cholesterol, or the importance of coenzyme Q10 for people taking statins. It explains why mainstream doctors continued to make Premarin®, with its conjugated horse estrogens, a top-seller for decades although many types of human estrogens (estradiol, estriol) were available.

It explains why, despite hundreds of studies in medical journals, most doctors don't know anything about magnesium's essential role for normal blood vessel functioning or that 80% of westerners are deficient in magnesium. By balancing calcium, magnesium is a safer, natural, much less expensive way to help reduce blood pressure than the prescription calcium blockers for which doctors write $4 billion in prescriptions each year, yet few mainstream doctors know about it.

WHAT YOU CAN DO

If you are doing well on a medication, that's good. That's the goal: receiving benefit without side effects. But if medications are causing problems, or if the next time you need a medication you want to minimize the risk, you need to inform yourself about the lowest, safest doses. Do not reduce doses without your doctor's guidance. Undertreatment can have serious medical consequences.

Hopefully, you have a doctor who recognizes the importance of precision prescribing. Some do.

But if your doctor, like most doctors, isn't aware of the low-dose alternatives, what can you do? Inform yourself. The day when you could rely on doctors to provide all of the important drug information is long gone. Doctors have less time than ever to read medical journals or to search the medical literature. You can access it yourself at www.PubMed.org, established by the National Institutes of Health. People spend a lot of time researching an auto or stereo purchase; they need to do the same for their own bodies.

YOU HAVE A RIGHT TO BE INFORMED

The American Medical Association's Code of Medical Ethics states: "The patient's right of self-decision can be effectively exercised only if the patient possesses enough information to enable an intelligent choice."[60] What is "enough information?" Surely, if a lower dose is effective, you have a right to know about it. If you are prescribed a standard dose of a drug without being told about an effective lower dose, you haven't received informed consent. If the standard dose has done major harm, you may have grounds to sue.

Higher doses are certainly appropriate sometimes. Emergencies and acute situations demand immediate relief. However, 90% of office visits aren't for acute problems, but for minor or chronic conditions. There's time to match doses to individuals. There's time to start with a lower, safer dose and then to adjust upward, if necessary. You are paying the bill and taking the risk, so you have a right to be fully informed about the options.

The low-dose method is especially fitting for:

- Older people
- Small people
- People with multiple medical conditions
- People taking multiple medications
- People with histories of medication sensitivities
- People wanting to minimize costs
- People wanting to minimize risks

The "start low, go slow" approach may take a little more time initially, but it saves a lot of time (and money) in the long run. Some people will get surprisingly good results with a low dose and never need higher doses. Some won't, and the dose will need to be increased. Even then, they are assured that they are getting exactly what their bodies need.

Not everyone opts for the low-dose approach. Some people know that they aren't sensitive to medications. With such people, starting with standard doses is valid. Indeed, some people seem resistant to drugs and require very high doses. The key is to match the dose with the person. Ultimately it doesn't matter whether you need a low dose or a high dose—what matters is that you get the right dose for you.

Doing so requires good dose information and a range of drug doses. If anything, the drug industry is providing less of each. The irony is that other industries not only recognize the differences among people, they capitalize on it. They produce cars, clothes, cosmetics and all kinds of commodities in vast arrays to match individual sizes and needs. But with its monopolistic patents and sway over doctors, the drug industry can do what it likes and charge what it wants.

In 2001, 3.2 billion prescriptions were filled in America—12 prescriptions for each man, woman, and child. Forty-six percent of adult Americans take a prescription drug every day. Each year, drug sales increase 25%.[61] And medication side effects remain a top killer. How can we restore sanity to this system? It will have to begin with you.

You are paying the bill and taking the risk, so you have a right to ask questions and to request better information. You have a right to ask your doctor why he's selecting a specific drug at a specific dose. Are there lower doses that work? What is his source of information? We must require doctors to explain their decisions, to think about their choices, and to consider other sources of information.

Most people don't like taking medication. If they must take it, they want to use as little as possible. When I offered the low-dose approach to patients, most opted for it, side effects dropped dramatically, success rates climbed, patients were pleased and so was I. Most side effects are avoidable. The side effect epidemic can be halted. And everybody wins. But the current system is entrenched, so change is going to have to begin with us.

References

1. Lazarou, J, Pomeranz, BH, Corey, PN. Incidence of adverse drug reactions in hospitalized patients: a meta-analysis of prospective studies. *JAMA* 1998;279(15):1200–5.

2. Gilman, AG, Rall, TW, Nies, AS, Taylor, P. Goodman and Gilman's *The Pharmacological Basis of Therapeutics*. New York: Pergammon Press, 1990 and 1996.

3. Melmon, KL, Morrelli, HF, Hoffman, BB, Nierenberg, DW. Melmon and Morrelli's *Clinical Pharmacology: Basic Principles in Therapeutics*. (3rd Edition). New York: McGraw-Hill, Inc., 1993.

4. American Medical Association. *AMA Drug Evaluations, Annual 1994.* Chicago: American Medical Association, 1994.

5. Grady, D. Too Much of a Good Thing? Doctor Challenges Drug Manual. *New York Times,* Oct. 12, 1999:D1–2..

6. *Physicians' Desk Reference,* 57th Edition. Montvale, N.J.: Medical Economics Company, 2003.

7. Executive Summary of the Third Report of the National Cholesterol Education Program (NCEP) Expert Panel on Detection, Evaluation, and Treatment of High Blood Cholesterol in Adults. *JAMA* 2001;285(19):2486–97.

8. Nowrocki, J, Weiss, S, et al. Reduction in LDL Cholesterol by 25% to 60% in Patients with Primary Hypercholesterolemia by Atorvastatin, a New HMG-Co-A Reductase Inhibitor. *Arteriosclerosis, Thrombosis, and Vascular Biology* 1995;15:678–682.

9. Wolffenbuttel, BH, Mahla, G, Muller, D, et al. Efficacy and safety of a new cholesterol synthesis inhibitor, atorvastatin, in comparison with simvastatin and pravastatin, in subjects with hypercholesterolemia. *Netherlands Journal of Medicine* 1998;52 (4):131–7.

10. Bakker-Arkema, RG, Best, J, Fayyad, R, et al. A brief review paper of the efficacy and safety of atorvastatin in early clinical trials. *Atherosclerosis* 1997;131(1):17–23.

11. Cilla, DD Jr, Whitfield, LR, Gibson, DM, et al. Multiple-dose pharmacokinetics, pharmacodynamics, and safety of atorvastatin, an inhibitor of HMG-CoA reductase, in healthy subjects. *Clinical Pharmacology and Therapeutics* 1996;60(6):687–95.

12. Roberts, WC. The rule of 5 and the rule of 7 in lipid-lowering by statin drugs. *American Journal of Cardiology* 1997;80:106–7..

13. Elliott, WJ, Maddy, R, Toto, R, Bakris, G. Hypertension in Patients with Diabetes. *Postgraduate Medicine* 2000;107:29–38.

14. Cohen, JS. Adverse drug effects, compliance, and the initial doses of antihypertensive drugs recommended by the Joint National Committee vs. the Physicians' Desk Reference. *Archives of Internal Medicine* 2001;161:880–85..

15. Recchia, AG, Shear, NH. Organization And Function Of An Adverse Drug Reaction Clinic. *Journal of Clinical Psychiatry,* 1994; 34:68–79.

16. Smucker, WD, Kontak, JR. Adverse drug reactions causing hospital admission in an elderly population: experience with a decision algorithm. *Journal of the American Board of Family Practice* 1990;3(2):105–9.

17. Williams, RD. Medications and older adults. *FDA Consumer Magazine*, Sept.-Oct. 1997.

18. Montamat, SC, Cusack, BJ, Vestal, RE. Management of drug therapy in the elderly. *New England Journal of Medicine* 1989;321 (5):303–9.

19. Writing Group for the Women's Health Initiative. Risks and Benefits of Estrogen Plus Progestin in Healthy Postmenopausal Women. *JAMA* 2002;288:321–333.

20. Lacey, JV, Mink, PJ, Lubin, JH, Sherman, ME, Troisi, R, Hartge, P, et al. Menopausal hormone replacement therapy and risk of ovarian cancer. *JAMA* 2002;288:334–341.

21. Ettinger B. Personal perspective on low-dosage estrogen therapy for postmenopausal women. *Menopause*, 1999; 6(3):273–6.

22. Weinstein L. Efficacy of a continuous estrogen-progestin regimen in the menopausal patient. *Obstetrics and Gynecology* 1987;69(6):929–32.

23. Greendale, GA, Reboussin, BA, Hogan, P, et al. Symptom relief and side effects of postmenopausal hormones: results from the Postmenopausal Estrogen/Progestin Interventions Trial. *Obstetrics and Gynecology* 1998;92(6):982–8.

24. McNagny, SE. Prescribing Hormone Replacement Therapy for Menopausal Symptoms. *Annals of Internal Medicine*, 1999;131:605–16.

25. Snider S. The Pill: 30 Years of Safety Concerns. US Food and Drug Administration, Dec. 1990; www.fda.gov/bbs/topics/consumer/CON00027.html. Checked: Mar. 9, 2002.

26. Marks L. "Not just a statistic": The history of USA and UK policy over thrombotic disease and the oral contraceptive pill, 1960s-1970s. *Social Science and Medicine* 1999;49:1139–1155.

27. Vessey MP, Inman WH. Speculations about mortality trends from venous thromboembolic disease in England and Wales

and their relation to the pattern of oral contraceptive usage. *Obstetrics and Gynecology in the British Commonwealth* 1973;80:562–566.

28. Bottiger LE, Boman G, Eklund G, Westerholm B. Oral contraceptives and thromboembolic disease: effects of lowering oestrogen content. *Lancet* 1980;1:1097–1101.

29. Shapiro, SS, Diem, K. The effects of ibuprofen in the treatment of dysmenorrhea. *Current Therapeutic Research* 1981;30(3):327–334.

30. Wierzbicki AS, Lumb PJ, Chik G, Crook MA. High-density lipoprotein cholesterol and triglyceride response with simvastatin versus atorvastatin in familial hypercholesterolemia. *American Journal of Cardiology* 2000;86:547–549.

31. Ose L, Luurila O, Eriksson J, Olsson A, Lithell H, Widgren B. Efficacy and safety of cerivastatin, 0.2 mg and 0.4 mg, in patients with primary hypercholesterolaemia: A multinational, randomised, double-blind study. Cerivastatin Study Group. *Current Medical Research and Opinion* 1999,15:228–240.

32. Peters TK, Muratti EN, Mehra M. Efficacy and safety of fluvastatin in women with primary hypercholesterolaemia. *Drugs.* 1 994;47(Suppl2):64–72.

33. Leitersdorf E. Gender-related response to fluvastatin in patients with heterozygous familial hypercholesterolaemia. *Drugs.* 1994;47(Suppl 2):54–58.

34. Lewis CE. Characteristics and treatment of hypertension in women: a review of the literature. *American Journal of the Medical Sciences* 1996;31 1(4):193–9.

35. Israili, ZH, Hall, WD. Cough and angioneurotic edema associated with angiotensin-converting enzyme inhibitor therapy. A review of the literature and pathophysiology. *Annals of Internal Medicine* 1992;1 17(3):234–42.

36. Women Sufficiently Represented in New Drug Testing, but FDA Oversight Needs Improvement. Report to Congressional Requesters. US General Accounting Office, GAO-0 1–754, July 6, 2001 :www.fda.gov/womens/informat.html.

37. Exploring the Biological Contributions to Human Health: Does Sex Matter? Wizemann, TM, Pardue, ML, Editors, Committee on Understanding the Biology of Sex and Gender Differences, Board on Health Sciences Policy, Institute of Medicine, National Academy of Sciences, National Academy Press, 2001.

38. Kritz, FL. Mars and Venus and Drugs: Sex Differences Create Extra Risks for Women. *Washington Post*, Feb. 20, 2001 :T7.

39. Bowman, L. 51% Of US Adults Take 2 Pills or More a Day, Survey Reports (Scripps Howard News Service). *San Diego Union-Tribune*, Jan. 17, 2001:A8.

40. Zuger, A. Caution: That dose may be too high. *New York Times*, September 17, 2002:nytimes.com.

41. Dorothy L. Smith, *DTC Perspectives*, Jan.-Feb. 2002.

42. Reuters Health. Medical Journals Act to Limit Drug Firms' Influence. Reuters, Sept. 10, 2001 :www.reuters.com.

43. Davidoff, F, DeAngelis, CD, Drazen, JM, Hoey, J, Hojgaard, L, Horton, R, et al. Sponsorship, Authorship, and Accountability. *New England Journal of Medicine*, Sept. 13, 2001 ;345(11):825–27.

44. Schulman, KA, Seils, DM, Timbie, JW, Sugarman, J, et al. A national survey of provisions in clinical-trial agreements between medical schools and industry sponsors. *New England Journal of Medicine* 2002;347:1335–41.

45. Bodenheimer, T. Uneasy Alliance—Clinical Investigators and the Pharmaceutical Industry. *New England Journal of Medicine* 2000;342: 1539–44.

46. Herxheimer A. How much drug in the tablet? *Lancet* 1991;337:346–8.

47. Zuger, A. Caution: That dose may be too high. *New York Times*, September 17, 2002:nytimes.com.

48. Herxheimer, A. Dosage needs systematic and critical review. *BMJ* 2001 ;323.

49. Moore, TJ, Psaty, BM, Furberg, CD. Time to act on drug safety. *JAMA* 1998;279(19):1571–3.

50. Lasser, KE, Alan, PD, Woolhandler, SJ, Himmelstein, DU, Wolfe, SM, Bor, DH. Timing of New Black Box Warnings and Withdrawals for Prescription Medications. *JAMA* 2002;287:2215–2220.

51. Gaist, D, Jeppesen, U, Andersen, M, et al. Statins and the risk of polyneuropathy: a case-control study. *Neurology* 2002;58: 1333–1337.

52. Avorn, J. The prescription as final common pathway. *International Journal of Technology Assessment in Healthcare* 1995:11 (3):384–90).

53. Wood, AJJ, Stein, CM, Woosley, R. Making Medicines Safer: the Need for An Independent Drug Safety Board. *New England Journal of Medicine* 1998;339:1851–54.

54. Young, SA. Is Academic Medicine for Sale? *New England Journal of Medicine* 2000;343:508.

55. Vollmann, J. Gifts to physicians from the pharmaceutical industry. *JAMA* 2000;283:2656–8.

56. Angell, M. Is Academic Medicine for Sale? *New England Journal of Medicine* 2000;342:1516–18:

57. Hensley, S. When doctors go to class, industry often foots the bill. *Wall Street Journal*, Dec. 4, 2002:A1.

58. Cimons, M. Scientists Study Gender Gap in Drug Responses. *Los Angeles Times*, Sun. June 6, 1999: A-1,8–9.

59. Angell, M, Relman, AS. Prescription for Profit. The *Washington Post*, June 20, 2001:A27.

60. American Medical Association Council on Ethical and Judicial Affairs. *Code of Medical Ethics*. 1998–1999 Edition. American Medical Association, Chicago, IL.

61. Top 10 Drugs of 2001. *Pharmacy Times*, Apr. 2002;68(4):10–15.

Table 1

1. Clark, WG, Brater, DC, Johnson, AR. *Goth's Medical Pharmacology*. 13th Edition. St. Louis: The C.V. Mosby Company, 1992.

2. Gilman, AG, Rall, TW, Nies, AS, Taylor, P. Goodman and Gilman's *The Pharmacological Basis of Therapeutics*. New York: Pergammon Press, 1990 and 1996.

3. Martin, E.W. *Hazards of Medication: A Manual on Drug Interactions, Contraindications, and Adverse Reactions with Other Prescribing and Drug Information.* 2nd edition. Philadelphia: J.B. Lippincott Company, 1978.

4. American Medical Association. *AMA Drug Evaluations,* Annual 1994. Chicago: American Medical Association, 1994.

5. Herxheimer, A. Dosage needs systematic and critical review. *BMJ* 2001 ;323.

6. Heerdink, ER, Urquhart, J, Leufkens, HG. Changes in prescribed drug doses after market introduction. *Pharmacoepidemiology and Drug Safety* 2002; 11:447–453.

7. Rowland, M, Sheiner, L, Steimer, J. *Variability In Drug Therapy: Description, Estimation, And Control. A Sandoz Workshop.* New York: Raven Press, New York, 1985.

Table 3

1. Rochon, PA, Anderson, GM, Tu, JV, et al. Age-and gender-related use of low-dose drug therapy: the need to manufacture low-dose therapy and evaluate the minimum effective dose. *Journal of the American Geriatrics Society,* 1999 47(8):954–9.

2. Clark, WG, Brater, DC, Johnson, AR. *Goth's Medical Pharmacology.* 13th Edition. St. Louis: The C.V. Mosby Company, 1992.

3. Wolfe, SM, Hope, RE. *Worst Pills, Best Pills II: The Older Adult's Guide to Avoiding Drug-Induced Death or Illness.* Washington, DC: Public Citizen's Health Research Group, 1993.

4. Brawn, LA, Castleden, CM. Adverse drug reactions. An overview of special considerations in the management of the elderly patient. *Drug Safety* 1 990;5(6):421-35.

5. Williams, RD. Medications and older adults. *FDA Consumer Magazine,* Sept.-Oct. 1997.

6. Everitt, DE, Avorn, J. Drug prescribing for the elderly. *Archives of Internal Medicine* 1986;146(12):2393–6.

7. Rochon, PA, Gurwitz, JH. Optimising drug treatment for elderly people: the prescribing cascade. *BMJ* 1997;315(71 15):1096–9.

8. *United States Pharmacopeia, Drug Information (USP DI): Drug Information for the Healthcare Professional.* Taunton, MA: Rand McNally, 1994.

9. Gibian T. Rational drug therapy in the elderly, or, how not to poison your elderly patients. *Australian Family Physician* 1992;21 (12): 1755–60.

2002

The FDA Versus the American Consumer

by William Faloon

S INCE 1984, THE LIFE EXTENSION FOUNDATION HAS BATTLED against the high-cost of prescription drugs. We long ago predicted that a healthcare cost crisis would erupt if Congress did not reign in the artificially inflated prices that Americans pay for their prescription medications.

To expose the incestuous relationship that exists between the FDA and the pharmaceutical giants, we made hundreds of appearances on TV and radio shows, mailed out millions of pieces of mail, ran full-page newspaper ads and set up anti-FDA web sites. We did this for the purpose of encouraging consumers to act-up against blatant corruption that is bankrupting the nation's healthcare system.

Some people ask why our scientific organization, whose mission is to discover novel methods of preventing disease and controlling aging, is so concerned about prescription drug costs. The most compelling reason is that seriously ill people join the Life Extension Foundation seeking our medical expertise. Far too often, the elaborate drug cocktails we recommend to combat their disease are cost-prohibitive. Insurance companies frequently refuse to pay for our drug recommendations because the FDA does not officially sanction them. While the individual drugs we recommend may be FDA-approved, the agency does not recognize the off-label benefits these drugs can provide. Insurance companies then use the FDA's non-recognition as an excuse to deny coverage.[1]

The end result is that human beings are needlessly dying because of bureaucratic red tape that delays and denies them access to lifesaving medications.[2-4]

LIFE ACROSS THE BORDER

There is no inherent reason why prescription drugs cost so much. The identical medications can be purchased in Europe and Canada at far lower prices.[5] This price gouging has gone on since as early as 1959.[6] The trouble is that the FDA has attempted to deceive Congress into believing that drugs from other countries are counterfeit or contaminated. Life Extension has shown that the FDA's assertions are baseless, false and misleading.[7]

On June 7, 2001, the FDA told Congress that they wanted to halt almost all small shipments of foreign drugs mailed to consumers in the US.[8] The only exemption would be for compassionate use, so that seriously ill patients who have exhausted all approved treatments could order drugs from overseas. The FDA told Congress: "We need to be able to make a blanket assessment that these things are not safe for American consumers and should be turned back."

In response to the FDA's assertions, Life Extension sent Freedom of Information Act (FOIA) requests in June 2001 asking the FDA to substantiate their sworn testimony before Congress that drugs imported from other countries were dangerous.

Even though the FDA is legally mandated to respond to Freedom of Information Act requests, they have ignored our repeated written requests and phone calls to substantiate their sworn testimony about the supposed dangers of imported medications.

In 1991, Life Extension sued the FDA for failing to respond to Freedom of Information Act (FOIA) requests dealing with this same issue. The FDA capitulated on this lawsuit and had to turn over embarrassing records to Life Extension. Despite the FDA being forced to turn over documents to Life Extension in 1991, the FDA continues to ignore our legitimate requests to substantiate sworn testimony made to Congress that imported drugs are dangerous.

BATTLING THE DRUG CARTEL

When the FDA told Congress that drugs imported from other countries are not safe, they provided no evidence to substantiate this intimidating allegation. The fact that no one asked the FDA to validate their baseless assertion is an indication of official apathy and the effects of massive influence peddling by pharmaceutical giants.

Life Extension has meticulously exposed the charade of prescription drug pricing. Drug price comparison charts published in *Life Extension* magazine have been enlarged for presentation on the House floor to show Representatives how much more Americans pay for prescription drugs compared to Canadians and Europeans.

Despite lobbying efforts by the pharmaceutical industry, the Senate passed a bill by a vote of 69 to 30 on July 17, 2002 that would allow licensed pharmacists and drug wholesalers to import drugs that have been approved by the FDA from Canada.[9]

Large pharmaceutical companies are determined to use their political influence to block passage of this bill in the House of

Representatives. The *New York Times* reports that even if a drug importation bill is passed, the Bush Administration will refuse to carry out the provisions, thereby denying Americans access to lower cost medications.[10] In December 2000, the Clinton Administration blocked implementation of a similar bill passed by the House and Senate that permitted Americans to import lower cost medications from other countries.

A battle is being waged against a drug cartel that is determined to protect its monopoly. Drug companies work hand-in-hand with the FDA to force Americans to pay the highest prices in the world for their medications.

THE DEBATE IN CONGRESS RAGES ON

The number one issue before Congress today is the high cost of prescription drugs. Consumers have besieged Congress with complaints that drugs their doctors say are necessary to keep them alive are unaffordable.

Several bills were debated this summer in Congress that would appropriate tax dollars to subsidize prescription drug programs. The problem is that the cost of drugs has become so enormous, that even the Federal government cannot figure out how to fund the gargantuan expense. The debate involved spending between 370 and 564 billion tax dollars over the next 10 years on drug subsidies. These proposals would not solve the problem, but do shift some of the burden from consumers to taxpayers.

Since most drug consumers are also taxpayers, Congress was essentially proposing to take more tax dollars from American citizens in order to subsidize the artificially inflated prices of their prescription drugs. That means that the true beneficiary of the bills debated in Congress would have been the drug industry, which would have pocketed enormous profits directly from consumers, insurance companies and the Federal government.

Another problem with tax dollars being used to pay for prescription drugs is the inevitable waste, mismanagement and fraud that occurs when government bureaucracies try to regulate the marketplace. The Federal government has had to litigate against large drug companies after finding that Medicare and Medicaid sharply overpaid for dozens of drugs. Government officials have sought billions of dollars in restitution based on their contention that drug companies induced Medicare and Medicaid to pay inflated prices for prescription medications.

In election years, everyone in Congress tries to show their constituents that they want to make prescription drugs affordable. The problem is that it is impossible to circumvent the catastrophic effects that the current FDA-protected drug monopoly creates. In the first place, there are no surplus tax dollars available to

Comparison of US, European, and Canadian Drug Prices

Drug	Qty	Potency	US Price	European Price	Canadian Price
Augmentin®	12	500 mg	$55.50	$8.75	$12.00
Cipro®	20	500 mg	$87.99	$40.75	$53.55
Claritin®	30	10 mg	$89.00	$18.75	$37.50
Coumadin®	100	5 mg	$64.88	$15.80	$24.94
Glucophage®	100	850 mg	$124.65	$22.00	$26.47
Norvasc®	30	10 mg	$67.00	$33.00	$46.27
Paxil®	30	20 mg	$83.29	$49.00	$44.35
Pravachol®	28	10 mg	$85.60	$29.00	$40.00
Premarin®	100	0.625 mg	$55.42	$8.95	$22.46
Prempro®	28	0.625 mg	$31.09	$5.75	$14.33
Prilosec®	30	20 mg	$112.00	$49.25	$59.00
Prozac®	20	20 mg	$91.08	$18.50	$20.91
Synthroid®	100	0.1 mg	$33.93	$8.50	$13.22
Zestril®	28	20 mg	$40.49	$20.00	$20.44
Zocor®	28	10 mg	$123.43	$28.00	$45.49
Zoloft®	30	100 mg	$114.56	$52.50	$47.40

fund these proposed programs, meaning the government will go deeper into debt to fund them. Secondly, the proposed bills would not have sufficiently lowered the price of prescription drugs to the consumer.

By July 31, 2002, Congress rejected the proposed drug subsidy bills and the issue is not expected to be raised before the elections.

A REAL SOLUTION TO THE HEALTHCARE COST CRISIS

Congressman Gil Gutknecht of Minnesota has written an amendment to a Medicare bill that prohibits the FDA from blocking importation by individuals and pharmacies of FDA-approved drugs. If this amendment is passed, it will help solve the prescription drug crisis without the need for taxpayer subsidies.

Two years ago, Congress passed legislation to allow Americans to import wholesale quantities of lower-cost prescription drugs into the United States. But the promise of this legislation has gone unfulfilled. Even though the FDA largely wrote the bill, and Congress provided the $23 million the FDA requested to implement the bill, then-Secretary Shalala refused to implement the measure. The result? Drug prices in Europe and elsewhere are still 30% to 300% lower than in the United States. Prices have not equalized. Americans still pay the highest prices in the world to subsidize the "starving Swiss." Even former Secretary Shalala admits this fact.

But that's not all. The FDA refuses not only to allow wholesale importation, the FDA also maintains that personal importation is illegal. Yet, because the market for lower-cost drugs is so large, the FDA looks the other way when people import personal-use quantities of prescription drugs. That's right: the FDA today allows folks to carry drugs over the border, and apparently now even allows [them] to mail order drugs from abroad. Yet all the while, the FDA publicly maintains such importation is illegal, thus threatening importers with dire legal consequences.

This is wrong. The FDA can't have it both ways. Either personal use importation is illegal, or it's not. Last year, by a vote of 324 to 101, the House passed language explicitly allowing individual Americans to import lower-cost FDA-approved drugs from FDA-approved facilities. This is common sense, and it is the FDA's current policy.

Unfortunately the Senate refused to pass this amendment, so the FDA continues to hold a legal dagger over the heads of those who try to import FDA-approved drugs.

Fortunately, with the House drug coverage bill coming to the floor soon, we have an opportunity to codify current FDA practice, AND allow our nation's pharmacists to offer the same drugs. With this, all Americans can be sure they have the right to save money on their prescription drugs.

The Congressional Budget Office estimates prescription drugs will cost Medicare beneficiaries $1.8 trillion over the next 10 years. Americans could save $630 billion from this bill if they could be allowed access to the same drugs from FDA-approved facilities throughout the world.[11] Price, not coverage, is the real prescription drug problem. The FDA should not stand between American consumers and lower drug prices. The Gutknecht Amendment (H.R. 5186) prohibits the FDA from blocking importation by individuals and pharmacies of FDA-approved prescription drugs from FDA-approved facilities.[12]

THE SHOCKING TRUTH BEHIND PRESCRIPTION DRUG PRICES

Do you ever wonder how much it costs a drug company to obtain the active ingredient in a prescription medication? Life Extension did a search of offshore chemical synthesizers that supply the active ingredients found in drugs approved by the FDA.

A significant percentage of drugs sold in the United States contain active ingredients that are actually synthesized in other countries. Drug companies import these active ingredients into the United States where they wind up in the expensive drugs you buy at the local pharmacy. While the FDA says you cannot trust drugs from other countries, the facts are that most of the drugs sold in the United States contain active ingredients synthesized in the very countries the FDA says you cannot trust.

In our independent investigation of how much profit drug companies really make, we obtained the actual price of active ingredients used in some of the most popular drugs sold in America.

The astounding profit margin enjoyed by drug companies exposes several facts. First, it shows why the pharmaceutical industry is the most profitable of all businesses. But since large drug companies only make around 15% net profit margins, it also exposes the incredible cost drug companies bear to comply with today's burdensome drug approval system.* If the FDA relaxed its drug approval standards, the cost of bringing new patented drugs could be reduced.

These exorbitant profit margins also provide incentive for drug companies to get their patented molecules approved by the FDA, whether they kill people or not. Horror stories abound of how drug companies have egregiously falsified data to obtain FDA approval.†

Many consumers are nervous about the FDA becoming less stringent, but the facts are that today's regulatory system is allowing lethal drugs on the marketplace and also acting as a disincentive for drug companies to develop novel drugs to save lives.

Take the cholesterol-lowering drug Baychol®, for example, which was removed from the market after killing 100 people.‡

---

* Stephen S. Hall, "Claritin and Schering-Plough: A Prescription for Profit." http://senrs. com/a_prescription_for_profit.htm

† David Willman, "The Rise and Fall of the Killer Drug Rezulin," *Life Extension* magazine, September 2000.

‡ "More deaths linked to Bayer's Lipobay," January 18, 2002. http://news.ft.com/ft/ gx.cgi/ftc?pagename=View&c=Article&cid=FT3HZ3AFMWC &live=true&tagid=IX LHT5GTICC&subheading=heal

WHAT DRUGS REALLY COST

Brand Name	Consumer Price	Cost of Active Ingredient	Percent Markup
Celebrex® 100 mg	$130.27	$0.60	21,712%
Claritin® 10 mg	$215.17	$0.71	30,306%
Keflex® 250 mg	$157.39	$1.88	8,372%
Lipitor® 20 mg	$272.37	$5.80	4,696%
Norvasc® 10 mg	$188.29	$0.14	134,493%
Paxil® 20 mg	$220.27	$7.60	2,898%
Prevacid® 30 mg	$344.77	$1.01	34,136%
Prilosec® 20 mg	$360.97	$0.52	69,417%
Prozac® 20 mg	$247.47	$0.11	224,973%
Tenormin® 50 mg	$104.47	$0.13	80,362%
Vasotec® 10 mg	$102.37	$0.20	51,185%
Xanax® 1mg	$136.79	$0.024	569,958%
Zestril® 20 mg	$89.89	$3.20	2,809%
Zithromax® 600mg	$1,482.19	$18.78	7,892%
Zocor® 40mg	$350.27	$8.63	4,059%
Zoloft® 50mg	$206.87	$1.75	11,821%

Baychol® is a statin drug that works via a mechanism similar to that in Mevacor®, Zocor®, Lipitor®, Pravachol®, etc. Was there a need for tens of millions of dollars to be spent developing another statin drug? Drug companies think so, because the FDA readily recognizes statin drugs, so they are easy to get approved.

The problem is that no life was saved because of Baychol®. Anyone who may have benefitted from Baychol® could have obtained the same results from other statin drugs. So when drug companies justify the high price of drugs because of research costs, remember that most of the so-called novel compounds they develop will not save a single life, as they are no different than what is already available.

Now that you know the outrageous profit margins on prescription drugs, you can understand why drug companies do almost anything to prevent competition from developing. Large drug companies intensely lobby Congress to pass laws that give them extra time of exclusivity, file lawsuits to delay generic competition, petition the FDA to stop the importation of lower cost medications, and go as far as to pay off generic companies to not compete.

Drug companies spend big dollars protecting their illicit monopoly, all of which is reflected in the price consumers pay for their prescription drugs.

BREAKING THE DRUG MONOPOLY

The Gutknecht Amendment provides Americans access to FDA-approved prescription drugs made in FDA-approved facilities at world market prices. Passage of this amendment could abolish high prices of prescription drugs forever.

While drugs sold in Europe and Canada do cost less than their American counterparts, they are still artificially high because of regulations in these other countries that stifle competition. If Americans are allowed to freely import prescription drugs from FDA-approved manufacturing facilities in other countries, there will be a surge of new laboratories that will seek FDA-certification. The result will be a flood of super low-cost drugs into the United States as various FDA-certified laboratories compete fiercely on quality and price.

When Congressional leaders debate the prescription drug cost crisis, few of them understand the huge discrepancy that exists between the cost of the active drug ingredient compared to the price charged for the brand name or generic drug. For instance, consumers pay $360.00 for 100 capsules of the stomach-acid suppressing drug Prilosec®. The cost of the active ingredient for 100 capsules of Prilosec®, however, is only 52 cents. There will soon be a generic version of Prilosec® available, but because of FDA overregulation, the cost per 100 capsules will probably be around $80.00. In a free market environment, where many companies could offer generic Prilosec® products instead of the chosen few anointed by the FDA, a product whose active ingredient costs 52 cents (like Prilosec®) would be available to consumers for under $7.00 a bottle.

A free market environment would eliminate the prescription drug cost crisis because the FDA would not be allowed to protect a monopoly that enables both brand name and generic companies to charge extortionist prices for lifesaving medications.

Drug company lobbyists are inundating Congress to prevent any type of prescription drug importation bill from becoming law. Consumer groups are intimidated by the FDA's baseless assertions that imported drugs are somehow dangerous. The FDA has preyed on fear and uncertainty for decades, while American consumers are extorted into paying the highest prices in the world for their prescription drugs.

This is not just an issue for individuals to be concerned with. There are dire predictions of severe economic upheavals in the United States if a solution is not found for the high cost of prescription drugs. Some of the largest corporations in America cannot afford to fund health insurance benefits for current and retired employees. Health insurance companies are going bankrupt because of astronomical drug prices. Medicare itself is predicted to be insolvent as soon as 2007.

The United States has been economically deteriorating as prescription drug prices skyrocket. In order to counter the influence peddling of the pharmaceutical behemoths, American consumers must become politically active. Consumers vastly outnumber drug industry lobbyists. Regrettably, ignorance and apathy have silenced many Americans and enabled drug money to create laws that favor outlandish pharmaceutical company profits at the expense of the consumer.

If the Gutknecht Amendment is passed, it will liberate the American consumer from becoming an economic serf to the pharmaceutical cartel.

References

1. "We Need an FDA Leader, Not a Regulatory Czar Healthcare: AIDS, cancer and Alzheimer's are among the issues where David Kessler has compromised science and ethics." The *Los Angeles Times* (Pre-1997 Fulltext), Feb 10, 1993.

2. "A National Survey Of Emergency Room Physicians Regarding The Food And Drug Administration," by Gregory Conko. October 1, 1999. http://www.cei.org/gencon/025,02298.cfm

3. "A National Survey Of Neurologists And Neurosurgeons Regarding The Food And Drug Administration," by Gregory Conko. October 5, 1998. http://www.cei.org/gencon/025,01586.cfm

4. "Who Is Mary J. Ruwart?" *Life Extension* magazine, July 2001. http://www.lef.org/magazine/mag2001/july2001_cover_ruwart.html

5. "Claritin and Schering-Plough: A Prescription for Profit," by Stephen S. Hall. http://senrs.com/a_prescription_for_profit.htm

6. "What's New About Prescription. . .," by Morton Mintz. *Washington Post*, Page B1, February 11, 2001.

7. "Drugs The FDA Says You Can't Have," *Life Extension* magazine, July 2001.

8. Statement of William K. Hubbard, Senior Associate Commissioner for Policy, Planning and Legislation, Food and Drug Administration, before the Subcommittee on Oversight and Investigations Committee on Energy and Commerce, US House of Representative, June 7, 2001. http://www.fda.gov/ola/2001/drugimport0607.html

9. Greater Access to Affordable Phamacauticals Act of 2001. Senate, July 17, 2002. http://thomas.loc.gov/cgi-bin/bdquery/z?d107:H.R.1862:

10. "Thursday Plan to Import Drugs From Canada Passes In Senate, but Bush Declines to Carry It Out," by Robert Pear. Late

Edition, Final, Section A, Page 14, Column 4. *New York Times* National Desk, July 18, 2002.

11. CBO Testimony, statement of Dan L. Crippen, Director Projections of Medicare and Prescription Drug Spending, before the Committee on Finance United States Senate, March 7, 2002. http://www.cbo.gov/showdoc.cfm?index=3304&sequence=0

12. Drug Importation Act of 2002 (Introduced in House), HR 5186 IH 107th Congress, 2d Session H. R. 5186, to amend the Federal Food, Drug, and Cosmetic Act with respect to the importation of prescription drugs. In the House of Representative, July 23, 2002. http://thomas.loc.gov/

Supreme Court Roundup

by William Faloon

O N APRIL 30, 2002, DECLARING THAT "REGULATING speech must be a last-not first-resort," the Supreme Court invalidated a provision of the federal food and drug laws that banned pharmacies from advertising the availability of "compounded" pharmaceuticals, drugs that pharmacists make themselves by mixing ingredients to meet the specific medical needs of certain patients.

A 1997 federal law that barred such advertising reflected federal regulators' concern that compounded drugs did not go through the detailed screening for safety and effectiveness to which drug companies have to submit their mass-produced drugs. In Congress' view, the advertising ban would limit consumer demand for compounded drugs.

But the 5-to-4 decision on April 30th said that "the government simply has not provided sufficient justification here" for choosing a restriction on speech rather than other possible ways to restrict access to compounded drugs, which generally are not commercially available and which patients may receive only by a doctor's prescription.

"We have made clear that if the government could achieve its interests in a manner that does not restrict speech, or that restricts less speech, the government must do so," Justice Sandra Day O'Connor said for the majority.

The real debate on the court was not over drug policy but over the constitutional value to assign to commercial speech. While the majority opinion today did not break ground, it was a powerful indication that the value a majority of the court assigns to commercial speech is high and getting higher.

Justice O'Connor's majority opinion outlined alternatives that, in the court's view, Congress should have used before turning to an advertising ban, most dealing with limitations on the amount of compounded drugs an individual pharmacy could make or sell. Or the government could require warning labels advising consumers that the compounded drug had not gone through the usual approval process, Justice O'Connor said.

"The government has not offered any reason why these possibilities, alone or in combination, would be insufficient to prevent compounding from occurring on such a scale as to undermine the new drug approval process," she said, adding, "Indeed, there is no hint that the government even considered these or any other alternatives."

She continued: "If the First Amendment means anything, it means that regulating speech must be a last-not first-resort. Yet here it seems to have been the first strategy the government thought to try."

The legal status of compounded drugs after the decision today was not immediately clear. The government took the position that such drugs were not legal before the 1997 law, the Food and Drug Administration Modernization Act, which made their lawful sale contingent on the advertising ban and on other restrictions. The Ninth Circuit, holding that the various provisions of the law could not be considered separately, struck down the entire statute, an aspect of its ruling that the court did not address on April 30th.

2001

Dying from Deficiency

by William Faloon

N EW SCIENTIFIC STUDIES INDICATE THAT TOO MANY PEOPLE
are dying from simple nutrient deficiencies.

Dr. Bruce Ames recently published a paper stating that
a deficiency of folic acid, vitamins C, E, B6, B12, niacin or zinc
causes DNA strand breaks, oxidative lesions and increased susceptibility to cancer. Dr. Ames compared a deficiency of any one
of these micro-nutrients to the DNA damaging effects of radiation.[1] When DNA strands are damaged, the body becomes more
vulnerable to cancer.

Dr. Ames stated that a micro-nutrient deficiency may explain
why people who eat the fewest fruits and vegetables have about
double the rate for most types of cancer when compared to those
with the highest intake. Fruits and vegetables are a rich source
of the micro-nutrients that protect DNA against changes that
can lead to cancer. Dr. Ames' conclusion was:

> Common micro-nutrient deficiencies are likely to dam-
> age DNA by the same mechanism as radiation and
> many chemicals. . . . Remedying micro-nutrient defi-
> ciencies should lead to a major improvement in health
> and an increase in longevity at low cost.

Dr. Bruce Ames is a well respected expert on cancer. He is a Professor of Biochemistry & Molecular Biology at the University of California–Berkeley and developed the internationally recognized Ames Test that is used for determining if a chemical damages cellular DNA.

WEAKENED HEARTS

A group of British doctors just published a paper indicating that deficiencies of selenium, calcium and vitamin B1 lead directly to heart failure.[2] These doctors went on to point out that vitamin C, E and beta-carotene help protect the arterial system, vitamins B6, B12 and folic acid reduce homocysteine, whereas carnitine and CoQ10 help maintain energy output. The doctors concluded that malnutrition of certain micro-nutrients may play a role in the degenerative process humans undergo during heart failure.

There are a number of causes of heart failure. One of them is a viral attack on the heart muscle itself. A mouse study showed that selenium deficiency made hearts much more vulnerable to viral damage compared to mice with adequate selenium status.[3] Human studies consistently show that selenium exerts an immune-enhancing and anti-viral effect. Selenium has been shown to protect against the progression and lethality of HIV, hepatitis C and influenza viruses.[4–7] Scientific studies repeatedly attribute selenium deficiency as an underlying reason for viral disease progression, yet conventional doctors seem oblivious to this established fact.

PLANT EXTRACTS PROTECT AGAINST
PROSTATE CANCER AND ARTERY DISEASE

Lutein is a plant extract that Life Extension members have been taking in supplemental form since 1985. New reports indicate that in addition to protecting against macular degeneration, lutein also protects against atherosclerosis and prostate cancer.

One of these new studies conducted at the UCLA Center for Human Nutrition showed that lutein reduced prostate cancer cell growth by 25% while lycopene reduced cell growth by 20%. When lutein and lycopene were combined, prostate cancer cell growth was reduced by 32%. The UCLA scientists who conducted this study indicated that both nutrients together help protect against prostate cancer better than either nutrient alone.[8]

The UCLA scientists then looked at a region of China where the incidence of prostate cancer is very low. People in this region have minute intakes of lycopene, but high intakes of lutein. The study was then expanded to include Chinese Americans and Caucasian men in the United States. The UCLA researchers concluded "Lutein and lycopene in combination appear to have additive or synergistic effects against prostate cancer."

Another group of scientists looked at the effects of lutein in protecting against vascular disease.[9] Doctors at the University of Southern California conducted a human study over 18 months and found that the presence of high amounts of serum lutein reduced the progression of early atherosclerosis as measured by intima-media thickness of the carotid artery. These doctors then looked at mouse models of atherosclerosis and found that greater lutein consumption resulted in an inhibition of atherosclerotic lesion formation. When these animals received supplemental lutein, lesion size was reduced by 43%. The doctors then looked at LDL cholesterol damage to the arterial wall of these mice, and found that lutein conferred protection against a type of early injury that can lead to atherosclerosis. The doctors concluded:

These epidemiological, in vitro, and mouse model findings support the hypothesis that increased dietary intake of lutein is protective against the development of early atherosclerosis.

Commercial companies are advertising lutein supplements on national TV. The problem with some of these supplements is that they only provide 300 micrograms of lutein . . . an amount too low to provide benefit.

CONTINUED GOVERNMENT INACTION

Despite a wealth of new scientific studies showing the importance of micro-nutrients, the FDA continues to suppress this information by censoring health claims on the labels of dietary supplements.

The US government says that Medicare will run out of money in the year 2023.[10] Healthcare outlays could be reduced, and the date of Medicare insolvency postponed, if Americans obtained enough micro-nutrients everyday.

Educated Americans learn what they can do to reduce their risk of contracting a degenerative disease. Those who choose to believe the government's anti-supplement propaganda may be dramatically shortening their heathy life spans.

References

1. Ames BN. DNA damage from micronutrient deficiencies is likely to be a major cause of cancer. *Mutation Research* 2001 Apr 18;475(1–2):7–20.
2. Witte KK, et al. Chronic heart failure and micronutrients. *Journal of the American College of Cardiology*, 2001 Jun 1;37(7):1765–74.
3. Gomez RM, et al. Host selenium status selectively influences susceptibility to experimental viral myocarditis. *Biological Trace Element Research* 2001 Apr;80(1):23–31.
4. Baeten JM, et al. Selenium deficiency is associated with shedding of HIV-1—infected cells in the female genital tract. *J Acquir Immune Defic Syndr* 2001 Apr 1;26(4):360–4.

5. Baum MK. Role of micronutrients in HIV-infected intravenous drug users. *J Acquir Immune Defic Syndr* 2000 Oct 1;25 Suppl 1:S49–52.

6. Beck MA, et al. Selenium deficiency increases the pathology of an influenza virus infection. *FASEB J* 2001 Jun;15(8):1481–3.

7. Berkson BM. A conservative triple antioxidant approach to the treatment of hepatitis C. Combination of alpha lipoic acid (thioctic acid), silymarin, and selenium: three case histories. *Med Klin* 1999 Oct 15;94 Suppl 3:84–9.

8. Presented at the American Institute of *Cancer Rese*arch meeting on July 16 in Washington, DC

9. Dwyer JH, et al. Oxygenated carotenoid lutein and progression of early atherosclerosis: the Los Angeles atherosclerosis study. *Circulation* 2001 Jun 19;103(24):2922–7.

10. http://www.senate.gov/~breaux/aging/boombasics.html

Are Offshore Drugs Dangerous?

by William Faloon

I F YOU SUFFER FROM TYPE II DIABETES, YOU'RE LIKELY TO BE PRE-scribed a drug called Glucophage®. This drug lowers glucose and other blood risk factors that cause lethal diabetic complications.

Glucophage® works by enhancing cell sensitivity to the effects of insulin. Since type II diabetes is characterized by cellular insulin resistence, the fact that Glucophage® helps restore insulin sensitivity makes it a potent weapon against a disease that currently afflicts 16 million Americans. Clinical studies dating back to the 1950s demonstrate Glucophage's efficacy and safety when properly used.

For several decades, Americans could not legally obtain Glucophage®. That's because the FDA said it was toxic and banned its sale in the US. The Europeans did not agree that Glucophage® posed a health risk and approved its use decades ago.

The FDA was proven wrong about Glucophage® and the drug was finally approved in December 1994. It is difficult to calculate exactly how many Americans died while Glucophage® was kept out of the United States. It is very easy, however, to document that American consumers are being price gouged because of the FDA's error. A one-month supply of Glucophage® costs $4.12 in other countries, while Americans pay $32.83 for the same quantity.

The reason for this unconscionable price disparity is that Glucophage® is old news in Europe, where it has been used since the 1960s. The FDA's delay in approval has enabled Glucophage® to enjoy a virtual monopoly in the United States, causing US citizens to pay more than seven times the price this same drug sells for in other countries.

The number of people who die each year from diabetic complications is staggering. American diabetics perished while Glucophage® was being safely used throughout the world. Because of FDA ineptitude, US citizens pay grossly inflated prices to obtain a drug (Glucophage®) that is more than 30 years old.

THE FDA'S LATEST CHARADE

The FDA now has the audacity to ask Congress to ban just about ALL imports of medications from other countries under the guise of "protecting" Americans against dangerous drugs.

On June 7, 2001, the FDA told Congress that they want to halt almost all small shipments of foreign drugs mailed to consumers in the US. The FDA wants US Custom Service agents to send back all small foreign drug shipments they find. The only exemption would be for "compassionate use," so that seriously ill patients who have exhausted all approved treatments could order drugs from overseas that are unavailable in the US.

The FDA says it needs to turn away all foreign drug shipments because of the sheer volume of drugs being imported. More American consumers are learning they can obtain prescription drugs at a fraction of the price charged in the US. The FDA now admits that the number of shipments far exceeds the agency's ability to review them on a case-by-case basis. The FDA told Congress, "We need to be able to make a blanket assessment that these things are not safe for American consumers and should be turned back."

The fraud being perpetrated by the FDA is the assertion that medications imported from other countries are automatically illegal, counterfeit or contaminated. This is what the FDA would have said about Glucophage® before they approved it in 1994. The facts are that drugs from other countries cost far less and are sometimes more advanced than what is available on the American marketplace.

The FDA told Congress that an estimated 2 million packages containing drugs enter the United States through international mail each year. "The inescapable conclusion is these drugs are virtually all unapproved in the United States. . . . They may be counterfeit or worse," the FDA said to Congress.

The truth is that most of the drugs the FDA complains about are already FDA-approved and are manufactured by the same companies that sell them to American pharmacies. The FDA is using scare tactics to protect the profits of the pharmaceutical industry . . . not the health of the public.

Currently, the law says that Customs must contact recipients if it detains drugs at the border. The FDA's new proposal would waive that requirement. In other words, the FDA wants all drugs to be turned away without even providing the US citizen (who paid for the drug) with a notice and opportunity to explain why they need them.[1]

Drugs the FDA says are safe kill over 100,000 Americans every year, while the agency cannot demonstrate drugs imported from other countries are hurting anyone.

That's not to say that some day an American won't suffer an adverse reaction from an imported drug. After all, many of the drugs being imported are the same FDA-approved medications that are killing over 100,000 Americans every year.[2-4]

The FDA denied Glucophage® to Americans for decades, but rapidly approved Rezulin® to treat Type II diabetics. Rezulin® killed about 391 Americans before it was withdrawn, according to a tabulation done by the *Los Angeles Times*.[5] Those afflicted with Type II diabetes suffered and died waiting for the FDA's belated approval of the relatively safe drug Glucophage®.*

So while the FDA brazenly testified before Congress that all drugs imported from other countries are "dangerous," the facts show the agency's assertion is blatantly false and misleading.

The FDA preys on fear and uncertainty, while American consumers are extorted into paying the highest prices in the world for their prescription drugs.

UNDOING THIS TRAVESTY

The FDA lacks the moral and scientific legitimacy to deny Americans access to medications that are approved by health ministries in other countries. The FDA's delay in approving Glucophage® is a prime example of why this agency should not be allowed to embargo drugs from other countries.

Bureaucratic barriers at the FDA stifle the development of novel medicines, while drug company influence enables lethal drugs (like Rezulin®) to be "approved" by the agency as safe and effective.

---

* Note: Glucophage® is now available in the United States under the generic name metformin. Glucophage® is not for everyone. To read safety precautions about this drug, log on to www.glucophage.com.

References

1. Statement of William K. Hubbard, Senior Associate Commissioner for Policy, Planning and Legislation, Food and Drug Administration, before the Subcommittee on Oversight and Investigations Committee on Energy and Commerce, US House of Representatives, June 7, 2001. http://www.fda.gov/ola/2001/drugimport0607.html

2. Lazarou J, et al. Incidence of adverse drug reactions in hospitalized patients: a meta-analysis of prospective studies. *JAMA* 1998 Apr 1 5;279(1 5): 1200–5.

3. Bates DW. Drugs and adverse drug reactions: how worried should we be? *JAMA* 1998 Apr 15;279(15):1216–7.

4. Cimons M. "FDA Moves to Reduce Accidental Drug Deaths." *LA Times* May 10,1999. Home Edition Section: PART A Page: A-1.

5. Willman David "Rise and Fall of the Killer Drug Rezulin," *Life Extension* magazine, Sept. 2000, p. 3 1–39.

JULY 2001

Drugs the FDA Says You Can't Have

by William Faloon

AMERICANS SUFFER AND DIE EVEN THOUGH EFFECTIVE DRUGS to treat their diseases are approved in other countries. The public is generally aware that novel drugs are sold in Europe and Japan, but intense lobbying by the pharmaceutical industry has blocked the wide-scale availability of these better medications.

Drug companies don't want Americans to shop the world for more effective therapies. They prefer the current FDA-protected system where large companies enjoy a virtual monopoly over the American marketplace. This archaic system earns record profits for drug companies at the expense of US citizens, who pay inflated prices for the medications the FDA does allow them to have.

The FDA deceives the public and Congress into believing that drugs approved in other countries are somehow "dangerous," despite having no evidence to support this. What the FDA conveniently ignores is the fact that drugs they say are "safe" kill over 106,000 Americans every year.[1-3]

THALIDOMIDE STILL KILLS

Proponents of today's drug approval system have to go back 41 years to the thalidomide debacle to find an example of an offshore drug causing a serious side effect. Thalidomide still kills because the FDA is using this old issue as an excuse to embargo life-saving drugs that are approved by health ministries in other countries. Furthermore, these drugs have been used in other countries for years without serious side effects.

Few people remember that it was not the FDA who discovered the thalidomide problem. It was a German scientist who identified thalidomide's dreadful power to halt limb development in the early stages of pregnancy. The FDA's sole contribution to avoiding this problem in the United States was a delay by a junior FDA officer in reviewing the original application.

There is tragedy on the other side of the thalidomide ledger, too. Thalidomide has been shown to halt the proliferation of blood vessels, an effect that may help starve certain cancers and protect against blindness induced by wet macular degeneration. In 1998, the FDA finally approved thalidomide to treat a complication related to leprosy. That means that doctors can legally prescribe thalidomide to patients with other diseases. The FDA, however, has put up so many restrictions on its off-label use, that few physicians or patients are willing to fight the red tape.[4]

The rare disease the FDA approved thalidomide to treat only occurs in about 50 Americans every year. The FDA, however, says the company that makes thalidomide cannot promote its use in treating cancer and macular degeneration. Recent First Amendment losses the FDA has suffered in the courts may enable thalidomide to be advertised,[5] but that would mean the company making the drug would incur the wrath of the FDA and be subjected to retaliation against other drugs it might want to get approved.

FEARING FDA RETALIATION

The FDA has taken science out of the practice of medicine and replaced it with an incompetent and biased bureaucracy. To win FDA approval of a new drug, it takes a lot of political influence.

The committees who advise the FDA whether or not to approve a new drug are largely comprised of individuals who are beholden to the pharmaceutical giants.[6] Small biotech companies who cannot afford to put their own people on these advisory committees are at a significant disadvantage. There are FDA-staffers who appear unusually friendly to large drug companies, but find every excuse imaginable to delay the approval of novel drugs from smaller companies.[7-12]

The FDA intentionally delayed the approval of ribavirin for decades while this anti-viral drug was saving lives in just about every civilized country on earth. The company who made ribavirin committed the terrible "sin" of holding a press conference to extol the virtues of this drug before the FDA approved it. Another victim of FDA retaliation was the immune-enhancing drug isoprinosine. While isoprinosine has been prescribed by doctors throughout the world for nearly two decades, the FDA will never approve it here because the manufacturer helped promote the fact that Americans could import it from other countries for their own personal use. The sad fact is that when effective drugs are not approved because of FDA retaliation, American citizens die.[13, 14]

The FDA has put up so many restrictions on its off-label use, that few physicians or patients are willing to fight the red tape.

LIFE-SAVING OFFSHORE DRUGS

An example of a drug that may never be approved in the United States is thymosin alpha-1, which is an immune boosting agent produced in the thymus gland.[15] Unfortunately, the small company making the drug lacked the resources to win FDA approval. Thymosin alpha-1 did gain approval in Europe. Published studies show that when used in combination with cancer chemotherapy, it helps mitigate bone marrow toxicity.[16, 17] When thymosin alpha-1 is combined with interleukin-2 or alpha interferon, it enhances immune response against cancer cells and the hepatitis C virus.[18-23] Thymosin alpha-1 should be available to Americans, but the FDA says no!

Another drug that could be of benefit to hepatitis C and certain cancer patients is polaprezinc. This ultra-safe Japanese drug has been shown to reduce viral load and induce complete response in Type 1b hepatitis C (when combined with interferon).[24] It may also be effective as an adjuvant therapy in cancer cells that up-regulate a growth factor called nuclear factor kappa beta. If you don't live in Japan, it is very difficult to obtain polaprezinc, a unique compound of carnosine and zinc.

Neurodegenerative diseases such as Alzheimer's have no effective treatment. A drug called memantine may delay the progression of Alzheimer's and Parkinson's disease. Memantine works by a different mechanism than current FDA-approved drugs such as Aricept® and Tacrine. Memantine has been used in Germany for the last ten years, but it remains bogged down in FDA-mandated clinical trials. Four million American Alzheimer's disease patients anxiously await.[25-33]

IT'S TIME TO REVOLT

Today's flawed system of drug approval needs a major overhaul or Americans will continue to perish while effective therapies exist in other countries. As more Americans learn that they are not getting the best that science has to offer, we believe the citizenry will rebel against the medical establishment, who place their monopolistic profits ahead over the wellbeing of the patient.

The world is rapidly changing and information about non-FDA approved therapies can easily be found on the Internet. The problem for consumers is separating real science from charlatans who prey on those seeking a solution for a serious medical problem.

WHERE ARE THE BEST DRUGS?

The most advanced drugs in the world are right here in the United States, but remain bogged down in the FDA's approval quagmire. The profit potential in the American marketplace is so large that drug companies are not seeking quick approval in other countries as much as they used to.

Pharmaceutical companies spend gargantuan sums of money on clinical trials before they can earn a penny on the sale of the drug. The inordinate delay created by the FDA not only causes the needless death of those in desperate need, but it makes the cost of drugs astronomical once they finally get approved.

A better approach would be to allow pharmaceutical companies to sell new drugs before they are officially "approved." This change would result in a renaissance of new medications becoming available at far lower prices. Those doctors and people who desire FDA protection could use only FDA-approved drugs, while individuals who think the FDA moves too slowly could gain immediate access to medications they believe could help them. Wouldn't it be wonderful if nonprofit groups competed to provide unbiased advice about unapproved drugs that could save lives?

Some argue that the FDA approves new drugs too fast and should mandate more stringent testing. The facts are that the dangerous drugs the FDA approves are often the result of drug company manipulation of the already-flawed approval process.

Those who think they need the FDA forget that scientists established the efficacy of vaccines, antiseptics and antibiotics long before lawyers arrived to supervise their work. Medical science does not require the Federal government's rules or approvals to know whether a drug works. The superposed political layer of review on research has been the major roadblock that prevents scientists from finding real cures for diseases that have too long plagued modern man.

Some pessimists are concerned that unethical companies would sell dangerous drugs in an unregulated environment, yet no private company prospers for long selling products that kill, maim or injure in an era when trial lawyers abound.

The following is an excerpt from the *Wall Street Journal* of an editorial entitled "FDA Caution Can Be Deadly, Too":

> Most ordinary, healthy people probably still take some comfort in the thought that a diligent, generally competent, well-meaning federal agency is keeping an eye on the contents of their medicine cabinets. But we live in an age of enormously rapid progress in medical science. Impelled by genetic science, we are progressing toward ever more individualized, customized therapies. Some therapies already depend on extracting, modifying and cultivating cells, tissues or organs from the patient's own body, or from close relatives. General-issue tailoring of your medicines is fine if you happen to stand smack in the statistical middle of everything, but few real people do. And in the direst circumstances, the best therapies will often be the ones on the edges of science, well outside the bounds of the truths that have been fully certified in Washington.[34]

EDITOR OF *THE LANCET* SAYS THE FDA IS FAR TOO COZY WITH DRUG INDUSTRY

According to a May 19, 2001 editorial published in *The Lancet*, patients taking a controversial new drug for irritable bowel syndrome may have died because the FDA has become a "servant of [the drug] industry."

This devastating editorial reveals that although Glaxo-Smith Kline voluntarily withdrew the drug Lotronex® from the US market last November after the deaths of five patients, senior FDA officials are now seeking to reintroduce it.

This editorial goes on to say:

> This story reveals not only dangerous failings in a single drug's approval and review process but also the extent to which the FDA, its Center for Drug Evaluation and Research (CDER) in particular, has become the servant of industry.

This two-page editorial is entitled "Lotronex® and the FDA: A Fatal Erosion of Integrity." It accuses the FDA of receiving hundreds of millions of dollars in funding from industry.

The editorial claims the views of FDA scientists who raised safety questions about the drug were dismissed by FDA officials and that these scientists were excluded from further discussion about the drug's future. It goes on to allege that negotiations between the FDA and the Glaxo on the drug's future involved a "two-track process, one official and transparent, one unofficial and covert."

The FDA approved Lotronex® in February 2000 but it was never approved by the European Medicines Evaluation Agency. The company withdrew the product in the United States in November 2000 after 49 cases of ischaemic colitis and 21 of severe constipation, including instances of obstructed and ruptured bowel. In addition to five deaths, 34 patients had required admission to hospital and 10 needed surgery.

The Lancet says that as early as July 2000, it was known that seven patients had developed serious complications. The clinical data confirmed "substantial and potentially life-threatening risks." Instead of withdrawing Lotronex®, the FDA issued a medication guide. "This decision was to prove fatal," according to *The Lancet*.

The editorial states that FDA scientists knew that the warning advising patients to stop taking Lotronex® if they felt "increasing abdominal discomfort" was impractical. The reason is that abdominal pain can be confused as a classical symptom of an irritable bowel.

FDA scientists argued that it was unreasonable to expect patients or physicians to know if this type of pain was an early warning of possibly fatal ischaemic colitis. Their view was dismissed by FDA officials. According to *The Lancet*, "The scientists who raised these issues felt intimidated by senior colleagues and were excluded from further discussions about Lotronex®'s future."

In a memorandum dated November 16, 2000, FDA scientists said, "Early warning of the dire side effects of this drug is clearly not feasible" and added a "risk management plan cannot be successful." FDA officials choose to ignore this warning.

By the time of a key November 28th, 2000 meeting between Glaxo and FDA officials, rather than reject the company's proposal to withdraw Lotronex®, the FDA offered several conciliatory options including voluntary withdrawal pending further discussion.

The Lancet claims "many within the FDA's leadership now want to bring Lotronex® back. An advisory committee meeting set up to do so is being planned for June or July."

The reason this highly critical editorial against the FDA was published is because *The Lancet* previously published some of the trial data that led to the FDA approving the drug. As increasing reports of adverse effects became known, the editor of *The*

Lancet became "more intrigued about what was happening, it opened up into an issue of how science is dealt with by the FDA and how, because of industry funding, it has fatally compromised its independence."

The Lancet editor went on to say that "The scientists within the FDA who analyze and interpret adverse drug reactions have been largely ignored after the drug was approved and marketed. That is where there has been a terrible failure in evaluating the safety of this drug."

References

1. Lazarou J, et al. Incidence of adverse drug reactions in hospitalized patients: a meta-analysis of prospective studies. *JAMA* 1998 Apr 1 5;279(1 5): 1200–5.

2. Bates DW. Drugs and adverse drug reactions: how worried should we be? *JAMA* 1998 Apr 15;279(15):1216–7.

3. Cimons M. "FDA Moves to Reduce Accidental Drug Deaths." *LA Times* May 10, 1999. Home Edition Section: PART A Page: A-1.

4. Thalidomide Information. "FDA Announces Approval of Drug for Hansen's Disease (Leprosy) Side Effect—Imposes Unprecedented Authority to Restrict Distribution" http://www.fda.gov/cder/news/thalinfo/thalidomide.htm.

5. Faloon W. "What's Wrong with the FDA?—FDA Suffers Massive Defeats." May 2001 issue *Life Extension* magazine.

6. Cauchon Dennis. "FDA advisers tied to industry." *USA Today*; Arlington, Va.; Sep 25, 2000.

7. William David. "Scientists Who Judged Pill Safety Received Fees." *LA Times*, October 29, 1999. PART A Section.

8. William David. "2nd NIH Researcher to Become Part of Conflict Probe." *LA Times*, September 4, 1999. Home Edition PART A Section.

9. William David. "Researcher's Fees Point to Other Potential Conflicts at NIH."

10. "Deadly Medicine" by Thomas J. Moore.

11. A Letter from Roderic Dale, PhD May 2000 issue *Life Extension* magazine.

12. Driscoll J.P. "Perspective on Drug Policy—FDA's 'Caution' Is Killing People; Unnecessary delays in approval for vital drugs and medical devices are more dangerous than thalidomide." *LA Times*, June 4, 1995. Home Edition Section: Opinion Piece Page: M-5.

13. FDA vs ICN Pharmaceuticals, Drug: Ribavirin.

14. FDA versus Newport Pharmaceuticals, Drug: Isoprinsoine.

15. Anti-Aging News Vol. 1 No. 11 November 1981 "Thymosin: The Immunity Hormone."

16. Ohta Y, et al. Thymosin alpha 1 exerts protective effect against the 5-FU induced bone marrow toxicity. *Int J Immunopharmacol* 1 985;7(5):761-8.

17. Ohta Y, et al. Immunomodulating activity of thymosin fraction 5 and thymosin alpha 1 in immunosuppressed mice. *Cancer Immunol Immunother* 1983; 15(2): 108–13.

18. Moscarella S, et al. Interferon and thymosin combination therapy in naive patients with chronic hepatitis C: preliminary results. *Liver* 1998 Oct;18(5):366–9.

19. Sherman KE, et al. Combination therapy with thymosin alpha1 and interferon for the treatment of chronic hepatitis C infection: a randomized, placebo-controlled double-blind trial. *Hepatology* 1998 Apr;27(4):1 128–35.

20. Garaci E, et al. Thymosin alpha 1 in the treatment of cancer: from basic research to clinical application. *Int J Immunopharmacol* 2000 Dec;22(1 2): 1067–76.

21. Beuth J, et al. Thymosin alpha(1) application augments immune response and down-regulates tumor weight and organ colonization in BALB/c-mice. *Cancer Lett* 2000 Oct 16;159(1):9–13.

22. Moody TW, et al. Thymosinalpha1 is chemopreventive for lung adenoma formation in A/J mice. *Cancer Lett* 2000 Jul 31;155 (2):121–7.

23. Pica F, et al. High doses of Thymosin alpha 1 enhance the anti-tumor efficacy of combination chemo-immunotherapy

for murine B 16 melanoma. *Anticancer Res* 1998 Sep-Oct; 1 8(5A):3571-8.

24. Nagamine T, et al. Preliminary study of combination therapy with interferon-alpha and zinc in chronic hepatitis C patients with genotype 1b. *Biol Trace Elem Res* 2000 Summer;75(1–3):53–63.

25. Winblad B, et al. Memantine in severe dementia: results of the 9M-Best Study (Benefit and efficacy in severely demented patients during treatment with memantine). *Int J Geriatr Psychiatry* 1999 Feb;14(2):135–46.

26. Schneider E, et al. [Effects of oral memantine administration on Parkinson symptoms. Results of a placebo-controlled multicenter study]. *Dtsch Med Wochenschr* 1984 Jun 22;109(25):987–90.

27. Fischer PA, et al. [Effects of intravenous administration of memantine in parkinsonian patients (author's transl)]. *Arzneimittelforschung* 1977 Jul;27(7): 1487–9.

28. Jain KK. Evaluation of memantine for neuroprotection in dementia. *Expert Opin Investig Drugs* 2000 Jun;9(6):1397–406.

29. Androsova LV, et al. [Akatinol memantin in Alzheimer's disease: clinico-immunological correlates]. *Zh Nevrol Psikhiatr Im S S Korsakova* 2000; 1 00(9):36–8.

30. Wenk GL, et al. No interaction of memantine with acetylcholinesterase inhibitors approved for clinical use. *Life Sci* 2000 Feb 11 ;66(12):1079–83.

31. Mobius HJ. Pharmacologic rationale for memantine in chronic cerebral hypoperfusion, especially vascular dementia. *Alzheimer's Dis Assoc Disord* 1999 Oct-Dec;13 Suppl 3:S172–8.

32. Parsons CG, et al. Memantine is a clinically well tolerated N-methyl-D-aspartate (NMDA) receptor antagonist—a review of preclinical data. *Neuropharmacology* 1999 Jun;38(6):735–67.

33. Ditzler K. Efficacy and tolerability of memantine in patients with dementia syndrome. A double-blind, placebo controlled trial. *Arzneimittelforschung* 1991 Aug;41 (8):773–80.

34. Huber Peter, "FDA Caution Can Be Deadly, Too." The *Wall Street Journal* 07/24/1 998 Page A14.

What's Wrong with the FDA

by William Faloon

*"That whenever any form of government becomes
destructive of these ends, it is the right of the people
to alter or abolish it."*

Thomas Jefferson, Declaration of Independence,
July 4, 1776

CONGRESSIONAL COMMITTEES AND INVESTIGATIVE JOUR-
nalists have exposed massive incompetence, neglect and
fraud at the FDA. In the Courts, the agency continues to
lose critical cases as Federal judges rule that FDA policies are blatantly unconstitutional.

For the past 21 years, the Life Extension Foundation has compiled evidence indicating that the FDA is the number one cause of
death in the United States. The FDA causes Americans to die by:

- Delaying the introduction of life-saving therapies
- Suppressing safe methods of preventing disease
- Causing the price of drugs to be so high that some Americans do without
- Denying Americans access to effective drugs approved in other countries
- Intimidating those who develop innovative methods to treat disease
- Approving lethal prescription drugs that kill
- Censoring medical information that would let consumers protect their health
- Censoring medical information that would better educate doctors
- Failing to protect the safety of our food
- Misleading the public about scientific methods to increase longevity

The greatest threat the FDA poses to our health is the fact that the agency functions as a roadblock to the development of breakthrough medical therapies. Innovation in medicine is stifled by FDA red tape, which is why Americans continue to die from diseases that long ago might have been cured if a free marketplace in drug development existed.

FDA Suffers Second Massive Legal Defeat in "Pearson vs. Shalala II"

Court to FDA? The First Amendment Must Be Followed

by William Faloon

N 1999 THERE WAS AN UNPRECEDENTED LEGAL VICTORY AGAINST the FDA in a landmark Federal Appellate Court ruling. The title of the case was *Pearson v. Shalala*. For the purposes of this article, we will refer to the 1999 case as "Pearson I." When discussing the most recent triumph over FDA tyranny, this case will be called "Pearson II."

The historical significance of Pearson I cannot be overstated. By an 11–0 margin, an appellate court mandated that the FDA abide by the First Amendment (free speech) provisions of the United

States Constitution. Prior to this ruling, the FDA behaved as if the First Amendment did not apply to them.

Still reeling from the devastating loss in Pearson I, the FDA on February 2, 2001, suffered yet another massive legal defeat in the Pearson II case. Pearson I and II are significant victories for freedom of informed choice in the healthcare marketplace. They make it clear that the First Amendment to the United States Constitution disarms FDA of any power to ban nutrient-disease claims (so-called "health claims") unless FDA has solid evidence that the claims actually mislead. The Courts have ordered FDA to stop censoring science on dietary supplement labels and to let that science reach consumers. The Courts ruled that the only constitutional right the FDA has on the issue of health claims is to insist on reasonably worded disclaimers such as, "These statements have not been evaluated by the Food and Drug Administration."

WHAT THE FDA WANTED TO CENSOR

In Pearson II, Durk Pearson, Sandy Shaw, the American Preventive Medical Association, Dr. Julian M. Whitaker and Pure Encapsulations, Inc. appealed an FDA ruling that would have prevented the public from learning that synthetic folic acid is more effective than food folate in reducing neural tube defects. The specific claim the FDA wanted to ban was:

> 800 mcg of folic acid is more effective in reducing the risk of neural tube defects than a lower amount in foods in common form.

In the Pearson I decision, the Federal Appellate Court ruled that the FDA had unconstitutionally suppressed this health claim. Over two years later, FDA still suppressed the claim in disobedient disregard of the Pearson I ruling. The FDA's decision to suppress this health claim not only violated the First Amendment rights of the Pearson plaintiffs, it also deprived the public of health information vital to every fertile American woman.

THE FDA IGNORES THE COURT'S RULING

The fact that synthetic folic acid in amounts ranging from 400 mcg to 800 mcg is more effective than food folate in reducing neural tube defects is well-established in the scientific literature. The Institutes of Medicine of the National Academy of Sciences has determined that synthetic folic acid is twice as bioavailable as food folate and, thus, is more effective in reducing neural tube defect risk. Despite the ruling in Pearson I, and despite the overwhelming scientific evidence in favor of the claim, the FDA held for a second time that the claim would not be allowed. In the process, it once again denied American women information they need to save them and their future children from the horrible affliction of neural tube defects. It also proved that this agency continues to be willing to harm the public health to keep in place its regime of censorship over health claims.

Pearson II is an outgrowth of Pearson I. A landmark First Amendment decision, Pearson I struck down as unconstitutional four FDA rules that suppressed the health claims that Durk Pearson, Sandy Shaw, the American Preventive Medical Association and Citizens for Health wanted to make. The four claims were:

1. Consumption of antioxidant vitamins may reduce the risk of certain kinds of cancers.
2. Consumption of fiber may reduce the risk of colorectal cancer.
3. Consumption of omega-3 fatty acids may reduce the risk of coronary heart disease.
4. 800 mcg of folic acid in a dietary supplement is more effective in reducing the risk of neural tube defects than a lower amount in foods in common form.

The Court also held FDA's interpretation of its health claims review standard unconstitutional. It ordered FDA to allow the four claims even if they failed to satisfy that review standard.

The Court ruled the FDA's health claim standard to be arbitrary and capricious because it was so subjective that no one could determine precisely what level of scientific evidence FDA expected in order to approve a claim. It ordered FDA to define a new standard comprehensibly—something that FDA has still not done. It told FDA that even in the presence of a defined standard the agency would be expected to allow health claims except in the narrowest of circumstances: when it proved with empirical evidence that a health claim was not only misleading to consumers but also that it could not be rendered nonmisleading through the addition of a disclaimer. Pearson I made disclosure over suppression the order of the day. FDA was supposed to implement the decision immediately, fully and faithfully. FDA did not. In fact, FDA still has not done so.

FDA DRAGGED INTO COURT AGAIN

In Pearson II, Durk Pearson, Sandy Shaw and the other Pearson plaintiffs returned to federal court to force FDA to comply with Pearson I by allowing the plaintiffs' folic acid claim to enter the marketplace immediately. The Court granted the plaintiffs request for a preliminary injunction to the extent that it declared FDA's action unconstitutional. The Court held that "FDA acted unconstitutionally, and particularly in violation of the Court of Appeals decision in [Pearson I], in suppressing Plaintiffs' claim rather than proposing a clarifying disclaimer to accompany the Claim." FDA has sixty days to implement the decision but, rather than do that, it has asked the Court to reconsider its ruling, another delaying tactic.

Pearson II is a particularly bitter defeat for FDA because it comes at the hands of the very judge who ruled in favor of FDA in the case reversed by Pearson I: Judge Gladys Kessler of the US District Court for the District of Columbia. At oral argument before she ruled in Pearson II, Judge Kessler explained that she had been persuaded that her earlier decision had been incorrect.

She said that she believed that the Court of Appeals' decision in Pearson I was the proper resolution of the matter. She then issued a very well-reasoned decision that constitutional law experts who have studied the case believe will be very hard, if not impossible, for FDA to appeal successfully.

In Pearson II, Judge Kessler rejected FDA's arguments one by one. She found FDA's failure to comply with the Pearson I order inexcusable, writing, "There is no question that the agency has acted with less than reasonable speed in this case; for example, it waited for more than 18 months before revoking rules declared unconstitutional by the Court of Appeals." She found it "clear that the FDA simply failed to comply with the constitutional guidelines outlined in Pearson." She stated that "The agency appears to have at best, misunderstood, and at worst, deliberately ignored, highly relevant portions of the Court of Appeals Opinion." She found that "FDA has continually refused to authorize the disclaimers suggested by the Court of Appeals—or any disclaimer, for that matter" and "has simply failed to adequately consider the teachings of Pearson: that the agency must shoulder a very heavy burden if it seeks to totally ban a particular health claim."

In granting the injunction against FDA's decision to prohibit the folic acid claim, Judge Kessler found, "FDA's decision . . . was arbitrary, capricious and an abuse of discretion." She thought it "very clear that Plaintiffs are harmed by the FDA's suppression of the Folic Acid Claim," explaining that the continued violation of their First Amendment rights constituted "irreparable harm."

JUDGE SAYS FDA'S POSITION "HARMED THE PUBLIC INTEREST"

Indeed, Judge Kessler found the FDA's suppression of the claim inexcusable not only because it deprived the Plaintiffs of their "rights to effectively communicate . . . health message[s] to consumers" but also because it harmed the public interest. FDA's existing, allowable folic acid claims convey the false and misleading impression that folate in unfortified foods is effective in reducing neural tube defects when, in fact, it has never been proven effective. The only source of folic acid proven effective is synthetic, i.e. the kind of folic acid found in supplements. The only amounts shown to reduce neural tube defects consistently and reliably are above 400 mcg, with 800 mcg regarded as an ideal dose by many leading scientists. The only large-scale placebo controlled clinical trial corroborating a 100% reduction in neural tube defects in women with no prior history of neural tube defect births involved use of dietary supplements containing 800 mcg a day of folic acid.[1] The FDA rejected this study, but Judge Kessler did not. She ruled FDA's rejection of the study an abuse of discretion, finding the need for the information substantial. Here is what the judge said:

> The public health risk from neural tube defects (NTD) is undeniably substantial. NTDs occur in approximately 1 of every 1,000 live births in the United States. Approximately 2,500 babies are born every year with an NTD. Of the children born with NTDs, most do not survive into adulthood, and those who do experience severe handicaps. The lifetime health costs associated with spina bifida, the most common NTD, exceed $500,000, and the yearly costs in Social Security payments exceed $82 million.

> Given that the scientific consensus, even as acknowledged by the FDA, confirms that taking folic acid substantially reduces a woman's risk of giving birth to an infant with a neural tube defect, the public interest is well served by permitting information about the folic acid/NTD connection to reach as wide a public audience as possible. Plaintiffs' Folic Acid Claim . . . communicates this vitally important message.

IS THE FDA NOW IN CONTEMPT OF COURT?

Pearson II and Pearson I have profound implications for FDA's regulation of health information. These decisions establish beyond any legal doubt that the FDA must comply with the First Amendment. Those decisions make it clear that FDA cannot suppress health information on the basis that the agency disagrees with the message communicated. Instead, FDA must be in the business of fostering the dissemination of health information to the public, not censoring it.

Although the Pearson I and II decisions concern dietary supplements, they rest on broad First Amendment doctrines that are the supreme law of the land and have greater authority than any FDA regulation. As a consequence, the Pearson decisions are likely to cause the toppling of FDA's censorship of food and drug claims over time. If applied to their full extent, the First Amendment principles of Pearson mean that FDA has no constitutional power to prevent the public from receiving any truthful and nonmisleading health information about any product that agency regulates.

Those principles mean that FDA must rely on corrective disclaimers, whenever possible, as an alternative to its current practice of censorship. The days of FDA censorship are destined to come to an end. For the moment, however, the agency still (even after Pearson II) continues to censor health claims for supplements, health claims for foods and off-label claims for drugs. That would appear to be contempt of court. In one case now pending before the United States Court of Appeals involving FDA suppression of a vitamin B6, vitamin B12, folic acid and vascular disease claim, plaintiffs represented by attorney Jonathan Emord have asked the US District Court to hold FDA in contempt for its noncompliance with the Pearson decision. It may well be that in due time FDA and its officers will be made to account personally for FDA's unlawful refusal to comply with the First Amendment.

Reference

1. "Prevention of the first occurrence of neural-tube defects by periconceptional vitamin supplementation," *New England Journal of Medicine* 1992 Dec 24; 327(26):1832–5

FDA Loses Case against Compounding Pharmacies on First Amendment Grounds

by William Faloon

MOST AMERICANS DON'T KNOW THAT THEY CAN LEGALLY obtain certain drugs that are not FDA-approved at compounding pharmacies. The cost of these "compounded" drugs is often lower than what it costs to buy finished drugs made by pharmaceutical companies. The reason most Americans don't know about drugs available at compounding pharmacies is that up till now, the FDA said it was "illegal" for compounding pharmacies to promote the drugs they offered.

A Federal appellate court has just ruled that the FDA cannot restrict advertising by pharmacists who sell compounded drugs.

The decision pitted the free speech rights of pharmacists against a Federal law aimed at restricting advertising of compounds that require a doctor's prescription, but aren't subject to the FDA's approval process.

In citing previous cases, the US Court of Appeals for the Ninth Circuit Court (San Francisco) stated that "government prohibitions of truthful commercial messages are 'particularly dangerous' and deserve 'rigorous review.' "

In this case, the FDA contended that restrictions on ads for compounds were an attempt to balance the needs of individual patients with the protection of the broader public by "preventing widespread distribution of compounded drugs."

In an opinion (that upheld a lower court ruling), Judge Cynthia Holcomb Hall wrote that "the government neither explains nor supports" its contention that wider distribution of compounded drugs would endanger the public. "In fact, most of the evidence runs to the contrary," she wrote, noting that "compounding is not only legal under state law, but most states require their pharmacists to know how to compound."

Judge Hall went on to say that the government offered "no evidence demonstrating that its restrictions would succeed in striking the balance it claims is a substantial interest, or even protect the public health."

Two years ago, the FDA lost a similar case when they challenged the right of drug company representatives to promote the use of approved drugs for uses that were not approved by the FDA. In both of these cases, the FDA was trying to censor the promotion of a legal activity. Since both drug compounding and using approved drugs for unapproved uses is legal, the FDA did not have a right to ban it, so say the Courts.

Need to Reform the FDA

by William Faloon

I N A SERIES OF BLATANT ABUSES OF POWER, THE FOOD AND DRUG Administration unwittingly offers the public compelling reasons for its immediate reform. Their actions show that the FDA and the multibillion dollar pharmaceutical industry have one goal in common: Increasing profits from prescription drug sales.

Not only do the FDA and the drug lords daringly loot the pockets of the American consumer, they do so without any regard to the laws and regulations designed to ensure fairness and honesty. As a comparison, imagine you are in court, suing a large company (call it the Megabig Corporation.) The evidence is clearly in your favor, but when you reach the courtroom, half of the jurors work for Megabig! In addition, the judge is the president of Megabig! Guess who wins? Unfair? Unconstitutional? Undemocratic? Yes, but that is exactly the situation that exists today when the FDA makes a decision about a prescription medication.

The FDA exercises its power through 18 different "Expert Committees," made up of scientists with the experience needed to examine varying classes of drugs. These panels evaluate and recommend actions regarding medications that are worth millions, even billions of dollars to the pharmaceutical houses that invented, imported or modified them. Any one decision by a panel can move a drug company's stock up or down quickly, and the committee members are well aware of the significance of their choices. Obviously, the drug lords are also knowledgeable as to how each panel can influence their careers and their collective fortunes. Because of these factors, there are government regulations in place to protect the American public from biased or even corrupt panel members. The rules state that a person cannot sit on a committee if he or she has an obvious conflict of interest, defined as a situation in which a ruling could make a significant financial impact on that person. This seems to guarantee a relatively unbiased decision making process, but never underestimate the power of a greedy corporation and a corrupt government agency.

Despite all the safeguards, over 50% of the FDA's Expert Committee members are people with direct financial ties to the pharmaceutical industry. This astounding disregard for federal regulations was first uncovered and published in *USA Today* on September 25, 2000. Their investigative report showed that 54% of all those serving on FDA committees have a direct financial interest in their own decisions. These conflicts include receiving direct fees from the drug company, owning its stock, having a spouse employed by the company up for review or having their research funded by the same company whose drugs they are evaluating. Even participating "consumer representatives" were found to be on the drug lords' payrolls.

How does the FDA get away with a behavior that the Ralph Nader-founded Public Citizen's Health Research Group calls "outrageous"? They accomplish this modern highway robbery through the generous practice of granting "waivers." The FDA is permitted to waive the conflict of interest rules if an expert's value outweighs the potential financial conflict. This sounds reasonable until you learn that 803 waivers were granted over a two-year period starting in 1998. In fact, the report determined that there were financial conflicts in 146 of 159 FDA advisory meetings during this time.

With the escalation of drug prices, health plans drop their sickest patients or go bankrupt, more and more people go without insurance and small businesses disappear because they cannot afford the increased cost of employee benefits.

The FDA's rationale for these incestuous relationships is that the most qualified experts for their committees are those people within the drug companies doing the research and testing on that drug. This is patently ridiculous. No reasonable person would believe that there are no other qualified chemists, biologists, pharmacists, cardiologists or other specialists available except for those obligated to the drug manufacturers. But the FDA, in its arrogance, expects the public to believe whatever it says. A case can be made that the FDA experts are exactly the wrong people to be placed in such important positions.

Unfortunately, this corruption is deep seated and unlikely to change without direct congressional action. To prevent additional publicity that might damage their cozy, lucrative system, the FDA plans to stop revealing financial conflicts on their committees in the name of "personal privacy."

The FDA pretends to carefully investigate new drugs for safety and efficacy. The reality is that those responsible for recommending FDA approval often have a financial interest in the very drugs they are supposed to be independently evaluating. Is it any wonder that drugs the FDA declares "safe" kill more than one hundred thousand Americans every year?

When it comes to determining whether a drug is "effective," this provides an even greater opportunity for drug company insiders (who sit on FDA committees) to make biased decisions. This means that bad drugs can get approved by those with the right connections, while more effective medications are sometimes never allowed to be sold in the United States.

In deciding what new drugs are to be christened with FDA approval, scientific objectivity is replaced by the economic influence of large pharmaceutical companies. The consumer is thus denied access to innovative medications offered by smaller biotech companies, while large drug companies can push their products through FDA committees comprised of people who have a significant financial interest in the drug gaining FDA approval.

The drug approval system in the United States is riddled with corruption, causing Americans to pay inflated prices for mediocre medications. Despite this economic pillage suffered by the consumer, the public has remained surprisingly apathetic to this abusive drug approval process. At the end of this article, we propose several ways to reform this disgraceful system that is causing Americans to needlessly suffer and die from bad medicine while being forced to pay the highest prices in the world for their healthcare.

FDA OPPOSES FAIR MARKET PRICING

In contrast to its public role as a consumer watchdog, the FDA has done everything possible to support higher and higher drug prices, ensuring record profits for the pharmaceutical industry. The House Commerce Committee recently estimated that the American public and the governmental agencies which purchase medications (Medicare and Medicaid) are overpaying by an astronomical one billion dollars yearly.

Certainly, if any Medicare prescription plan becomes law, there must be a major revision in the way prices are determined. The primary problem, however, remains the anti-consumer stance of the FDA. Their policies have resulted in skyrocketing drug prices, the driving force behind the yearly 15–20% increases in healthcare costs. Senator Paul Wellstone (D-Minn.) stated that the drug industry looks only "to make huge profits on the misery and illness of consumers." This misery reaches well beyond the actual struggle to afford critical medications. With the escalation of drug prices, health plans drop their sickest patients or go bankrupt, more and more people go without insurance and small businesses disappear because they cannot afford the increased cost of employee benefits. The *New York Times* reports that basic health insurance premiums could be raised by as much as 30% in certain regions of the country.

The FDA has shown fanatical opposition to the free market reimportation of prescription drugs, one way in which overall drug spending might be lowered. ("Reimportation" refers to the consumer purchase of legitimate drugs from foreign pharmacies. The medications are sold by US manufacturers at lower prices to other countries because of the buying power of such large group entities.) The FDA finds any reason to block a US citizen's right to buy back medications at that cheaper price from these countries, including nations with standards equal to ours, such as Canada and England. They are opposed even if the drug is exactly the same as sold in the United States, is made by the same company and was approved by the FDA the day before it was shipped. They have gone to the extreme of having 11 former FDA commissioners write personal letters to Congress, urging Representatives to vote against reimportation. Fortunately, Congress has seen through these efforts and has supported reimportation. Some House members have even arranged for their constituents to travel to Canada to make prescription purchases. In response, the FDA has waged a media campaign warning the public about possible "counterfeit" or spoiled drugs, though no such cases have been found. Had the FDA found evidence of spoiled or inferior medications, they would have trumpeted the news to bolster their fragile position.

Despite both Houses of Congress voting to allow Americans to purchase lower-cost prescription drugs from overseas sources, Donna Shalala at the very end of year 2000 used a loophole and announced that she was declining to implement this new law or to submit a budget justification for the $23 million Congress made available specifically for this purpose. This enabled the FDA to declare the law unworkable and effectively killed the legislation that was so overwhelming supported by the House, Senate and the American public. The drug companies got their way because the FDA refused to implement the law passed by Congress. This means that the American consumer continues to be raped by having to pay the highest prescription drug prices in the world.

The FDA continues to argue (without providing any evidence) that drugs from other countries are somehow "dangerous." A close look reveals that the true danger lies in the neglect and incompetence of the FDA itself. The agency is charged with ensuring the purity and safety of the raw ingredients used in the manufacture of approved drugs. These ingredients often come from foreign sources, and are supposed to be inspected by the FDA. Shockingly, the *Wall Street Journal* published a report on September 12, 2000 showing that at least 57 separate companies had shipped "misbranded" ingredients to American drug manufacturers. Rep. Thomas Bliley (R–VA) called the FDA's efforts "ineffective" and "limited." In other words, the FDA says it is "dangerous" for an American to obtain a finished drug product sold at a Canadian pharmacy, but the FDA shows little concern with "misbranded" raw materials being imported into the United States that wind up in the expensive drugs that are sold in American pharmacies. So while they were alarming the public about the hazards of buying the medications from foreign sources, the FDA was falling down on the job by allowing the wrong raw materials to be used in the manufacture of "safe" American drugs.

What is obvious is that the FDA's concern for the American public is simply lip service. Their neglect of true drug safety, their public campaign against cheaper drug prices and their tainted expert committees show their true priorities to be preserving their own bureaucracy and protecting their allies in the drug industry.

WE PAY, THEY PROSPER

The combined efforts of the FDA and the drug lords are aimed at an enormous prize. Spending for medications has become the nation's bottomless pit. When a 20-tablet bottle of the allergy medication Claritin® costs $8.75 in Europe, but $44.00 in the United States, it becomes extremely obvious that there is no actual cost-basis for drug pricing. Certainly, the drug lords would not sell at a cheaper price in Europe if they were losing money. Why is the United States the "cash-cow" of the pharmaceutical industry? The sad answer is that they know their actions are insulated and protected by the FDA.

The drug companies defend their unfair pricing by claiming that they need more research funds. This is an attempt to play on our fears of death and aging. There always will be tremendous financial motivation to develop new, more effective and safer drugs. It is easier, though, to attempt to extend the expiring patent rights on drugs such as Claritin®, a huge profit center for its manufacturer, than to worry about research and development. Fortunately, the FDA's efforts to achieve such an unfair advantage for their drug friends were thwarted by an increasingly alert Congress. However, patents for drugs are complicated issues involving multiple components. As a result, the drug companies are able to delay the expiration of many profitable patents for indefinite periods of time.

FAILING TO PROTECT THE FOOD SAFETY

The General Accountability Office (GAO) issued a report to Congress on February 13, 2001 indicating that the FDA was not adequately inspecting seafood for potentially lethal bacterial contamination. According to this report, more than half the seafood firms are failing to follow food safety standards and FDA inspectors are not cracking down on these violations.

Even when FDA inspectors found a serious violation, they failed to move quickly to make the company correct the problem. As far as imported products, when the FDA finds a problem at foreign seafood firms, it does not automatically check the food that is entering US ports from these very same companies. The FDA moved to block food from being imported from nine foreign companies only after GAO investigators raised the issue. The GAO report to Congress stated that, "The potential health risks associated with these violations are significant."

Americans suffer an estimated 114,000 seafood poisonings each year and the FDA is failing to comply with a food inspection program it announced in 1997 that was supposed to cut this number in half.

The FDA track record on food safety inspections grows more appalling each year. According to FDA records there were 21,000 food inspections in 1981, but by 1996, the number dropped to only 5,000. This 76% reduction in food safety inspections occurred during a time when the FDA admits there is a lot more food to inspect.

The FDA attributes its failure to adequately inspect food to "budgetary constraints," yet the agency is squandering millions of dollars a year in litigation expenses in a futile attempt to suppress the free flow of information to the consumer. While the FDA suffers one defeat after another in Federal Court, 9,000 Americans die each year from food poisoning that FDA inspections are supposed to prevent.

THE TIME TO REFORM THE FDA IS NOW

With the backbreaking cost of medicine threatening to destroy our healthcare system, with the potential of Medicare prescription abuse and with the very life of many citizens at stake, solving the FDA/pharmaceutical company dilemma must begin now. Any reform has to begin with the FDA, since it maintains and supports the "robber baron" practices of the drug companies. As a government agency, it can and should be held accountable to the Congress and its various committees. There are several possible ways to improve the situation, the most severe of which is to simply abolish the FDA. The best argument for abolition is the thorough and deep-rooted corruption described in this article. This leads to a search for the FDA's necessity for existence, and whether it does more harm than good. It is possible that other agencies could assume the more beneficial functions of the FDA.

The second possibility is FDA reform, though it may be asked if this is possible, given its present, well-entrenched structure. Certainly, if the FDA is allowed to exist, consumers must demand a complete investigation of the abuses being uncovered on a regular basis, as well as a new and reputable Commissioner to enforce ethical guidelines. This would be a lengthy and expensive process, and might allow the current regime and its friends too much time to wring even more undeserved profits.

A third option is far simpler and much less expensive: Make the FDA a voluntary organization. Allow a free market economy to thrive by converting the FDA into a consumer-information agency. Those people desiring the FDA stamp of approval could choose to purchase only those medications that receive such an acknowledgment. Others could seek out other sources from this country and reputable foreign prescription and non-prescription suppliers. It would be expected that other organizations would arise to offer different evaluations of the same drugs, providing alternative educational health statements for the consumer to weigh. This is the same situation that consumers find themselves in when they look to purchase almost everything other than medicine. Considering the number of deaths associated with FDA-approved drugs, it is difficult to see the negatives in such a democratic drug marketplace. Consumers are smarter than the FDA thinks. They can only do well without a corrupt FDA controlling their health and their lives.

FDA reform is crucial because our very lives are at stake. If we don't tear down FDA barriers against new drug development, those of us alive today may not benefit from the breakthrough therapies that are being discovered in research laboratories. We are also facing an economic healthcare crisis because FDA policies are denying Americans access to lower cost medications.

2000

Life Extension Wins in the House and Senate

by William Faloon

N A STARTLING SETBACK TO THE **FDA** AND THE DRUG CARTEL, a bill that enables Americans to legally obtain lower cost prescription drugs from other countries passed the House of Representatives on June 29, 2000. This is great news for consumers who have been paying inflated prices for their medications because the FDA inappropriately blocked the importation of less expensive drugs from other countries.

The pharmaceutical industry's panicked response has been to run full-page newspaper ads stating that prescription drugs from Mexico and Canada are somehow "counterfeit" and cannot be trusted. This is a truly remarkable allegation when one considers that the lower priced drugs from Canada and Mexico are often manufactured by these very same pharmaceutical companies.

The drug industry is using scare tactics that have no basis in fact to block Americans from gaining access to lower-cost prescription medications, and the FDA wholeheartedly supports the drug companies. American citizens, on the other hand, are revolting against outrageously high drug prices.

On July 20, 2000, the Senate passed a similar bill—by a vote of 74 to 21—that allows pharmacists and wholesalers to import US-approved drugs available at lower prices overseas. The House bill, on the other hand, lets individuals buy drugs abroad, so a compromise measure is now being crafted.

CONVENTIONAL MEDICINE FAILS MOST AMERICANS

You might think that since US citizens pay the highest healthcare prices in the world, that the quality of medicine would be commensurate with the cost. According to the World Health Organization, this is not the case. A recently released study from the World Health Organization showed that the United States ranked 37th in overall healthcare quality, meaning that 36 countries are doing a better job than the US at keeping their citizens healthy. The fact that countries who are ahead of the United States pay significantly less in healthcare costs indicates that there is something fundamentally flawed about the present FDA-protected healthcare monopoly. According to a health economist at Princeton University, the United States is very good at employing heroic expensive procedures, but poor at low-cost preventative care that keeps citizens of other countries healthier. This is not surprising when one looks at the FDA's 80-year reign of terror against those involved in preventive medicine.

NEW ENGLAND JOURNAL OF MEDICINE ATTACKS PHARMACEUTICAL INDUSTRY

Anyone who reads the *New England Journal of Medicine* knows that this publication derives almost all of their advertising revenue from prescription drug advertising. That's what makes their blunt editorial against the pharmaceutical industry so credible.

This editorial, written by Dr. Marcia Angell, and published in the June 22, 2000 edition, accuses the pharmaceutical industry of hiding behind a cloak of "exaggerated or misleading" claims to justify high drug prices. Drug companies state that they need high prices to develop new cures and better treatments. But Angell argues that many of the new drugs that companies produce add little to therapeutic innovation except expense and confusion.

The *New England Journal of Medicine* editorial depicts the industry as one in which top companies rake in huge profits, spend enormous amounts on questionable marketing and advertising practices and are free to charge inflated prices as a result of government-sanctioned monopolies. "The pharmaceutical industry is extraordinarily privileged. It benefits enormously from publicly funded research, government-granted patents and large tax breaks, and it reaps lavish profits," says Dr. Angell.

Dr. Angell said that she is speaking out because the prices of drugs are rising so fast and the use of drugs is so great that it's becoming a real problem for consumers. She also worries that the ongoing Congressional debate on a Medicare prescription drug benefit has largely focused on who will pay and the breadth of coverage instead of the price of the drugs themselves.

It should not be surprising that the Pharmaceutical Research and Manufacturers of America, which represents drug companies, issued a prepared statement blasting Dr. Angell's point of view as "a complete distortion of the facts."

WALL STREET JOURNAL EXPOSES DRUG COMPANY PROPAGANDA

The July 6, 2000 issue of the *Wall Street Journal* also featured an article critical of the drug industry's claims that high drug prices are needed to fund research. According to this article, the pharmaceutical industry is not delivering the kind of break-throughs that were once promised. The *Wall Street Journal* pointed out that the drug industry still spends far more on sales-men than it does on scientists and that overall, the industry's marketing and administration expenses are generally more than twice those of research and development. At Pfizer, for instance, marketing and administration make up 39% of expenses, com-pared with 17% for R&D.

WHY THESE ATROCITIES CONTINUE

Americans pay the highest prices in the world for substandard medical care. It's easy to point fingers at the drug companies, but it is the FDA who provides the pharmaceutical giants with the immoral monopoly that allows them to rape the American consumer's health and pocketbook. If the FDA were abolished, drug companies would have to get back to aggressive research and cut prices dramatically if they were to compete against the small biotech companies that are being held back by FDA red tape.

With the FDA out of the way, large and small companies would be free to offer novel therapies without having to spend hun-dreds of millions of dollars on FDA "approval." New drug effi-cacy would be determined by allowing private organizations to test drugs on volunteer terminally ill patients without first hav-ing to obtain FDA approval. In today's heavily regulated climate, on the other hand, terminally ill patients are denied access to promising therapies unless they meet the rigid criteria set by the FDA. This bureaucratic obstacle often dooms a drug to fail-ure because the agency first demands the patients fail grueling rounds of toxic conventional therapy before being allowed to try the novel approach.

Some people still think the FDA protects us against dangerous drugs. Instead, when humanitarian FDA employees tried to alert the public about a dangerous drug, the FDA launched an internal affairs investigation and threatened these honorable people with imprisonment.

The FDA's primary focus is on protecting the profits of the large drug companies and not in safeguarding the consumer against dangerous drugs. It is encouraging that a growing number of judges, members of Congress and the media are recognizing the health fraud being perpetrated against the American public by the FDA.

No Consumer Protection

by William Faloon

THE FDA REMAINS BIASED AGAINST ALTERNATIVE MEDICINE, and this can be seen in the agency's proposal to seek ten million tax dollars a year to regulate Internet pharmacies and health sites. As we reported three months ago, one of the FDA's excuses for seeking this annual tax payer subsidy is to keep Americans from being able to order Viagra® without a prescription. A new report, however, shatters the FDA's argument that Viagra® can be safely used when prescribed by a physician.

This study shows a higher number of deaths and serious cardiovascular events associated with Viagra® than what were previously thought. These findings were presented at the March 14, 2000 meeting of the American College of Cardiologists in Anaheim, CA. In this analysis of 1,473 major adverse events related to Viagra®, 522 people died, the majority due to cardiovascular causes. According to the study's senior author, the majority of deaths were associated with standard Viagra® dosages (50 mg) and were due to cardiovascular causes that appeared to be clustered around the time of dosing (most deaths occurred within four to five hours of taking Viagra®). These 522 deaths are sharply higher than previous estimates.

What is most striking is that the majority of deaths occurred in patients who were less than 65 years of age, and who had no reported cardiac risk factors. You may remember that after men started dropping dead after taking nitrate drugs and Viagra®, the FDA responded by mandating new labeling that warned against prescribing Viagra® to those whose underlying cardiovascular disease might predispose them to an adverse reaction. However, this new study showed that most deaths (88%) actually occurred in patients who were not taking nitrates, leading investigators to speculate whether there are some susceptible individuals who are vulnerable to Viagra's lethal side effects even if they don't take nitrate drugs.

The question begging to be answered is how the FDA could have missed these lethal side effects after spending so many years and dollars evaluating Viagra® for safety. As a consumer, you are paying $8 to $10 a tablet for Viagra®, and the drug company justifies this outrageous price by factoring in the high FDA-approval costs. The FDA, however, failed to detect Viagra's lethal side effects, 522 people have died to date and Americans are still being deceived into believing that the FDA "protects" the public's health.

While the FDA has no plans to restrict sales of Viagra®, it still classifies natural testosterone as a "scheduled drug," which makes it more difficult for physicians to prescribe it. Natural testosterone is more effective in restoring lost libido than Viagra®, and is completely safe (for men who do not already have prostate cancer)[1]. Alternative medicine has been extolling the virtues of natural testosterone replacement therapy for years, while misguided FDA policies have suppressed this safe, non-patented libido-enhancing therapy.

It is difficult to ascertain how the FDA can claim to be guarding the public against dangerous drugs when 522 men have died after taking Viagra® and many more have encountered "major adverse events." Under the guise of protecting the consumer from unsafe products, the FDA has instead created a multibillion dollar monopoly for the manufacturer of Viagra®. The consumer pays for this non-existent "protection" every time they buy an exorbitantly priced FDA-approved drug.

There are free market solutions that would allow Americans to safely and quickly gain access to new life saving therapies. As a health consumer, your best protection lies in a free market environment, as opposed to the current system whereby giant pharmaceutical companies work hand and hand with the FDA to ensure that Americans pay the highest drug prices in the world. Under existing rules, Americans are denied access to life saving therapies while the FDA pretends to protect consumers against dangerous and ineffective products. The facts are that the FDA approves dangerous drugs that kill over 125,000 Americans a year while simultaneously suppressing innovative therapies that could save many lives. Despite these abysmal facts, the FDA continues to put forth a charade that it functions as a "consumer protection" agency. The FDA acts to protect the financial interests of the large drug companies, at the expense of the American consumer's health and pocketbook.

Reference

1. Safety and efficacy of natural testosterone discussed in *Maximize Your Vitality and Potency* (Jonathan V. Wright, MD), *The Testosterone Syndrome* (Eugene Shippen, MD), and *Disease Prevention and Treatment* (Life Extension Foundation)

MAY 2000

Americans are Getting Healthier—But the FDA Remains a Major Impediment

by William Faloon

A CCORDING TO A NEW STUDY, LIFE IS NOT ONLY BECOMING longer in the US, it appears to be getting better. People over age 84 in 1993 were shown to be healthier and more independent compared with those the same age in 1986. This new report was published in the *Journal of the American Medical Association* (January 26, 2000).

The study also showed that fewer men and women over age 84 used healthcare services and entered into nursing homes during the last year of their lives. According to a co-author of the report, Dr. Richard S. Cooper, "There have been substantial changes over the last generation in terms of health-related behaviors and we are beginning to see the impact of that among the elderly."

New studies are likely to continue to show significant prolongation of a healthier life span based on the aggressive measures Americans are taking to prevent the diseases of aging. One example of how Americans are taking better care of themselves can be seen in the explosive growth of vitamin supplements. Sales of dietary supplements in the United States in 1982 were only two billion dollars. By 1999, dietary supplement sales topped fifteen billion dollars. Based on the health and longevity effects that supplements confer on human populations, there should be increasing numbers of Americans who live independently, relatively free of the common degenerative diseases that have afflicted previous generations.

WHY THESE STATS ARE NOT GOOD ENOUGH

Improving the overall quality of life is a short-term objective of the Life Extension Foundation. Our ultimate goal is the indefinite extension of the healthy human life span. There is strong scientific reason to believe that the eradication of killer diseases and control of human aging may be right around the corner. The problem is that an entire generation of Americans may perish waiting for the FDA to approve these breakthrough therapies.

There are biotech companies making revolutionary medical discoveries, but the FDA's regulatory quagmire prevents many of these potential life saving therapies from making it to market. We reprint on the next page an unsolicited letter that exemplifies the problem that small drug companies have in dealing with the FDA. This exceptionally well stated letter, detailing how the FDA stifles medical innovation, was sent to me by a biotech company president.

The solution to the FDA's bureaucratic obstruction of advancement in medicine is to radically restructure or abolish the agency. The dilemma is that the average person still thinks the FDA does what it is supposed to, i.e., "protect and promote the health of the American public." The unfortunate facts are that science is moving ahead too rapidly for any central bureaucracy to keep up with it all. The FDA roadblock against progress has to be dismantled or many more will die from a disease that could have been prevented or cured if free enterprise was allowed into the medical science arena.

A LOGICAL PROPOSAL TO END FDA TYRANNY

The letter here provides an inside look at how the FDA inhibits innovation and how simple it would be to restructure the agency in a way that would allow for a medical renaissance to occur in the United States.

From the Desk of
RODERIC M.K. DALE, PHD

February 25, 2000

William Faloon
Life Extension Foundation
PO Box 229120
Hollywood, FL 33022

Dear Mr. Faloon:

I have read with great interest of your battles with the FDA. It would appear that the FDA believes that it is above the US constitution and that it can intimidate, threaten and enforce inherently flawed authoritarian regulations and even regulate what people can say. This last point was of course, documented in court in the lawsuit that was brought by Pearson and Shaw charging that the FDA was guilty of suppressing truthful and non-misleading information. As you know, the courts agreed with Pearson and Shaw and the appellate court voted 11 to zero not to hear an appeal by the FDA.

The frustration that our company has experienced stems from yet another aspect of the FDA's activities. Our company, Oligos Etc. Inc., is a contract manufacturer that has established itself as a premier source for the highest quality nucleic acids for research, diagnostics, nucleic acid arrays, cosmetics, nutritional supplements and therapeutics. Over the past several years we have been pursuing a research program using internally generated funds. These studies have led to the development of several truly innovative formulations based on our extensive experience with nucleic acid synthesis as well as novel chemistries and processes for the manufacture of nucleic acids that we have developed (patents pending). Therapeutic formulations of these compositions could be extremely valuable in inflammatory conditions such as psoriasis, asthma, arthritis, rosacea and eczema. Other compositions could be easily developed for issues ranging from hair loss, ED, IBD, cardiovascular function and cancer, to aging.

Originally we thought that we might pursue the development of clinical formulations of some of our compositions. However, we discovered that the therapeutic approval process that the FDA has created is extremely expensive ($200 to $500 Million) and incredibly time-consuming (8–12 years) for a single product. It is a process that allows only the large multinational drug companies to participate. Ultimately, a small company like ours would have to sell off its ideas to one of the pharma giants to get a product through the new drug application process (NDA). However, the large pharmas are resistant to new approaches. Even if they express interest in a new drug, they are as likely to bury it as they are to develop it, especially if it threatened to compete with one of their existing product lines. We spoke to numerous consultants including former FDA lawyers, business lawyers and officers of other biotech companies who recommended that from a business perspective we would be better off if we considered looking at cosmetic or dietary supplement formulations. This view was confirmed after seeing what happened to companies like Shaman Pharmaceuticals and Procyte. Both of these excellent biotech firms initially pursued clinical development of their products only to be frustrated, and eventually, after spending tens of millions of dollars, opted for nutritional supplement and cosmetic formulations, respectively.

As we began to look into the possibilities of other approaches we encountered the FDA regulations concerning cosmetics and nutritional supplements that essentially prevent the presentation of scientific research in support of product claims. We were astounded to find a US agency openly violating the first amendment right of free speech. The FDA has seemingly made itself the sole arbiter of what may be said in the US regarding food and drugs. As we began to read about healthcare in the USA it became apparent that the situation involved other players as well as the FDA.

The FDA working with the drug companies and the medical establishment has become a major impediment to both disease prevention and novel drug development and the principal cause of the horrendous medical costs both the country as a whole, as well as individuals, must bear. It is necessary to develop legislation to totally revamp the way we approach healthcare in the USA. The current medical system is basically not functioning well in disease prevention or drug development, and has flaws in the area of treatment while still costing a fortune. We do not need to spend more on healthcare. Those payments are basically subsidies for the major drug companies. The medical establishment has become largely an insensitive entity more interested in treating disease than in preventing or curing it. Please consider the following points.

As discussed above, the FDA has made the new drug approval process so expensive in both dollars and time as to preclude all but a small private club of very large and wealthy multinational pharmaceutical companies. The costs for drug development in Japan are reportedly about 10% of those in the US. This is not impossible to believe given that the cost for development of a new drug for the US veterinarian market is between $0.25 and $2.0 million. This is 1% or less of the cost to develop a drug for human use. It should be possible to develop new drugs for human use for similar costs.

At one time the documentation for a new drug application (NDA) would fill one or two 3-ring notebooks. Today, because of the FDA's approach that more data is always better, it is possible to fill an entire tractor-trailer with FDA mandated documentation.

Despite the exponential increase in all this expensive documentation, the number of adverse drug reactions (ADRs) to new drugs has remained essentially constant for the past 32 years according to an article in the April 14th, 1998 issue of the Journal of American Medical Association. The authors Bruce H. Pomeranz, MD, PhD and his colleagues at the University of Toronto, observed that ADRs to FDA approved drugs account for more than 100,000 deaths a year and are between the 4th and 6th leading cause of death in the United States. If one includes errors of administration the death toll may be 140,000 people per year (*JAMA* Vol.277, No. 4, January 22/29 1997, pp.301–306). According to the *New England Journal of Medicine* (Vol. 339, No. 25, December 17, 1998, pgs. 1851–1854), "Overall 51% of [FDA] approved drugs have serious side effects not detected prior to approval." Clearly, the FDA has succeeded in driving up the costs for new drug development while providing no more safety than existed when the costs were a fraction of today's costs.

Unfortunately, a triumvirate has developed among the FDA, multinational drug firms and the established medical community that benefits from perpetuation of the current situation. The large pharmaceutical companies begin giving "gifts" to future doctors while in medical school. (When is a Gift Not a Gift?,

JAMA, January 19, 2000, Vol. 283, No. 3, pgs. 373–380). According to the *New York Times* (January 11, 1999, A1 "Fever Pitch: Getting Doctors to Prescribe is Big Business") over 6 billion dollars
are spent every year to "educate" doctors about the new drugs
developed by the large drug firms. The multinational drug companies also pay nearly $1 billion annually, in user fees to the FDA
(The Durk Pearson and Sandy Shaw Life Extension News, Vol. 3
No. 1, February 2000). As mentioned above, the costs for the
studies required by the FDA can really only be covered by the big
drug companies ensuring that the circle is complete.

The structure of the triumvirate is also such that what is
addressed is the treatment of disease—not prevention or cure.
The ideal drug product from the perspective of the large drug
companies is one that is used daily for the rest of a person's
life. For example, developing vaccines, unless needed yearly, is
not interesting financially. There has also been a major effort by
all the members of the triumvirate to restrict both information
about alternative and preventive medical approaches as well as
products such as nutritional supplements in the form of vitamins
and herbal products. Long before it became open knowledge that
the daily use of aspirin could lessen the chances of a heart attack
it had been documented in clinical studies that this was the case.
However, the FDA forbade manufacturers of aspirin from making
those claims. It has been estimated that as many as 800,000 lives
could have been saved over a 10 year period if this information
had not been kept hidden by the FDA (Interview with Durk and
Sandy, online at http://irc.lycaeum.org/~maverick/p&s.htm).

Another area that is truly absurd is the limitation the FDA
places on the claims that can be made for supplements that
pass through the intestinal tract. Although it has been shown
that there is often better adsorption of nutritional supplements
through the mucosal tissue in the mouth and nasal passages,
according to the FDA, these routes of administration turn a

dietary supplement into a drug. This goes under the heading of magic or perhaps madness. Likewise, although administration of many herbal remedies over the centuries has involved topical application of extracts, it is also forbidden by the FDA to make any claims if a supplement is applied to the skin. Again this regulation is clearly counterintuitive, but then the rules of logic do not seem to apply to FDA regulations.

The FDA, many doctors and the drug companies object to herbal and nutritional supplements arguing either that the herbalists and others are dishonest or that the reports are all anecdotal and have not been rigorously and scientifically shown to be beneficial. The FDA has therefore decreed that before any therapeutic claims can be made an herbal or supplement must be run through the FDA controlled $200—$500 million dollar drug approval processes. They also argue that people might forgo FDA approved medical treatment if they had ready access to alternative sources of medicinal treatment. Given the Adverse Drug Reaction data it could easily be argued that a person has a better chance at recovery and avoiding death if he or she avoids many of the FDA approved drugs. The former head of the FDA, Dr. Kessler asserted that, "The FDA should be the sole authority on health and nutrition." He also is reported to have said that if people were allowed to make health choices themselves there would be no need for the FDA. Exactly, and at that point people would have free access to information about ways to prevent many diseases, herbal and supplement therapies as well as novel approaches developed by innovative biotech firms, all for a fraction of the current healthcare costs. This brings up other points.

There are charlatans in every field, but that is hardly a reason for denying access to an entire area that has shown successes for several thousand years. Most medicines were initially derived from herbal remedies. After that most drugs were synthetic analogs of the compounds found in nature that appeared to be the

active component. Unfortunately, pulling out one specific ingredient from a complex mixture can result in a toxic medicine.
Many beneficial effects seen with herbal treatments may be the
result of the interactions of several components. It is only relatively recently that the central approach to new drug development has lost all touch with botanical and other natural sources
of medicines. The principal method of finding new drugs is to
screen tens of thousands of chemically synthesized compounds
in the hope of finding one that has the desired effect. As seen
above, however, they frequently have other undesirable effects,
such as death.

People are looking for non-allopathic medicinal solutions because
modern medicine has become insensitive and distant to the people
it ostensibly serves. Anyone knows this who has had the misfor-
tune of either being in a hospital or having a loved one in a hospital.
The alternatives frequently offered to people are a modern day
version of the pit and pendulum. Given the large number of
deaths due to adverse drug reactions, doctors, the FDA and the
large drug companies' assertion that people need to get these
treatments has a hollow self-serving ring. By contrast, there are
very few deaths that can be attributed to nutritional supplements
or herbal remedies.

If the costs for getting substances approved for medicinal use
were not so exorbitant it would be economically feasible to take
herbal treatments through the process. As it is, there are numerous excellent scientific studies showing both safety and efficacy
that have been done outside the FDA arena. However, the FDA
does not permit the inclusion of that data with the supplements.

There is a need for a new structure to handle drug development
in the 21st century, one that is more open and far less costly. It
might be well to restrict the FDA's activities to monitoring the
food supply. A variety of ideas have been put forth. Perhaps the
NIH and/or the CDC would establish standard tests for toxicity

and a toxicity scale of 1 to 10 that would be included on every drug/supplement. The NIH could review the results of the studies, and assign a score to the particular drug. The company sponsoring the drug would then be able to conduct clinical efficacy studies. The cost of taking a new compound or herbal through the pipeline could be reduced to 1% or less of the current costs.

If it were possible to freely pursue alternative approaches to medicinal therapies that would include a healthy dose of preventive efforts, and include herbal and other supplements, and also to develop and market new drugs at lower costs, the entire crisis in healthcare costs could fade away. To restructure the current system will require formation of a coalition of the various groups involved in non-traditional approaches, as well as those opposed to the current drug regulatory process. These groups must pool their resources and efforts, join together and work with those members of congress interested in addressing the healthcare crisis to pass the appropriate legislation. If this happens we could see a new age of reduced healthcare costs coupled with improved health and longer more productive lives.

SUMMARY

The FDA, Drug Companies and the medical community derive mutually rewarding financial and control benefits from the current system. The triumvirate seems determined to fight any changes that would jeopardize their respective positions.

The current system has proven to be ineffective and counterproductive. It fails to address prevention and seeks treatments rather than cures for diseases, treatments that are often more dangerous than proven alternatives.

The costs associated with the system do not afford protection of the public from dangerous drugs but simply serve to ensure control of the system by the large pharmaceuticals, the medical community and the FDA.

The system has and continues to cost the lives of over 100,000 people per year in the USA.

The FDA, large drug companies and the medical community are the principal reason for the enormous healthcare costs that threaten the financial and physical health of the country.

While offering no solutions, the trio aggressively opposes freedom of individuals to pursue their own healthcare and the dissemination of truthful non-misleading scientific information about alternative and traditional medicines.

The current FDA drug approval process is so outrageously expensive that it prevents all but the inner circle of large drug companies from developing new drugs as well as making it too expensive to demonstrate the value of traditional medicines not covered by patents.

RECOMMENDATIONS

- Limit the FDA's authority to monitoring the safety of food and delete all drug regulatory activities from their charter.
- Ask the National Institutes of Health to establish a standardized series of toxicity studies with relative toxicity ratings from 1 to 10. All dietary supplements and drugs would be required to be evaluated and rated by independent labs and marked on labels.
- Let the FTC continue to judge whether the claims made for a product are properly substantiated.

BENEFITS

- Reduced healthcare costs—through reduced development costs of drugs and the use of alternative herbal and nutritional supplements.
- Improved health through prevention of disease. This also reduces costs and improves the quality and length of people's lives.

■ A greater number of innovative drugs made available at far lower costs addressing not only the major diseases, but the aging process itself.

Sincerely,

Roderic M. K. Dale, PhD
CEO, Oligos Etc., Inc.

FDA Seeks to Destroy Alternative Health Websites

by William Faloon

THE FDA'S HISTORY IS ONE OF INCOMPETENCE, FRAUD, DECEIT and the continuous striving for more power. Over the past 25 years, the Food and Drug Administration has sought to gain authoritarian control that Congress never intended it to have. In every attempt to seize this kind of power, the FDA has been beaten back by a swell of public protest.

The FDA has just launched a disinformation campaign to deceive Congress into believing that the agency needs to "protect" the public from health information on the Internet. The FDA is seeking ten million tax dollars a year to attack alternative health and pharmacy websites. If the FDA convinces Congress to give it the power and money to do this, American consumers will be denied access to innovative therapies, and will be forced to pay a good deal more for the nutrient and drug therapies the FDA allows them to buy over the Internet.

One of the FDA's proposals is to be able to fine Internet pharmacies $500,000 every time they dispense a drug without a prescription authorized by the agency. With this kind of excessive fining power, the FDA will be able to bankrupt any online pharmacy it targets. To make it easy for them to shut down large numbers of websites, the FDA wants the power to issue subpoenas without first obtaining a court order, a totalitarian tactic the American public revolted against when the agency proposed it in 1990. Finally, the FDA says it wants to set up a "rapid response team" to identify, investigate and prosecute websites. In other words, the FDA is seeking to establish an army of cyberspace storm troopers to enable it to shut down large numbers of websites quickly.

The FDA is using the free-flowing popularity of the Internet in a ploy to deceive Congress into appropriating ten million tax dollars a year to fund an unconstitutional witch hunt against free speech. The new powers the FDA is seeking are blatantly un-American and resemble the kinds of police-state tactics employed by totalitarian regimes such as communist China.

The alleged purpose of these new powers is to "target and punish those who engage in illegal drug sales over the Internet." This may sound reasonable to the average person, but as members of the Life Extension Foundation well know, the FDA's history is one of ineptitude and corruption that has caused millions of Americans to suffer and die needlessly. In 1994, the FDA Museum was established to document FDA malfeasance, and show that the agency hasn't the scientific legitimacy to be allowed to police the healthcare of the American people.

A flagrant example of FDA deception can be found in their current attempt to control the Internet. The FDA has identified one person who died after obtaining Viagra® from a web pharmacy without a prescription. The FDA is using this one death as an example of why the FDA needs to impose dictatorial power over all health websites. One problem with this position is that, as of November 1998, at least 130 Americans died from taking Viagra® legally prescribed by their doctors. (The total number of Viagra®-related deaths for 1999 has not yet been calculated.) The FDA approved Viagra® as being safe, even though many Americans have died when the drug has been legally prescribed. The FDA failed to detect the lethal side effects of Viagra®, yet it is now seeking gestapo-like power to attack any Internet health company it wishes to, without due process.

WHY INTERNET REGULATION IS DOOMED TO FAIL

The powers the FDA is seeking are unconstitutional, and the agency has neither the competence nor the integrity to police the Internet, but even if it did, it would be impractical for the agency to do so. There are currently an estimated 8,000 health sites on the Internet. If Congress gives the FDA $10 million a year, the best the agency could do is shut down a couple of hundred sites a year. Within a few years, the FDA would create a litigation monster whose appetite would far exceed their $10 million annual budget. The FDA would be bogged down in a quagmire of judicial proceedings, while thousands of new health websites would be springing up that the agency would be at an utter loss to control.

The end result of the FDA's war against the free flow of information on the Internet would be tens of millions of tax dollars wasted, with less so-called consumer "protection" than exists today.

THE FDA ALREADY HAS THE LEGAL POWER IT NEEDS

The charade the FDA is parading before Congress is that they need more money and stricter laws to regulate e-commerce. The facts are that the FDA already has the regulatory structure to "protect" the consumer on the Internet. Much of what the FDA wants is already covered by existing Federal and State law, but the agency is seeking to add another bureaucratic layer of law and money to suppress the dissemination of health information.

AN ALTERNATIVE PROPOSAL

The FDA has its own website (www.fda.gov). For a fraction of the cost of becoming the health police of the Internet, the agency could post its own evaluation of alternative health websites that it thought were promoting fraudulent or dangerous products. Americans would then be free to make their own decisions about whether to believe what the FDA says about health websites. However, the FDA has no interest in trying to persuade Americans with evidence. It wants (and has always wanted) authoritarian powers and as much money as possible from Congress because it is a political organization rather than a scientific one. As a result, FDA suppression of information has been, historically, the leading cause of death in the United States, while adverse reactions to FDA approved drugs is currently the 4th to 6th leading cause of death. Clearly, the FDA lacks the constitutional authority, the competence, the integrity or the scientific credibility to be given additional power and money to police the Internet.

1999

Encore! The FDA Suffers Another Legal Defeat

by William Faloon

THE FDA'S NINE-YEAR STRING OF LOSSES IN THE FEDERAL Courts continues unabated. In a First Amendment lawsuit filed by the Washington Legal Foundation, a US District Court ruled that drug makers can give doctors copies of published medical studies that highlight the use of their drugs for diseases not approved by the Food and Drug Administration. The FDA had sought to severely restrict drug companies from doing that.

This July 28, 1999 ruling gives pharmaceutical companies the ability to promote drugs for unapproved uses. The FDA should not be allowed to suppress the dissemination of information that appears in peer-reviewed scientific journals. While this is considered a major victory for drug companies, it's also great news for American citizens who may now learn more quickly about innovative therapies that could be used to save their lives.

US District Judge Royce Lamberth ruled that the Food and Drug Modernization Act illegally restricts the free speech of drug companies. He termed government arguments defending the limits "preposterous." Under the judge's ruling, the studies the companies provide to doctors cannot be false or misleading and drug company salespeople must disclose any association between the company and researcher. Further, the company must disclose whether the treatment detailed in the studies are FDA approved.

The FDA wanted the authority to review (i.e. censor) published studies before companies could give them to doctors. Regulators also wanted the power to require drug makers to give doctors additional studies on the drug. And, the FDA wanted companies to only distribute studies of drugs when the firms were already in the federal review process for the additional uses. The Court made it clear that censorship of free speech will not be tolerated.

The FDA has previously filed criminal indictments against Foundation leaders William Faloon and Saul Kent alleging that they committed "criminal acts" by promoting both approved and unapproved drugs for "unapproved uses." While these criminal indictments were eventually dismissed by the government, the fact that the FDA is willing to jail its political opponents sends a chilling message to pioneering doctors and scientists who are seeking to make major medical advances available to dying Americans.

This ruling represents a major victory for the free speech provisions of the First Amendment and against FDA censorship.

Cancer-Causing Drug Tamoxifen Approved for Healthy Women

by William Faloon

D ESPITE WHAT YOU MIGHT HAVE HEARD, THE USE OF TAMOXI-
fen for breast cancer prevention is highly controversial. Its
long term effects on healthy women are unknown, while
tamoxifen's cancer-causing properties raise considerable concern.

In a stunning move, the Food and Drug Administration
approved the use of tamoxifen (Nolvadex®) chemotherapy for
healthy women with no evidence of breast cancer. The approval
came after almost two decades of wrangling over research that
cost American taxpayers hundreds of millions of dollars, created
fraud, prompted a congressional hearing, and spanned great controversy. The FDA's decision—announced on October 30, 1998—
allows Zeneca Pharmaceuticals to tap into a market potentially

worth 36 billion dollars annually. The decision allowing the drug to be sold for breast cancer prevention was made despite objections from women's health organizations and researchers around the world. When the advisory committee recommending approval was asked whether the tamoxifen prevention study demonstrated that the drug had "a favorable benefit-risk ratio for the prevention of breast cancer in women at increased risk as defined by the study population," it said "no" unanimously. Yet, the FDA approved tamoxifen for healthy women anyway.

Tamoxifen is a synthetic estrogen blocker—one of many that have been around since the early '70s that once had potential as birth control pills. Like diethylstilbestrol (DES) tamoxifen blocks estradiol, but also like DES, it has estrogenic properties that cause cells to grow. Despite its dual personality, tamoxifen has been successfully used to prevent recurrence of breast cancer in women who are estrogen-receptor positive.

Using tamoxifen in cancer patients is one thing; using it in healthy women is another. Tamoxifen is a well-known carcinogen which causes DNA strand breaks. This is an accepted feature of standard chemotherapy where the overriding concern is to keep cancer cells from growing. Carcinogens have not traditionally been an accepted part of preventive medicine, however. The FDA's decisions to allow the sale of tamoxifen and certain cholesterol-lowering drugs (notably the peroxisome inhibitors clofibrate and gemfibrozil) to healthy people marks the first time that drugs with cancer-causing potential have been approved as health enhancements. This marks a dangerous new trend in drug approval.

The paucity of data makes the approval of tamoxifen for prevention particularly questionable. Approval was based on a single study run at various hospitals around the United States under the auspices of the National Cancer Institute (NCI). An outgrowth of the "National Surgical Adjuvant Breast and Bowel Project"

(NSABP) begun in the '80s, the study was about 10 years shy of producing any meaningful information, according to one expert. Two similar European studies reported no preventive effect of tamoxifen. The FDA rejected these studies as irrelevant because they were too small (3500 people combined).

THE HYPE

There was no statistical difference in survival for the women taking tamoxifen versus women taking placebo in the NCI study. The justification for Zeneca's claim of a 50% reduction in breast cancer lies in the difference between a 1.4% incidence of cancer in women taking tamoxifen versus a 2.7% incidence in those taking placebo. The price of that 1.3% difference was very dear. Tamoxifen doubled the risk of endometrial cancer for women under 50. It quadrupled it in women over 50.

In short, what a healthy woman over 50 got when she took tamoxifen was a proven four times higher risk of endometrial cancer in return for an unknown amount of risk reduction for breast cancer in the short term. And that's not all. Thirty-five tamoxifen-takers developed blood clots in the lung, and three of them died. The risk of cataracts was doubled, and almost half the women participating rated the side effects as "quite a bit or extremely bothersome." Technically, tamoxifen also doubled the risk of suicide (two on tamoxifen versus one on placebo). Worth it? Well, there was a 0.4% reduced risk of a certain type of bone fracture.

OTHER STUDIES FIND NO BENEFIT

Two European studies reported interim findings about the same time as the NCI study, which wrapped up early. Both found no preventive effect of tamoxifen in healthy women. The authors of the NCI study devoted considerable space to discrediting these two European trials. One of the studies was conducted at the Royal Marsden Hospital in England; the other at the European

Institute of Oncology in Italy. Together, these two studies had more women on tamoxifen much longer than the American study where only 25% of the participants took the drug five years or longer. Unlike the American study which was halted before long-term effects could be discovered, these studies are ongoing so as to get a picture of what tamoxifen does in the long run. Although both the advisory committee and the FDA dismissed them as unimportant, the studies have in fact produced new information about tamoxifen.

It appears that women who take hormone replacement therapy plus tamoxifen may have some benefit. However, some of the data indicate that if a woman took hormone replacement therapy before she entered the study, she is at higher risk for breast cancer. This hints at the yet unexplored interaction between tamoxifen and synthetic estrogens in the environment, including synthetic hormone replacement therapy. At present, no one knows what happens when a synthetic estrogen blocker with estrogenic potential is given to women exposed to synthetic estrogens.

TAMOXIFEN-INDUCED CANCER

While no conclusions can be drawn from the study on whether tamoxifen can prevent breast cancer, conclusions can be drawn about tamoxifen's ability to cause endometrial cancer. About a thousand published studies deal with tamoxifen and endometrial (or uterine) cancer. An analysis of several large studies shows that tamoxifen approximately doubles a woman's risk for uterine cancer when used for one to two years, and quadruples it at five years. While this may be an acceptable risk for women diagnosed with breast cancer (or a woman without a uterus), it is an unacceptable risk for healthy women with no evidence of cancer.

Tamoxifen is also associated with stomach and colorectal cancer. Some data indicates that prior treatment with hormones adds to this risk. What is especially chilling is the likelihood that the risk of cancer with tamoxifen may be a function of total life-time dose. In other words, the longer you take it, the higher the risk. Women taking tamoxifen longer than five years are reported to have a high incidence of various cancers. Despite the statistics Dr. Norman Wolmark, head of the study, advises women to start taking tamoxifen as soon as they discover they are at high risk for breast cancer. Don't wait, he urges. Age thirty-five has been designated as the age to start worrying.

PUTTING A FACE ON APPROVAL

One might ask why tamoxifen was approved when so many serious questions remain. The FDA didn't approve tamoxifen by itself. It had help from a group known as an "advisory committee." By law, advisory committee members are not supposed to have financial interests in the company that manufactures the drug they're advising on. In addition, advisory committees are supposed to be made up of people with "diverse professional education, training and experience." This is so that they bring different points of view to the table. In recent years, advisory committees have recommended approval for a number of dangerous drugs. The public should be aware that participants in the approval process are frequently paid consultants to drug companies.

The committee that endorsed tamoxifen was composed of 11 people, eight of whom are doctors who routinely test emo-therapies. Some, including Richard L. Schilsky, Derek Raghavan and Robert F. Ozols, accept grants from drug companies. Others such as Kim A. Margolin, Kathy S. Albain and Janice P. Dutcher test chemotherapeutic drugs with taxpayer money through the National Cancer Institute (NCI).

The tamoxifen committee represented very little diversity. Its role as an independent body was also questionable. Ozols and Schilsky have both collaborated on studies with doctors who conducted the tamoxifen study. One of the committee members,

Richard Simon, works at the National Cancer Institute, which conducted the study.

Simon is a typical example of the type of person currently sitting on advisory committees. A statistician by training, Simon's forte is number crunching—not breast cancer.

In the past, Simon argued for not stopping trials early. In an editorial published in the *Journal of Clinical Oncology*, he used the example of clofibrate to illustrate his point. (Clofibrate is a cholesterol-lowering drug whose effects appeared promising during the early stages of the Coronary Drug Project. If the study had been prematurely stopped, as the tamoxifen study was, the real picture would not have emerged: clofibrate is no better than placebo in reducing heart-related mortality. By the end of the study it was shown that clofibrate caused a 44% increased mortality from cancer and other causes). Studies must not be stopped early, Simon argued. His pen-and-ink arguments melted away, however, when it came to tamoxifen, which he supported.

The public expects committee members to be impartial. Yet before he ever sat on the tamoxifen committee, Simon had attacked data showing tamoxifen causes increased risk of colorectal and stomach cancer. The motivation for the attack is not known. He failed to respond to a request to clarify his position.

FRAUDULENT STUDIES

The study on which tamoxifen was approved for healthy women has a lurid history. A surgeon named Bernard Fisher was the driving force behind tamoxifen's approval as a preventative agent. Fisher began conducting studies on tamoxifen in the early '80s under the taxpayer-funded NSABP. The project, which he headed, was receiving about $18M a year in federal money when NCI decided to spend $68M to see whether tamoxifen would prevent breast cancer. Fisher was to coordinate the massive project which began in 1992.

In 1990, it was discovered that a doctor participating in NSABP trials had falsified data for 99 people enrolled in 14 breast cancer studies that preceded the prevention trials. Fisher was accused of not reporting the falsification, then using the data in an article published in the *New England Journal of Medicine*. In 1993, it was discovered that secretaries in charge of enrolling women at a hospital participating in the breast cancer prevention trial had manufactured data. One of them was receiving $250 a head for each woman she enrolled. The fraud was discovered during a routine audit, and Fisher's office was notified. Apparently Fisher buried the report and never told NCI. A few months later, a woman named Hazel Cunningham, who wanted to enroll in the tamoxifen prevention trial, discovered that the consent form being used by Fisher didn't inform women about the true number of uterine cancer deaths occurring in the cancer trials. She filed a petition to stop the trials.

Representative John Dingell began congressional hearings into the NSABP, and Fisher was stripped of his position. The trials were halted. Although Fisher refused to appear at hearing—citing medical problems—he had enough fortitude to file lawsuits against five federal agencies, their directors, and the University of Pittsburgh. A federal judge threw out the case against the agencies in 1996. After much wrangling Fisher, who admitted knowing about the fraudulent data but felt the study would have been hurt if he eliminated it, was exonerated by an investigative arm of the Department of Health and Human Services which has been accused of favoring bigwig researchers. His case against the University of Pittsburgh was settled, and he was ultimately paid money and reinstated on the study. A judge also ordered the NCI to quit flagging his research as unreliable.

FDA REVIEW FALLS SHORT

In light of all that had occurred, the FDA had valid reasons to carefully review all the data from the prevention trial. It did not.

In fact, the agency may have set a record for fast review. According to Dr. Susan Honig who was in charge, the FDA received the final data on tamoxifen on August 4th, four weeks before the advisory committee hearing on September 2nd. Originally, the FDA was sent submissions missing crucial data. According to the transcript of the advisory committee hearing, the agency reviewed 625 of the 6681 case report forms of the women who got tamoxifen. (Case report forms are the actual record of what occurred to the patient, as filled out by healthcare workers who actually interacted with her. This is distinct from data summaries created by the drug manufacturer). Reviewing case forms is important, as numerous investigators on drug trials have been caught falsifying data. Given that it was already known that data had been falsified in tamoxifen trials, it would seem crucial for the FDA to review a substantial number of the case report forms. Instead, it held a committee meeting four weeks after receiving data from the trial, and announced its approval four weeks later.

COMMITTEE REJECTS MONITORING OF WOMEN ON TAMOXIFEN

One might wonder how a committee that refused to endorse the statement that tamoxifen has a favorable risk/benefit ratio for the prevention of breast cancer would ultimately approve tamoxifen for the prevention of breast cancer. The answer lies in semantics. A review of the record shows that the committee refused to use the word "prevention" but reframed the issues until they could recommend approval. The actual recommendation of the committee is that tamoxifen be approved for the "risk reduction of the short-term incidence of breast cancer in women at increased risk as defined by the study population." Despite the refusal of the committee to recommend tamoxifen for prevention, the American Cancer Society and the media immediately hailed tamoxifen as a breast cancer prevention drug.

And despite evidence that tamoxifen causes endometrial cancer, the committee rejected advising women to undergo endometrial testing while on tamoxifen. During the discussion among committee members, George W. Sledge Jr., a drug researcher, stated his belief that such testing would be nothing more than an employment act for OB-GYNs. The committee agreed with Sledge and voted not to warn women to have endometrial testing. They also nixed yearly eye examinations for cataracts. The issue of warning women about blood clots never came up, although the committee felt the FDA should ask someone to look into it further.

After the committee finished with tamoxifen, they went on to another hearing about the drug, Herceptin. Drs. Schilsky and Raghavan's conflicts-of-interest were duly noted for the record.

Further Reading

Bern HA. "The fragile fetus" in Chemically-induced alterations in sexual and functional development: the wildlife/human connection. Theo Colborn and Coralie Clement, Eds., part of Advances in modern environmental toxicology, M.A. Mehlman, Ed. (1992, *Princeton Scientific*: Princeton).

"Code of Federal Regulations," Title 21, Volume 1, Part 14, Subpart E, Sec. 14.80 and Subpart A, Sec. 14.1.

Comoglio A, et al. 1996. Effect of tamoxifen feeding on metabolic activation of tamoxifen by the liver of the rhesus monkey: does liver accumulation of inhibitory metabolites protect from tamoxifen-dependent genotoxicity and cancer? *Carcinogenesis* 17:1687–93.

Fisher B, et al. 1994. Endometrial cancer in tamoxifen-treated breast cancer patients: findings from the National Surgical Adjuvant Breast and Bowel Project (NSABP) B-14. *J Natl Cancer Inst* 86:527–37.

Fisher B, et al. 1998. Tamoxifen for prevention of breast cancer: report of the national surgical adjuvant breast and bowel project p-1 study.

J Natl Cancer Inst 90:1371–1388. Gail MH, et al. 1989. Projecting individualized probabilities of developing breast cancer for white females who are being examined annually.

J Natl Cancer Inst 81:1879–86. Guillot C, et al. 1996. Alteration of p53 damage response by tamoxifen treatment. *Clin Cancer Res* 2:1439–44.

Hemminki K, et al. 1996. Tamoxifen-induced DNA adducts in endometrial samples from breast cancer patients [see comments]. *Cancer Res* 56:4374–7.

Kedar RP, et al. 1994. Effects of tamoxifen on uterus and ovaries of postmenopausal women in a randomised breast cancer prevention trial [see comments]. *Lancet* 343(8909):1318–21.

Li D, et al. 1997. Effects of chronic administration of tamoxifen and toremifene on DNA adducts in rat liver, kidney and uterus. *Cancer Res* 57:1438–41.

McGonigle KF, et al. 1998. Abnormalities detected on transvaginal ultrasonography in tamoxifen-treated postmenopausal breast cancer patients may represent endometrial cystic atrophy.

Am J Obstet Gynecol 178:1145–50. Nephew KP, et al. 1996. Tamoxifen-induced proto-oncogene expression persists in uterine endometrial epithelium. *Endocrinol* 137:219–24.

Ogawa Y, et al. 1998. Tamoxifen-induced fatty liver in patients with breast cancer [letter]. *Lancet* 351(9104):725.

Okubo T, et al. 1998. DNA cleavage and 8-hydroxydeoxyguanosine formation caused by tamoxifen derivatives in vitro. *Cancer Lett* 122:9–15.

Powell-Jones W, et al. 1975. Influence of anti-oestrogens on the specific binding in vitro of (3H)oestradiol by cytosol of rat mammary tumours and human breast carcinomata. *Biochem J* 150:71–5.

Powles T, et al. 1998. Interim analysis of the incidence of breast cancer in the Royal Marsden Hospital tamoxifen randomised chemoprevention trial see comments]. *Lancet* 352(91 22):98–1 01.

Rutgvist LE, et al. 1995. Adjuvant tamoxifen therapy for early stage breast cancer and second primary malignancies. *J Natl Cancer Inst* 87:645–51.

Shuibutani S, et al. 1997. Miscoding potential of tamoxifen-derived DNA adducts: alpha-(N2-deoxyguanosinyl) tamoxifen. *Biochem* 36:13010–17.

Simon R. 1995. Discovering the truth about tamoxifen: problems of multiplicity in statistical evaluation of biomedical data. *J Natl Cancer Inst* 87:627–29.

Smith MA, et al. 1997. Role of independent data-monitoring committees in randomized clinical trials sponsored by the National Cancer Institute.

J Clin Oncol 15:2736–43. Vancutsem PM, et al. 1994. Frequent and specific mutations of the rat p53 gene in eptocarcinomas induced by tamoxifen. *Cancer Res* 54:3864–7.

Veronesi U, et al. 1998. Prevention of breast cancer with tamoxifen: preliminary findings from the Italian randomised trial among hysterectomized women. Italian tamoxifen prevention study [see comments]. *Lancet* 352(9122):93–7.

Wilking N, et al. 1991. Breast cancer prevention with tamoxifen: results from a randomized trial in early breast cancer (meeting abstract). *Proc Annu Am Soc Clin Oncol* 10:A58.

Zimniski SJ, et al. 1993. Induction of tamoxifen-dependent rat mammary tumors. *Cancer Res* 53:2937–39.

MAY 1999

The Plague of FDA Regulation

by William Faloon

EW PEOPLE REALIZE HOW LONG IT TAKES BEFORE A SCIENTIFIC breakthrough turns into a life-saving therapy. The bureaucratic process is so burdensome that the total time from discovery to market approval has more than doubled since 1964, from 6.5 years to 14.8 years.[1]

One might think that this delay is at least providing Americans with safe medicines. The facts tell otherwise. This month's issue exposes a drug-approval system riddled with incompetence and corruption that results in the death of over 125,000 Americans every year from drugs the FDA says are safe. The current system provides a protected market for pharmaceutical giants who can afford to pay top dollar to get their drugs legalized in this country. As in any market that is artificially protected, innovation is stifled and the consumer pays a grossly inflated price for the final product.

The United States government officially endorses unfettered competition in the marketplace, yet when it comes to medicines, there is no free market. The revolving door between the FDA and multinational drug companies creates a system that excludes outsiders, and virtually ensures that Americans only have access to drugs guaranteed to make billions for large companies. The recent trend is for companies to develop "life-enhancing" drugs, such as Viagra®, at the expense of life-saving drugs that may return less profit. The FDA takes extraordinary steps to keep out foreign competition, even if the offshore drug is safer, cheaper, and more effective than its American counterpart. The net result is that Americans pay the highest prices in the world for pharmaceuticals. At the same time, we suffer the highest rate of drug-induced adverse reactions, in as much as deaths from prescription drugs are the fifth or sixth leading cause of death in the United States.[2] Inflated prices for bad products reflect a system that is corrupt and must be changed if Americans are to live healthier and longer.

Drug manufacturers criticize the FDA for the delay and high cost of getting new drugs through the system. One statistic drug companies point to is that from 1977 to 1996, they increased spending on new pharmaceutical compounds 15-fold, yet FDA approval of new drugs remained relatively flat.[3] Additional problems cited by the drug industry include turnover of FDA personnel, limitations of drug reviewers' technical knowledge and communication problems between the FDA and the drug companies.[4] However, large pharmaceutical companies are by no means innocent victims of FDA red tape.

All of this points to a bureaucratic quagmire that enables large drug companies to dominate the market, making it far too expensive for smaller companies to compete. But in a deregulated market, where economic success is predicated on a company developing effective products at a fair price, companies that make unsafe or ineffective products would be driven out of business, and Americans would soon gain access to more advanced medicines to prevent and treat the degenerative diseases of aging.

References

1. Advancing Medical Innovation: Health, Safety and the Role of Government in the 21st Century. *The Progress and Freedom Foundation,* 1996.

2. The *Journal of the American Medical Association (JAMA),* April 15, 1998.

3. *Science* (1998:May).

4. University of California at San Diego study (1997).

The FDA Versus Folic Acid

by William Faloon

THE FDA ARGUES AGAINST FOLIC ACID SUPPLEMENTATION because the presence of folic acid in the blood could mask a serious vitamin B12 deficiency. But the *Journal of the American Medical Association* (Dec. 18, 1996) noted that folic acid supplements fortified with vitamin B12 would be a prudent way of gaining the cardiovascular benefits of folic acid without risking a B12 deficiency. In addition, the April 9, 1998, issue of the *New England Journal of Medicine* endorses folic acid as a means of reducing the incidence of heart attack and stroke. Nevertheless, the FDA refuses to accept that folic acid has any benefit other than preventing a certain type of birth defect.

In fact, it took the FDA more than 30 years to even acknowledge that folic acid prevents neural tube birth defects. Tens of thousands of deformed babies have been born because the FDA prohibited claims that pregnant women should take folic acid. When former Commissioner David Kessler was confronted with overwhelming evidence that women of childbearing age should supplement with folic acid, he responded in an NBC interview, "The quandary we're in at the Food and Drug Administration is how to make folic acid available to women of childbearing age, but not put it in excessive amounts in the food supply for other populations such as teenage boys or elderly people."

A newly released study shows just how fatally flawed the FDA's position is. Data from the famous Nurses' Health Study conducted at the Harvard Medical School show that long-term supplementation with folic acid reduces the risk of colon cancer in women by an astounding 75%. The fact that there are 90,000 women participating in the study makes this finding especially significant. The authors explain that folic acid obtained from supplements had a stronger protective effect against colon cancer than folic acid consumed in the diet.

The Nurses' Health Study also demonstrates that the degree of protection against cancer is correlated with how long a dna-protecting substance (such as folic acid) is consumed. The women who took more than 400 micrograms of folic acid a day for 15 years experienced the 75% reduction in colon cancer; short-term supplementation produced only marginal protection.

There now exists a massive body of evidence that supplementation with folic acid can prevent both cardiovascular disease and cancer, yet the FDA has proposed rules that would prohibit the American public from even learning about these benefits. Colon cancer will kill 47,000 Americans this year. Too bad the FDA didn't allow these colon cancer victims to learn of folic acid in time.

Further Reading

Folate prevents colon cancer: *Annals of Internal Medicine*, 1998; 129:517–524

Folate prevents cardiovascular disease: *JAMA*, 1993, Dec 8: 2693–2698 & 2726–2727

Folate protects against DNA damage: *Proc of the Nat Academy of Sciences*, 1997 94(7):3290–5

Folate protects against dna damage: *Baillieres Clinical Hematology*, 1995, 8(3):461-78

Folate protects against birth defects: "Folates and the Fetus." *Lancet*, Feb 26, 1977, p 462

Folate metabolism in pregnancy: *Am J Obstetrics and Gynecology*, 1967 99:638–648

Folate deficiency & oral contraceptives: *JAMA*, 1970 214:105–1 08, 1970

Folate deficiency in mental patients: *British J Psychiatry* 113:241–251, 1967

1998

FDA Regulation: At Odds—*Again*—with Your Health Freedom

by William Faloon

THE FDA HAS NOW PROPOSED NEW RULES, DESIGNED TO enforce DSHEA, that would prohibit Americans from learning about certain types of medical information.

The FDA's proposed rules say that consumers can be told about how a vitamin affects the "structure or function" of the body, but that any reference to how the vitamin affects specific diseases will be classified as illegal speech. If the FDA's proposed rules become law, most consumers will not be able to find out about the nutrients they need to prevent, mitigate or treat any disease.

Examples of what the FDA has proclaimed to be illegal speech include such descriptions of benefits as "reduces nausea associated with chemotherapy," "protects against cancer," and "treats hot flashes." In other words, specific treatments for specific ill-nesses. But that is often exactly why consumers turn to natural, alternative therapies.

For example, since the FDA contends it's illegal to suggest any-thing but drugs to reduce nausea associated with chemotherapy, it would also be illegal to recommend coenzyme Q10 and vitamin E to reduce chemotherapy-induced heart muscle damage, melatonin to reduce chemotherapy-induced immune system damage, and N-acetylcysteine to reduce chemotherapy-induced liver damage.

The FDA is proposing that cancer patients be denied informa-tion about how to protect their hearts, livers, guts and immune systems against the lethal effects of FDA-approved chemother-apy drugs. These new proposed rules mandate suffering for cancer patients. They are not only immoral, they are blatantly unconstitutional.

Life Extension vs. the FDA a Hollow Victory: Why the Agency's Approval of Ribavirin is Inadequate

by William Faloon

THE US FOOD AND DRUG ADMINISTRATION HAS JUST approved ribavirin for the treatment of hepatitis C. Ribavirin is a drug that could save about 5,000 lives a year. However, 60,000 hepatitis C victims already have died while waiting for this drug to be approved, and many more Americans will perish because the FDA has only approved it for limited use. This is not the typical story about the FDA being too slow to approve lifesaving drugs. The circumstances surrounding this drug include several criminal investigations, felony indictments, stock market manipulation, squandered tax dollars, FDA agents traveling to Europe, contamination of the nation's blood supply and lots of dead Americans.

The events began in the early 1980s, at a Southern California research laboratory, where scientists made the unique discovery that ribavirin, then sold in Mexico, could cure feline leukemia. Since ribavirin was able to eradicate the feline leukemia virus, the scientists began taking ribavirin themselves when they contracted the flu and, in most cases, their flu symptoms disappeared within 24 to 48 hours.

This was no ordinary research laboratory. It was partially funded by the Life Extension Foundation, which meant that when the discovery was made, Foundation members learned about it quickly. In 1986, the Foundation recommended that members with serious viral diseases travel to Mexico to buy ribavirin, or order it from offshore mail order companies. The FDA did not like this (and similar recommendations we made) and, in 1991, the Foundation's officers were indicted on 28 criminal counts of conspiring to import unapproved drugs into the United States.

About the same time, the FDA also launched a criminal investigation against the New York Stock Exchange company, ICN Pharmaceuticals, that owned ribavirin, for the "crime" of promoting the use of ribavirin in adults. The FDA viewed this action as criminal because at that time it had approved ribavirin only to treat a viral infection that affects infants. Thus, ICN was charged with promoting an "unapproved" (for adults, that is) drug.

The FDA asked the Justice Department to impanel a federal grand jury to see if ICN officials should be charged with criminal misconduct. Shortly thereafter, the Securities and Exchange Commission also launched an investigation to determine if ICN had committed securities fraud by promoting ribavirin's antiviral effects.

To avoid a felony indictment and avert financial disaster, ICN entered into a consent agreement to stop promoting ribavirin.

The FDA scored a temporary victory by keeping ribavirin out of the hands of adults.

The FDA, however, was facing some serious problems of its own. Tens of thousands of Americans were contracting viral diseases from blood transfusions, and investigative reporters exposed the fact that the FDA had failed to protect the nation's blood supply. Of course, the media failed to appreciate that the FDA had kept itself busy by conducting record-breaking numbers of raids against vitamin companies, seizing personal-use shipments of drugs like ribavirin in the mails, and trying to throw people in jail for selling ribavirin to adults.

Not only was the FDA failing to inspect blood banks, but it also was dramatically reducing the number of food safety inspections. Meanwhile, tens of thousands of Americans continued to die from viral diseases that ribavirin was curing in other countries.

During this entire period, studies were appearing in major medical journals showing that ribavirin is effective against a wide range of viral diseases. Health ministries throughout the world were approving ribavirin as a broad-spectrum anti-viral drug. What made the FDA's stonewalling so serious was that there was no effective anti-viral drug approved in the US. Elderly people affected with influenza either got better on their own or died.

Influenza kills as many as 60,000 (mostly elderly) Americans in a bad year, and ribavirin stops many influenza viruses from replicating. While Third World countries were using ribavirin to treat their citizens infected with influenza, hepatitis and other viral diseases, American citizens were dying from these same diseases.

The irony is that many hepatitis C patients contracted their disease from contaminated blood that the FDA was supposed to have inspected. Rather than properly regulating blood banks, FDA bureaucrats choose instead to squander the agency's resources in an attempt to deny access to a drug (ribavirin) that could have saved the lives of hepatitis C patients.

Many of the hepatitis C patients who could have been saved by ribavirin are not dead yet, but their livers have suffered severe damage. While the FDA stonewalled the approval of ribavirin, these patients faced a significant risk of developing cirrhosis or liver cancer.

The Life Extension Foundation never stopped informing its members about the anti-viral benefits of ribavirin. The criminal indictments against the Foundation's officers were dismissed in 1995 at the request of the Justice Department, but the FDA continued to harass Americans who imported ribavirin for their own personal use.

In 1997, FDA agents managed to convince European health ministries to raid companies that were shipping ribavirin to Americans for personal use...even though ribavirin was approved for sale to European citizens. the Foundation responded by launching a massive communications campaign to inform the public that the FDA had taken draconian steps to deny hepatitis C patients access to a drug that was shown to be a highly effective treatment against the disease when combined with interferon.

The most significant study shows that ribavirin combined with interferon is 10 times more effective in treating hepatitis C than interferon alone. The FDA's response was to instigate more raids against companies in Europe shipping ribavirin to Americans, thus condemning many hepatitis C patients to the permanent liver damage that often results in disability and death. (Do not use ribavirin to treat HIV infection. While some studies show it to be effective, there are better anti-viral drug combinations that are specific to HIV.)

The economic cost to the Foundation for fighting for the approval of this one drug was enormous. Full page ads were taken out in newspapers, thousands of press releases were sent to the media, and hundreds of thousands of first-class letters were mailed urging Foundation supporters to protest the FDA's

actions. the Foundation went so far as to produce and repeatedly air a half-hour TV infomercial attacking the FDA for failing
to approve ribavirin and other lifesaving drugs that were already
approved in other countries.

After 12 long years of battling the FDA, and after the needless,
premature death of at least 430,000 Americans, ribavirin was
finally approved this past June. There still remains a significant
problem, however: The FDA has restricted the use of ribavirin
(sold in the US under the name Rebetol®) only to chronic hepatitis C patients who first fail to benefit from interferon alone.

Approximately four million Americans are chronically infected
with the hepatitis C virus, according to the Centers for Disease
Control. The CDC has estimated that 20 to 50 percent of chronically infected hepatitis C patients will develop liver cirrhosis,
and 20 to 30 percent of those will go on to develop liver cancer
or liver failure requiring a liver transplant. Hepatitis C infection
contributes to the deaths of 8,000 to 10,000 Americans every
year. This toll is expected to triple by 2010 and exceed the number of annual deaths due to AIDS.

Nevertheless, the FDA has mandated that hepatitis C patients
must first fail a grueling six month therapy period with recombinant interferon-alpha before they can try the ribavirin-plus-
interferon combination therapy that is proven to work 10 times
better than interferon by itself. The maker of ribavirin is peti-
tioning the FDA to allow more hepatitis patients to have access
to ribavirin.

The FDA's recent approval of ribavirin is a hollow victory. After
battling FDA bureaucrats for 12 years, most Americans are still
being denied access to this lifesaving drug. Some people are actually applauding the FDA for approving ribavirin so fast.

In December 1997, massive political pressure forced the FDA
to put ribavirin on the "fast-track," and seven months later, the
FDA said that some hepatitis C patients can now use the drug

legally. Somehow the 430,000 Americans who died waiting for FDA approval of the drug were forgotten.

A study published in the April 15, 1998, issue of the *Journal of the American Medical Association* (*JAMA*) showed that toxic side-effects from FDA-approved drugs are the fourth to sixth leading cause of death in the United States. This shocking fact exposes the FDA's failure to provide the public with safe medicines. The FDA-induced delay in approving ribavirin is irrefutable proof that the "drug lag" is causing Americans to die. Why is this irrefutable? Because, while the FDA itself now says that ribavirin is effective, history shows the FDA intentionally denied this lifesaving medicine to the public, to the point of spending millions of tax dollars trying to incarcerate those involved in promoting it.

FDA actions (and inactions) contribute to more premature deaths in the United States than any other cause. The agency routinely approves deadly, dangerous drugs that kill Americans, while failing to approve safe and effective lifesaving drugs for patients suffering from life-threatening diseases.

First Amendment Alert

by William Faloon

THE FDA'S PROPOSED RULES WOULD SEVERELY RESTRICT what you can learn about dietary supplements, and represents a new intrusion into your health freedom.

This is about the United States of America . . . not China, Iraq, Cuba or the other countries where free speech is unheard of. Citizens will be outraged when they learn about the FDA's new Orwellian endeavor to suppress the dissemination of truthful medical information.

Vitamin consumers won a major victory in 1994 when Congress passed a bill that took away the FDA's power to regulate dietary supplements as drugs. The FDA has now proposed new rules to prohibit Americans from learning about certain types of medical information.

The FDA's proposed rules say that consumers can be told about how a vitamin affects the "structure or function" of the body, but that any reference to how the vitamin affects diseases will be classified as illegal speech. If the FDA's proposed rules become law, most consumers will not be able to find out about the nutrients they need to prevent, mitigate or treat any disease.

Examples of what the FDA has proclaimed to be illegal speech include such descriptions of benefits as "reduces nausea associated with chemotherapy," "protects against cancer," and "treats hot flashes." Let's look at the effects the FDA's proposed new rules will have on the consumer.

FDA-MANDATED SUFFERING FOR CANCER PATIENTS

A study in *Environmental Toxicology and Pharmacology* (Netherlands) 1996 1/3 (179–184) showed that a combination of vitamin C, glutathione and vitamin E significantly reduced chemotherapy-induced vomiting in dogs. Other studies have shown that nutrients can reduce the side effects of toxic drugs in humans. However, the FDA's proposed rules say it is illegal to suggest that chemotherapy patients who suffer from nausea and vomiting take these nutrients to reduce their suffering. While it's OK to state that the nutrients "inhibit chemotherapy-induced free radical activity in the gut," it's illegal to cite the published study showing that these nutrients inhibit chemotherapy-induced vomiting.

Since the FDA contends it's illegal to suggest anything but drugs to reduce nausea associated with chemotherapy, it would also be illegal to recommend coenzyme Q10 and vitamin E to reduce chemotherapy-induced heart muscle damage, melatonin to reduce chemotherapy-induced immune system damage, and n-acetyl-cysteine to reduce chemotherapy-induced liver damage.

The FDA is proposing that cancer patients be denied information about how to protect their heart, liver, gut and immune system against the lethal effects of FDA-approved chemotherapy drugs. These new proposed rules mandate suffering for cancer patients. They are not only immoral, they are blatantly unconstitutional.

SUPPRESSING EVIDENCE ABOUT PROTECTION AGAINST KILLER DISEASES

Despite the many new human studies (and thousands of animal and laboratory studies) showing that nutrients protect against cancer, the FDA says it is illegal to inform the American public about these findings. Under the FDA's proposed rules, it would be permissible to say that selenium "increases serum glutathione peroxidase levels and reduces DNA damage," but it would be illegal to inform Americans about a placebo-controlled study in The *Journal of the American Medical Association* (*JAMA*) on Dec. 25, 1996, showing that 200 micrograms of supplemental selenium reduced cancer mortality in humans by 50 percent.

And since it is illegal (according to the FDA) to say that nutrients "protect against cancer," it is also illegal to say that they "protect against heart attacks." That means that folic acid can be promoted to "lower serum homocysteine levels," but not to protect against heart attacks-even though The *New England Journal of Medicine* (April 9, 1998) recommends the use of folic acid to lower heart attack risk.

The FDA would ban statements such as "treats hot flashes," but there are a wide variety of plant extracts that can be used to treat hot flashes in place of FDA-approved estrogen drugs that have been proven to cause breast, ovarian and uterine cancer. Under the FDA proposed new rules, American women won't get to hear about natural alternatives to estrogen drugs because the FDA has made it illegal to utter the phrase "treats hot flashes" for anyone who sells the plant extracts that are effective against hot flashes.

The FDA does provide some guidance as to what is permissible to say. "Helps maintain cardiovascular health" or "supports the immune system" would be permitted health claims under the agency's new proposed rules. The problem is that a person with dilated cardiomyopathy (heart muscle degeneration) will derive little benefit from therapies designed to treat coronary atherosclerosis. But under the FDA's proposed rules that the agency says are "designed to make claims for dietary supplements more informative, reliable and uniform," a person suffering from different forms of heart disease, peripheral vascular disease, transient ischemic attacks, stroke and so forth will have no idea whatsoever if a product that "helps maintain cardiovascular health" will be of value to them.

If all we are permitted to learn is that a nutrient "supports the immune system," does this mean it protects against immune deficiency associated with cancer and viral diseases? Or does the nutrient suppress an over-active immune system (autoimmunity) associated with rheumatoid arthritis, lupus, and multiple sclerosis? The FDA's proposed rules will force the consumer to guess about such life-or-death matters.

Here is another shocking example of the FDA's twisted Orwellian logic: According to the FDA, it is illegal to promote a product to lower cholesterol levels because everyone (purportedly) knows that high cholesterol causes heart attacks. Once knowledge of the fact that elevated homocysteine causes heart attacks becomes better known, the FDA will probably say it is no longer legal to claim that folic acid lowers homocysteine levels, and only grant approval to statements such as, "Folic acid facilitates the methylation of homocysteine into methionine and S-adenosylmethionine (SAMe)." But when the public learns the benefits of increasing SAMe levels, the FDA will then prohibit statements about SAMe as well.

In effect, the FDA's proposed rules only permit the dissemination of obscure, difficult-to-understand descriptions about nutrients that show lifesaving potential in studies published in medical journals. The rules would prohibit clear, accurate, truthful and easy-to-understand statements about these findings, and the publication of the studies (or their abstracts) themselves in conjunction with the sale of the nutrients used in these studies.

In short, the FDA's proposed rules are a deliberate attempt to keep lifesaving information from the American people and, by so doing, contribute to the premature death of millions of Americans.

Does the FDA have the legal right to keep Americans from learning about views contrary to its own? The FDA says yes, but the Supreme Court says no. With their proposed new rules, the FDA has defied the Supreme Court decision in a case called Daubert v. Merrill Dow.

Daubert replaced the "General Acceptance Test" (an equivalent phrase to "significant scientific agreement") with the Federal Rules of Evidence for admitting scientific testimony at a federal trial. The new standard mandated by the Supreme Court demands that there be "significant scientific evidence" to support a claim, instead of the "significant scientific agreement" standard proposed by the FDA. The difference between the two standards is enormous. The Supreme Court standard relies on scientific evidence rather than the opinions of FDA scientists and bureaucrats, who may be unaware of the evidence in favor of a claim, or may chose to ignore this evidence.

The FDA has shown a consistent pattern of bias against dietary supplements over the past 70 years. Moreover, the agency does no research of any kind itself. It depends entirely on evidence submitted to it by companies and individuals. As a result, the FDA is often ignorant of important scientific findings that no one has told it about.

According to the Daubert decision, the FDA should have recommended that it adopt Durk Pearson and Sandy Shaw's proposal to allow a gradation of label claims, depending on the amount of evidence to support the claim. Under Pearson and Shaw's proposal, the FDA would not be the sole arbiter of truth; a consumer could see at a glance whether or not the FDA had approved any given claim, but could also see how much support the claim has, based on the number ascribed to it (level 1 being the lowest threshold of evidence, and level 5 being the highest).

Because the Supreme Court's ruling on how to evaluate scientific evidence was made on June 28, 1993, after the passage of the Nutrition Labeling and Education Act of 1990 in which the FDA first thrust their "significant scientific agreement" standard upon us, there is no excuse for the FDA's proposed new rules. The FDA has chosen to defy the Supreme Court's ruling in its ongoing bias against dietary supplements.

DEFENDING FREEDOM OF CHOICE IN HEALTHCARE

Health activists often wonder why they have to keep battling the government to protect liberties supposedly protected under the Bill of Rights. The root of the problem is that, while citizens labor long and hard to pay their taxes, the federal government is given free rein to use taxpayer dollars to increase central government authority.

The ultimate solution is to reduce the size of, and gain control over, the government. Since no politician has the fortitude to implement such changes, it is up to us to protect our constitutionally guaranteed rights against illegal government intrusion.

An Archaic System

by Saul Kent

T HE IDEA OF THE FOOD AND DRUG ADMINISTRATION DETER-
mining which health and medical therapies should be made
available to Americans may have been serviceable 50 years
ago when far less medical research was being conducted, and
home computers and the Internet hadn't yet been invented.

Today, however, the idea of the FDA controlling the availability of new therapies is utterly absurd. There are thousands
of new health and medical studies published weekly, regular
breakthroughs in prevention and treatment, advances in aging
research, and a system that puts much of this information at the
fingertips of anyone with a computer and a modem.

We've written extensively about the harm caused by the FDA's
longstanding bias against dietary supplements, the agency's cozy
relationship with large pharmaceutical companies, and its illegal
and unconstitutional acts against Americans and (lately) citizens
of other countries as well.

It's important to understand, however, that even if the bias and corruption of the FDA were entirely eliminated, the system itself would remain archaic and obsolete. In order to better understand why this is so, let's take a look at how the system operates.

All health and medical therapies go through an extensive and complex FDA approval process—which costs vast amounts of money and a great deal of time—before the public is permitted access to the therapy. The costs of this process must be borne entirely by the company that wants to offer the therapy to the public. This makes it extremely difficult for small companies to obtain approval for therapies, and gives the large companies huge advantages. Yet, it is usually small, innovative companies that develop the most exciting breakthroughs.

Plus, there is the vast number of approval applications stemming from the explosion of new health and medical breakthroughs. The FDA has traditionally taken a leisurely, highly cautious approach to the approval of new therapies, but in recent years they've been overwhelmed by an onslaught of new applications for approval of therapeutic claims, causing long delays.

Also, the increasing percentage of health and medical breakthroughs with nutrients and other natural products simply don't fit into the current regulatory scheme. With the emerging availability of phytochemical and herbal extracts to add to vitamins, minerals, amino acids and essential fatty acids, there are now hundreds of natural therapies—often with a history of medical use that goes back thousands of years—which are being proved effective for a wide variety of conditions and diseases.

It is clearly in the public interest to have information about these therapies readily available so that doctors and their patients can decide for themselves if they want to try them.

Just this past autumn, for example, studies have been published showing that vitamin E can prevent heart attacks, ginkgo biloba can slow the progression of Alzheimer's disease, N-acetylcysteine can prevent flu symptoms, carotenoids such as lutein can prevent macular degeneration of the eye, and soy extracts can prevent various types of cancer . . . to name only a few recent findings.

These therapies are safe, have multiple health benefits, and can be purchased easily at affordable prices. It is both inappropriate and impractical to require government "approval" (or any other kind of approval) for the use of these therapies in preventing and treating diseases. To do so would be to sacrifice people's lives needlessly.

1997

OCTOBER 1997

Twelve Angry Jurors

Dr. Burzynski's Latest Victory Signals Citizen Revulsion at Federal Tactics

by Dean Mouscher

T HE LATEST CHAPTER IN THE FOOD AND DRUG ADMINISTRA-tion's 14-year-old war against cancer pioneer Stanislaw Burzynski ended abruptly on May 27, when a jury acquit-ted him on the lone remaining charge. Burzynski had originally stood trial on 75 federal felony counts, with most charges dismissed in March.

With the May acquittal of *Cancer Re*searcher Stanislaw Burzynski in his federal retrial of earlier charges, onlookers are arriving at a powerful consensus: That it is intolerable in a democratic country that the government prevents fully-informed citizens from healing themselves in the manner they choose.

Interviews and press conferences with Burzynski's highly articu-
late patients terrified that their own government would take away
their last hope for life brought that message home. Burzynski himself rejoiced that his 14-year persecution may have reached an end.

On this day after Memorial Day, I'm happy to be able to say
the FDA's war against us is over, said Burzynski, after the verdict. And hopefully it may mark the beginning of the end of the
war against cancer. The case ended as a major embarrassment for
the FDA. After devoting 14 years and untold millions of dollars
of public funds, prosecutors were unable to convince jurors that
Burzynski was guilty of even one of the 75 counts.

Congress is looking into the case as well . . . to examine the
behavior of the government. In a letter to Department of Health
and Human Services Secretary Donna Shalala, dated June 5, Rep.
Joe Barton (R-TX), chairman of the Investigations and Oversight
subcommittee of the House Commerce Committee, asked for all
documents from the FDAís associate chief counsel for enforcement Robert Spiller and the FDA's Office of Chief Counsel related
to Burzynski, and a detailed accounting of the resources expended
by the FDA related to investigating and prosecuting him. Barton
also asked Shalala to locate and preserve for safekeeping all material that may be reasonably related to this investigation.

Burzynski has been the target of federal regulators for years,
with his clinic raided continuously. The trial that ended in March
was a partial vindication for the doctor, with most of the charges
dismissed, and a deadlocked jury disposing of the rest for the
time being.

A MOOT POINT

Not lost on the jury in that trial was the fact that most of the
indictment was moot. The FDA already had approved 73 phase
II clinical trials of antineoplastons, under which Burzynski's
patients were being treated. Thus, Burzynski was treating out-

of-state patients, and even shipping the drug out of Texas (violations of interstate commerce were among the original charges)
with full FDA knowledge and approval.

Clearly, this made both trials a puzzlement to many, including jurors. But prosecutors apparently felt they had left themselves no way out. Negotiations broke down over the unresolved
charges, leading to the retrial in May. This time, however, there
was a marked difference in the jury pool. Everyone in Houston
now knew about the FDA's long harassment of Burzynski and
his patients. The judge said he didn't care if possible jurors knew
about the case, so long as they could put their opinions aside and
listen to the evidence.

The voir dire, where lawyers speak to prospective jurors in a
group, seemed at times as if it would deteriorate into an angry
mob scene. One prospective juror told prosecutors the FDA was
like the Gestapo. A 24-year career marine said the case made
him ashamed of his country, and that he found it very disturbing. When asked if they had any questions, one woman stood up
and asked, Why isn't the FDA being prosecuted for violating our
constitutional rights? In Roe versus Wade, the Supreme Court
determined that interfering in the doctor-patient relationship
is an unconstitutional invasion of the patient's right to privacy.

Prosecutors in the second trial dropped all counts (with prej-
udice, meaning they could not be retried) against Burzynski
Research Institute and all 40 interstate commerce counts against
Burzynski himself. Thus, all that remained of the original 75-count
indictment was a single count of contempt of court. Still, a con-
viction could have destroyed Burzynski's career, ended patients'
access to antineoplastons, and stopped research on the drug.

Testimony in the retrial lasted just three days, two for the
prosecution and one for the defense. As with the first trial,
the prosecution called witnesses who seemed to hurt its case.
Even the chief FDA witness admitted that Burzynski had been

trying to cooperate with the FDA for 14 years, that the data he had sent occupied fully 25 feet of shelf space at FDA headquarters, and that the FDA had never approved a drug for an individual, but only for large pharmaceutical companies with unlimited resources.

This time jurors took just two-and-a-half hours to find Burzynski not guilty on the remaining charge.

It was a Big Brother issue said juror Stephanie Shapiro afterward. The order was ambiguous, and the jurors felt Burzynski had made every good-faith effort to follow it. Moreover, we were disturbed that the government had not exhausted civil remedies before resorting to this very serious criminal trial.

THE TABLES TURNED

And the tables seemed to turn quickly. An investigative arm of the Justice Department, the Office of Professional Responsibility, is investigating possible prosecutorial misconduct in the Burzynski case. After the not-guilty verdict, prosecutor Michael Clark was seen on local news shows, sweating profusely as he told reporters that he will be exonerated of any wrongdoing.

What next for Burzynski? He continues to accrue patients to the clinical trials being conducted under Investigational New Drug exemptions filed with the FDA. Those trials are showing particularly promising results for patients with primary malignant brain tumors and non-Hodgkin's lymphoma.

Will the FDA now accept the scientific data on antineoplastons and approve the drug invented by a man they have been trying to jail for a decade and a half?

Stay tuned.

1996

Ozone Clinic Raided

by William Faloon

O N JAN. 4, 1996, AT 8:30 AM, TEN FDA AGENTS AND TWO state troopers with drawn guns burst into the Lazare Clinic and home of clinic officers Richard Harley and Jackie Kube in Shawnee on the Delaware, Pennsylvania.

Vice President Jackie Kube recounted the terrifying ordeal in which the armed agents burst into her home, yanked her son out of the shower, and herded everyone into the dining room, while they rifled through everything in the house, indiscriminately grabbing personal files, dietary supplements, and numerous other items not listed on the search warrant. Their warrant, which was signed by Magistrate Raymond J. Durkin of the US District Court for the Middle District of Pennsylvania, authorized the raiders to seize "ozone/oxygen therapy devices and all accessories, topozone oil and any materials used to manufacture it, records, files, documents, receipts related to the sale and promotion of ozone/oxygen therapy devices and/or topozone oil, and any other unapproved drug or device."

Ms. Kube complained that they took all her olive oil which she needs for cooking. They took the computer, peripherals, client records, all sales brochures—everything that wasn't nailed down!

NO CHARGES FILED, NO PROBABLE CAUSED REVEALED

Typically, no charges were filed and the clinic was not closed down. It reopened a few days later with equipment borrowed from friends. Though not owned by a medical professional, the staff includes a medical doctor and nurses.

Before opening in September 1995, Lazare had gotten approval from the Commonwealth of Pennsylvania and had a letter of assurance that they were operating legally dated Nov. 22, 1995, from the Department of Health and Human Services Center For Alternative Medicine Research In HIV/AIDS, under the review of Leanna Standish, ND, Director of Research at Bastyr University.

STAFF IS BEWILDERED AND ANGERED

Jackie Kube, Richard Harley, and their staff are bewildered because they had gone to great lengths to comply with all regulations. Their patients fear being cut off from all future treatment. Bastyr University of Seattle, Washington, which is respected internationally in the emerging field of alternative medicine, had been serving as the institutional review board for Lazare's research. Attorney Lord fails to see any way in which the Pennsylvania based clinic was engaged in interstate commerce, as is implied by the FDA's actions, and questions their jurisdiction in the matter.

1995

SEPTEMBER 1995

The FDA's Vendetta Against Dr. Burzynski

by Dean Mouscher,
Director, Clinical Trials
Burzynski Institute

S TANISLAW R. BURZYNSKI IS AN MD WITH A PhD IN BIOCHEM-
istry. In 1967, while studying blood as a graduate student,
he found certain peptides that had never been described
before. Comparing the blood of patients with different diseases,
Dr. Burzynski found that over 98% of cancer patients were deficient in the peptides he had found—often with blood levels of
only 2% of those of healthy individuals. This led him to suspect
that these compounds—or a lack thereof—were implicated in
the development of neoplastic (cancerous) disease.

Most cancer experts believe we all develop cancer cells hundreds if not millions of times in our lifetimes. Given the trillions
of developing cells, the millions of errors that can occur in the

differentiation (maturing) process of each cell, and our constant exposure to carcinogenic substances (smoke, car fumes, radiation, etc.), the laws of probability dictate that mis-developing cells must occur frequently in the life of each individual. It stands to reason that a healthy body has a corrective system to "reprogram" newly-developed cancer cells into normal differentiation pathways before the cancer can take hold.

Dr. Burzynski postulated that healthy organisms have just such a corrective mechanism, which he termed the "Biochemical Defense System." He called the substances produced by this system "antineoplastons." Their purpose is to "reprogram" cancer cells to die like normal cells. Healthy cells are not affected.

Dr. Burzynski continued his research at Baylor University until 1977, when he felt he was ready to begin treating advanced cancer patients with the peptides he had discovered. After getting a written opinion from his lawyer that doing so would not violate any state or federal laws as long as he treated patients only in Texas, Dr. Burzynski began to give antineoplastons to patients with hopeless cancers—often with dramatic results.

THE FDA SEEKS AN INJUNCTION

In 1983 however, the FDA went to court for an injunction to stop Dr. Burzynski from manufacturing or using antineoplastons in his practice. US District Court Judge Gabrielle McDonald turned them down. In an 18-page decision, Judge McDonald made it clear that Dr. Burzynski could continue to "manufacture, package, sell, and distribute antineoplastons, so long as it occurs wholly intrastate."

Ignoring Judge McDonald's decision, the FDA tried to stop Dr. Burzynski by writing dozens of letters to Senators, Congressmen, insurance companies and pharmaceutical firms. These letters contained lies and distortions so outrageous that on October 23, 1985 Judge McDonald issued a Cease and Desist order, commanding the FDA to stop issuing false and misleading information about Dr. Burzynski.

A SERIES OF RAIDS AND GRAND JURY INVESTIGATIONS

In 1985, FDA agents and armed Federal Marshalls raided Dr. Burzynski's clinic and seized all his patient records—200,000 documents in all. In order to continue treating patients with advanced cancer, Dr. Burzynski had to install a copier—at his expense—at FDA headquarters and hire someone to shuttle back and forth, making copies of his records and bringing them back to the clinic. Dr. Burzynski had to make appointments with the FDA to make copies of his own documents.

Later in 1985, Federal prosecutors representing the FDA presented everything they seized in the raid—plus another 100,000 documents subpoenaed shortly after the raid—to a Federal Grand Jury. Their investigation of Dr. Burzynski lasted nine months, but prosecutors couldn't convince the Grand Jury that there was probable cause to believe a crime had been committed. No indictment was returned.

In 1990, the US Attorney's office in Houston, representing the FDA, convened another grand jury to investigate Dr. Burzynski, again for alleged violations of Judge McDonald's order. To the FDA's dismay, this Grand Jury also refused to indict Dr. Burzynski.

MORE RAIDS AND GRAND JURIES

In 1993, the FDA again raided the Burzynski Research Institute because of alleged bacterial contamination of antineoplastons, but tests proved conclusively that there was no contamination.

In 1994, US Attorneys—again representing the FDA—convened a third Grand Jury to investigate Dr. Burzynski. And for the third time, a skeptical Grand Jury refused to return an indictment. The main casualty this time was the Assistant US Attorney on the case, who was removed for prosecutorial misconduct involving abusive and improper use of subpoenas.

The latest chapter in the FDA's twelve-year campaign to stop Dr. Burzynski from treating patients with antineoplastons kicked off on March 24, 1995 with another raid on the clinic. Seven federal agents herded employees into a room and kept them there until they filled out forms with personal information. They then spent seven hours rifling through file cabinets and drawers, leaving with boxes of patient records and other documents.

Shortly thereafter the FDA began serving clinic employees with subpoenas commanding them to testify before a Federal Grand Jury investigating Dr. Burzynski. To date, federal prosecutors representing the FDA have subpoenaed nine employees including Dr. Burzynski. In addition, they have ordered him to turn over tens of thousands of pages of documents, including more patient records and diagnostic films.

AN ARBITRARY FISHING EXPEDITION

The law prohibits Grand Juries from "arbitrary fishing expeditions." Yet that is exactly what federal prosecutors are engaged in. Besides patient records—many of which have already been presented four times to various government investigators—prosecutors have subpoenaed "any and all agreements, draft agreements, proposals, correspondence, notes, memos, tape recordings, notes of conversations, telephone messages, reports, raw data, studies or other items to, from, or with any foreign or domestic pharmaceutical company or university, including contact person's name, title and phone number."

While this information is of no use in investigating criminal activity, it gives the FDA the opportunity to write letters to everyone they uncover, letting them know that Dr. Burzynski is the target of a federal investigation and to issue subpoenas to some of these people. This is more than just speculation. It is the exact behavior that sparked a 1985 "Cease and Desist" order against the FDA by US District Court Judge Gabrielle McDonald.

And so, on June 15 1995, prosecutor Amy LeCocq subpoenaed a huge Dutch pharmaceutical conglomerate—which has conducted negotiations with Dr. Burzynski—for all correspondence, memos, documents or other records it had regarding Dr. Burzynski or anyone associated with him. The obvious purpose of this subpoena was to frighten the company—which does a large business in the US—into having no further contact with Dr. Burzynski.

Prosecutors have also subpoenaed all patient billing records, again with no time limitation whatever. Dr. Burzynski has been treating patients since 1977. They have subpoenaed his accountants for every conceivable document an accountant can possess (again with no limitation on time), a classic fishing expedition. Prosecutors have even subpoenaed the names and addresses of every person who has ever received a brochure from Dr. Burzynski! As if that weren't enough, the subpoena went on to demand "Any other lists of persons," an absurdly general and burdensome request.

FDA HARASSMENT, ILLEGAL ACTIONS, AND TERRORISM

Besides throwing the entire clinic into chaos, wasting thousands of hours of employee time, and terrifying advanced cancer patients who don't know whether they will be able to continue getting the only medicine that has been able to help them, the grand jury's actions have severely threatened Dr. Burzynski's ability to practice medicine. Without patients' previous MRIs and CAT scans, Dr. Burzynski has nothing to which he can compare new scans, and no way of knowing if patients' tumors are growing or shrinking.

Moreover, the FDA has been careful to seize films and medical records of Dr. Burzynski's most successful cases, crippling his ability to defend himself by confiscating his single most valuable asset—proof of the anti-cancer activity of antineoplastons.

In the current case there has been illegal use of subpoenas as well. Dr. Ralph Moss, an award-winning journalist and author of books about cancer, was subpoenaed and ordered to produce every document in his possession—electronic, magnetic, printed or otherwise—relating to Dr. Burzynski. Dr. Moss has written favorably about Dr. Burzynski in the past.

Unfortunately for Amy Lecocq, the prosecutor in charge of this case, her subpoena of Dr. Moss violated at least six federal laws governing subpoenas of journalists. Such violations carry a penalty of administrative reprimand or other disciplinary action. When Dr. Moss pointed this out to Lecocq and gave her the opportunity to withdraw the subpoena, she did so with alacrity.

It's been said that a prosecutor can get a Grand Jury to indict virtually anyone. But despite the avalanche of documents supplied by the government to four Grand Juries, it has yet to convince any of them of probable cause to believe Dr. Burzynski has committed a crime. And so, unable to stop him legally, the FDA seems determined to harass him to death.

THE NCI REPORT ON DR. BURZYNSKI

The FDA's actions are all the more outrageous because their own oncology division has granted Dr. Burzynski permission to conduct Phase II clinical trials! In addition the National Cancer Institute (NCI)—following a visit by seven NCI experts to Dr. Burzynski's Houston clinic for a review of patient records—confirmed several remissions in patients with "hopeless" brain tumors after treatment with antineoplastons. Their report states that "The site visit team documented anti-cancer activity in this best-case series and determined that Phase II trials are warranted to determine the response rate."

In other words, the question is no longer "Do antineoplastons work?" but rather "How consistently do they work?"

And yet, despite the NCI report, despite the fact that the FDA's own scientists wish to see antineoplastons tested, the FDA's "enforcers" remain obsessed with shutting Dr. Burzynski down.

Index

A

Abbreviated New Drug Application (ANDA) 54–55
ABC News 274
Abela Pharmaceuticals, Inc. 149
Abigail Alliance for Better Access to Developmental Drugs 125–136
 Citizen Petition 127, 130, 133
abnormal platelet aggregation 153
ACCESS (Access, Compassion, Care, and Ethics for Seriously Ill Patients) Act 130
Accupril 297
Accutane 222
acetaminophen 117–122, 237–241
 and cataracts 239

and kidney cancer 238–239
and liver damage 117–120
overdoses of 119–120, 239
acetylcholine 241
Acthar 71
Adderall 71
ADHD 59
adverse drug reactions (ADRs) 305, 312, 353, 363
 deaths from 250, 397, 406, 409
Advil 55
AIDS. *See* HIV/AIDS
Albain, Kathy S. 425
Allegra 298
Altace 57, 297
Alzheimer's disease 9, 15, 145, 149, 173, 241
 ginkgo biloba and 458
 memantine and 240, 358
AMA Code of Medical Ethics 310

Ambien 71
American Association for Health Freedom (AAHF) 74
American Cancer Society 183, 428
American College of Cardiologists 397
American Heart Association 81
American Journal of Cardiology 295
American Journal of Clinical Nutrition 154
American Journal of the Medical Sciences 300
American Medical Association (AMA) 153, 290, 293, 310. *See also Journal of the American Medical Association* (JAMA)
American Preventive Medical Association 370–371
American Society of Clinical Oncology 270
Ames, Bruce 343–346
amlodipine 57
Angell, Marcia 307, 309, 393
anthocyanins 187
antidepressants 221, 222, 292, 294. *See also* specific antidepressants by name
antihistamines 118
antihypertensive drugs 296–297, 300
anti-inflammatory drugs 145, 189, 216, 290
antineoplastons 465–466, 474–479

anxiety 111–113, 290
apoptosis 265, 268–269
Archives of Internal Medicine 296, 299
Argentina 51–52
Arias, Ursula 11
Aricept 241, 358
Arizona 12–13, 229
arrhythmia 81
arthritis 146, 173, 188–189, 192, 216, 231, 404, 454
aspirin 118, 147, 216, 407
Associated Press 68–69
asthma 222, 404
AstraZeneca 206
atherosclerosis 81, 152, 345–347, 454
AT&T 93–95
Attorney's Office, US 11, 22
Augmentin 327
Australian Family Physician 299
autoimmune diseases 83
autologous blood banking 163–166, 169
Avandia (rosiglitazone) 143–144
Avorn, Jerry 306

B

Barton, Joe 464
Bastyr University 470
Baychol 331
Baycol 309
Benazepril 57
benign prostate enlargement 42, 54–55
beta-carotene 344

Bextra 223, 309
Big Pharma 32, 69
Biochemical Defense System 474
bioequivalence 54
bioidentical hormone debate 33–36, 68
BioMed Plus 212
birth control pills 300, 422
birth defects 83, 222, 284, 437
Bishop, Helen 5
Bliley, Helen 384
blood transfusions 163–165, 167, 447
   and hepatitis 164–166, 168, 447
Bodenheimer, Thomas 304
bone marrow toxicity 358
brain tumors 466, 478
Bristol-Myers Squibb Company 146
British Medical Journal (*BMJ*) 218, 293, 299
Bupropion 57
Burroughs, Abigail Kathleen 99, 125–128, 262
Burroughs, Frank 127, 132–135, 262
Burzynski Research Institute 465, 475
Burzynski, Stanislaw 463–466, 473–479

C

Calan 297
calcium 190, 309–310, 344
cancer 35, 44–45, 47–49, 59, 69, 71–72, 83, 99–100, 107–108, 125–126, 131–132, 135, 137–138, 145, 153, 155–156, 173, 181–183, 188, 206, 210–212, 261–264, 267, 271, 275, 285, 300, 343–346, 356, 358, 404, 443–444, 452–454, 459, 463–464, 473–475, 477–478
   bladder 265
   breast 68, 82, 421–431
   colon 82, 128–130, 168, 187
   colorectal 282, 371, 424
   endometrial 423–424, 429
   head 129, 139
   kidney 130, 238–239, 265
   liver 448–449
   lung 129, 139, 206
   neck 129
   ovarian 268–271
   pancreatic 97
   prostate 42, 54, 82, 141, 199–203, 265–266, 345, 398
   skin 181–183
   stomach 426
   vaccine 264–266
Cancer Gene Therapy 264
Cancer Patients' Alliance for Clinical Trials 131
Cannell, John Jacob 83
Capoten (captopril) 296–297
carboplatin 268
cardiomyopathy 81, 254, 453
Cardizem 297
Cardura 297
Carlow, Michael 211–212
carnitine 344

carnosine 358

carotid artery 345

Celebrex 216, 223, 331

Celexa 292

cell carcinomas 126, 182

Center For Alternative Medicine Research In HIV/AIDS 470

Center for Human Nutrition, UCLA 345

Center of Drug Development Science 301

Centers for Disease control and Prevention (CDC) 165, 167, 409, 449

Centex 146

chemotherapy 100, 126, 264, 267–268, 358, 421–422
    nausea from 443–444, 452

cherries 185–192

chlorophyll 154

chondroitin sulfate 190

Cialis 59

cirrhosis 448–449

Citizens for Health 371

Clarinex 309

Claritin 298, 327, 330–331, 385

Clark, Michael 466

Cleveland Clinic 144, 268

clinical pharmacology 306

clinical trials 54, 70, 125, 128–130, 138–139, 148–149, 249, 254, 262, 267, 269, 302, 358–359, 465–466, 478

clofibrate 422, 426

coenzyme Q10. *See* CoQ10

cognitive dysfunction 276

Cohen, Jay S. 117, 122–123, 289

colitis 361–362

Commerce Committee, US 382, 464

Committee on Government Reform and Oversight, US 166

compounded estriol-based creams 31–32

compounded medications 230

congestive heart failure 81, 143, 254

Congressional Budget Office, US 329

Conspiracy of Silence: How the FDA Allows Drug Companies to Abuse the Accelerated Approval Process 206

constipation 361

Consumers' Access to Health Information Act (H.R. 2352) 202

Cooper, Richard S. 401

CoQ10 95–96, 253–257, 309, 344, 444, 452

coronary atherosclerosis 81, 453

coronary thrombosis 81

Cosmegen 71

Coumadin 327

COX-2 inhibitors 216, 223

Cozaar 297

Crawford, Lester M. 234

Crestor 222

Critical Path Initiative (CPI) 130

Cross, James 304

Crown Zellerbach 146

Cunningham, Hazel 427

Current Therapeutic Research 146

Cutler, Richard 24

cyanid 187

cyclooxygenase-2 (COX-2) 216

D

Dale, Roderic M.K. 403, 412

Dangerous Doses: How Counterfeiters Are Contaminating America's Drug Supply 209

Daubert v. Merrill Dow 455–456

de la Torre, Jack 147

dementia 47, 276–277

dendritic immune cells 264

Depakote 57

Department of Justice, US 23, 446, 448, 466

depression 83, 111–112, 173, 292

Detroit Free Press 256

Deutsch, Peter 222

DHA (docosahexaenoic acid) 173, 234

DHT (dihydrotestosterone) 55

diabetes 83, 143, 285, 349, 352

diabetic neuropathy 240

Dietary Supplement Health and Education Act (DSHEA) 191, 287, 443

diethylstilbestrol (DES) 422

digoxin 291

Dilacor (diltiazem) 297

Dimethyl sulfoxide (DMSO) 145–149

Dingell, John 427

Divalproex 57

DNA strand breaks 343, 422

doxepin 292

Drug Enforcement Agency (DEA) 23

drug importation bill 326, 333

Drug Safety 120, 188, 217–218, 220, 293, 299

Duke University 265

Duract 309

Durkin, Raymond J. 469

Dutcher, Janice P. 425

E

Eban, Katherine 209

ECG (epicatechin gallete) 154–155

Effexor 292

EGCG (epigallocatechin gallate) 154–155

eiscosopentaenoic acid 234

Elavil 292

Eli Lilly 99

Emord, Jonathan 234, 282, 286–287, 375

Environmental Toxicology and Pharmacology 452

EPA (eiscosopentaenoic acid) 173, 234

Erbitux 126, 129–130
erectile dysfunction 295
Eschenbach, Edward von 104, 106, 270–271
estradiol 30–31, 34–35, 309, 422
estriol 30–35, 68, 309
estrogen
    blockers 422, 424
    drugs 30–31, 35, 68, 453
    equine 30–31, 34–35.
        See also Premarin and Prempro
estrone 34–35
European Institute of Oncology 423–424
excitotoxicity 241

F

Faloon, William 3–6, 10, 13–14, 403, 420
FDA (Food and Drug Administration, US)
    and blood supply 163–170
    and dietary supplements 112–113, 190–191, 256–257, 281, 284–287, 375, 455–456
    and experimental drugs 69–70, 262
    and fish oil 172–173, 231–235
    and food safety 386, 447
    and pharmaceutical industry 32, 36, 68, 145–146, 171, 189, 220, 224–226, 239, 251, 304–305, 309, 325, 330, 351, 361–363, 379–385

approved drugs, dangerous 32, 35, 37, 46, 68, 72, 99, 104, 143–144, 191–192, 207–214, 215–226, 237–242, 249–252, 253–257, 274, 359–363, 397–399, 416, 421–429
bans 30–32, 68, 185–192, 217, 223, 232, 257, 282–283, 350–352, 370, 373, 378, 453
"Better Health Information for Consumers" initiative 280, 286–287
censorship 185, 189–190, 233, 235, 256, 280, 282, 371, 375, 420
Center for Drug Evaluation and Research (CDER) 308, 361
compassionate use exemption 267, 324, 350
drug approval process 69, 107, 125, 130–133, 137–138, 140, 205–206, 224–225, 261, 265–266, 271, 338, 359, 378, 382, 404–406, 411, 425, 458
drug embargos 12–13, 257, 352, 356
illegal actions by 5–6, 13, 17–20, 229–230, 276, 280, 351, 478
lawsuits 9, 12–16, 19, 130, 133, 231–235, 240–241, 261–262, 325, 403, 419–420
Office of New Drugs 218, 224–225

reform 45, 66, 70, 74, 140–
141, 215, 221–226, 270–
271, 379–388
unapproved drugs 14–16,
186, 273–274, 359, 420,
446
warnings 143–144, 186–188,
191–192, 217, 305, 362,
383
failures to warn 239–241,
253–255, 429
"FDA Caution Can Be Deadly,
Too" 360
Fda Holocaust Museum 20
Federal Bureau of Investigation
(FBI) 23
Feldschuh, Joseph 163–170
Fen-Phen 309
"Fever Pitch: Getting Doctors
to Prescribe is Big Busi-
ness" 407
finasteride (Proscar) 42–43,
53–56
Fisher, Bernard 426–429
fish oil 171–174, 231–235. *See
also* omega-3 fatty acids
folic acid 154, 343, 372–373,
438
and neural tube defect risk
reduction 189–190,
282–284, 370–371, 374
cardioivascular benefits of
344, 375, 437, 453–454
Food and Drug Administration
Modernization Act 338
Food, Drug, and Cosmetic Act
70
Freedom of Information Act
(FOIA) 324–325

Friske Orchards 187
Frontline 249–252

G

Gabapentin 57
gastroenteritis 118–119
gemfibrozil 422
General Accountability Office
(GAO), US 62, 303, 386
generic drugs 42, 51–62
genomics 105–106
Geron Corporation 264–265
GlaxoSmithKline 251
Glucophage 327, 349–352
glucosamine 190
glutathione 121–122, 452–453
GMP-certified (Good Manufac-
turing Practices) 42, 53,
56, 59–60
Goldstein, Allan 24
Goth's Medical Pharmacology
293, 299
Goyan, Jere 256
Graham, David 188, 215–226
Grand Jury 10–11, 23, 475–
476, 478
Grassley, Charles 143, 220
Graveline, Duane 294–295
green tea 151–156, 199–202
Gutknecht Amendment (H.R.
5186) 329, 332, 334
Gutknecht, Gil 328–329

H

Hall, Cynthia Holcomb 378
Hall, Stephen S. 330
Hammell, John 8

Harley, Richard 469–470
Hauptmann Institute 16
Hazards of Medication 293
Health and Human Services
(HUD), US Department
of 130, 133, 201, 261,
270, 427, 464, 470
health freedom 8, 74, 98, 108,
451
Health Freedom Protection Act
(H.R. 4282) 189–191
heart attack 81, 147, 151–153,
173, 188, 190–192, 216–
218, 223, 231–232, 234,
407, 437, 453
heart disease 81, 83, 100, 123,
232–234, 254, 282, 285,
300, 371, 454
hemophilia 212
hepatitis 164–168, 344, 358,
445–449
Herceptin 429
Herschler, Robert 146
Herxheimer, Alexander
304–306
high blood pressure 222,
295–296. *See*
also hypertension
HIV/AIDS 43, 165, 165–166,
168, 211, 448–449, 470
HMG CoA reductase inhibitors.
See statin drugs
homocysteine 344, 453–454
Honig, Susan 428
hormone replacement therapies (HRT) 300
hot flashes 300, 444, 452–453
Hotze 230

House Commerce Committee,
US 382, 464
human immunodeficiency
virus. *See* HIV/AIDS
human T-cell lymphotropic
virus (HTLV) 168
Hurley, Daniel 3, 22
hypertension 83, 178,
295–296

I

ibuprofen 54–55, 216, 300
ICN Pharmaceuticals 446
Idant Laboratories 166, 169
Inderal (propanolol) 297
influenza 344, 446–447, 459
Ingram, Don 24
inositol hexanicotinate 309
insomnia 112, 290
insulin 291, 349
interferon 358, 448–449
interleukin-2 358
Internal Revenue Service (IRS),
US 23
International Conference on
Pharmacoepidemiology
218
Investigations and Oversight
subcommittee 464
Iressa 206
irritable bowel syndrome 361
isoprinosine 357
Isoptin 297

J

Jacob, Stanley 146–149
Joint National Committee 296

Journal of Clinical Oncology 426

Journal of the American Geriatrics Society 299

Journal of the American Medical Association (JAMA) 151, 289–290, 302, 305, 307, 401, 406–407, 437, 450, 453. *See also* American Medical Association (AMA)

Joyal, Steven V. 181

K

Kaiser Permanente 217

Katz, Martin 5–6, 17, 23

Keflex 331

Kent, Saul 3, 10, 13, 14, 420, 457

Kerlone (betoxolol) 297

Kessler, David 23–24, 106, 408, 437

Kessler, Gladys 281, 372–374

Ketek (telithrmycin) 66–68, 75

Kiefer, Dale 143

Kovach, Sue 125, 145, 163

Kube, Jackie 469–470

L

Laifer, Stephen 229

Lamberth, Royce 420

Lamictal 57

Lamotrigine 57

Lancet, The 218, 220, 302, 304, 361–363

Latham and Watkins, LLP 130

Lazare Clinic 469

LDL-C (low density lipo-protein-cholesterol) 294–295

LDL (Low-density lipoprotein) 152–154, 294, 345

LeCocq, Amy 477

Lee, William 119

Lescol 294

leukemia 265
  feline 446

Levatol (penbutolol) 297

Life Extension Foundation (LEF) 39, 98, 256, 276–277, 281, 323–324, 367, 402–403, 414, 446, 448
  and FDA 3–26, 51, 74, 232–235, 241–242

Life Extension Report 4–6, 12, 14, 24

Lipitor 81, 212, 294–295, 331

Lister, Joseph 79–80, 84

liver
  damage and failure 66–67, 117–123, 123, 237–238, 243, 254–255, 291, 295, 444, 448–449, 452
  transplant 66, 118, 449

Longevity Institute 16

Lopressor 57, 297

Lorenzen Cancer Foundation 130

Los Angeles Times 222, 352

Lotensin 57

Lotronex 309, 361–362

lupus 454

lutein 345–347, 459

lycopene 345

M

macular degeneration 345, 356, 459
magnesium 47, 309–310
Margolin, Kim A. 425
Markey, Edward J. 205–206
McCallion, Joe 208
McDonald, Gabrielle 474–475, 477
McNeil Consumer Health 122
McNellie, Jennifer 127–129
Medicaid 40, 43–45, 62, 99, 211, 213, 327, 382
Medicare 45–48, 54, 56, 58, 62, 71, 82, 99, 202, 328–329, 333, 335, 346, 382, 387, 393
    fraud 40–44, 327
Medicare Prescription Drug Act 41–42, 56, 58, 71
meditation 297
medroxyprogesterone acetate 35
melanocytes 182
melanoma 182–183, 265
melatonin 19, 444, 452
Melmon and Morrelli's Clinical Pharmacology 290
memantine
    and Alzheimer's disease 240–241, 246, 358, 365, 458
    and Parkinson's disease 240, 358
Merck & Co., Inc. 146, 192, 216–219
Meridia 222

metformin 352
methionine 454
methylcobalamin 241
metoprolol 57, 297
Mevacor 294, 331
micro-nutrient deficiencies 343–344
Miller, Clinton Ray 8
Mosholder, Andrew 221, 222
Moss, Ralph 478
Mouscher, Dean 463, 473
multiple sclerosis 130, 454
muscle weakness and wasting 83, 305
myopia 147

N

N-acetylcysteine 239, 444, 458–459
Namenda 240
National Academy of Sciences (NAS) 148, 301, 371
National Association of Boards of Pharmacy 209
National Cancer Institute (NCI) 270–271, 422–427, 478–479
National Cancer Institute (NSABP) 422
National Institutes of Health 131, 270–271, 310, 409–411
National Institutes of Health (NIH) 131, 270–271, 310, 409–411
National Library of Medicine 201

National Specialty Services 212

neural tube defects (NTDs) 189–190, 282–283, 370–371, 374

National Surgical Adjuvant Breast and Bowel Project (NSABP) 422–423, 426–427

Neurontin 57

New Drug Application (NDA) 54, 139, 187, 404, 406

New England Journal of Medicine 46, 121, 144, 298, 302, 307, 309, 392–393, 406, 427, 437, 453

New York Times 146, 326, 383, 407

Nexavar 130

Nexium 298, 309

niacin 343

nitrate drugs 398

Nolvadex. *See* tamoxifen

non-Hodgkin's lymphoma 466

nonsteroidal anti-inflammatory drugs (NSAIDs) 216

Norpramin 292

nortriptyline 57

Norvasc 57, 296, 327, 331

nuclear factor kappa beta 358

nucleic acids 404

Nurses' Health Study 438

nutrient deficiencies 343–346

Nutrition Labeling and Education Act 456

O

obesity 112

O'Connor, Sandra Day 338

Office of Professional Responsibility, US 466

Oligos Etc. Inc. 404

omega-3 fatty acids 47, 172, 174. *See also* fish oil and coronary heart disease 190, 231–235, 282, 371

omeprazole 57

Oncogene 268

osteoarthritis 83, 146, 190

osteomalacia 84

osteoporosis 83, 173

over-the-counter (OTC) drugs 54, 113, 118–122, 239, 300

oxcarbazepine 57

Oz, Mehmet 33

Ozols, Robert F. 425

ozone/oxygen therapy 469

P

Pamelor 57, 292

Paracelsus 293

Parkinson's disease 240, 358

Paxil 75, 112, 292, 308, 327, 331

PDR (Physicians' Desk Reference) 292–297, 307–308

Pearson, Durk 231, 234, 403, 407, 455

Pearsons I and II 281–284, 369–375

Peck, Carl 301

penbutolol 297

peptides 473–474

periodontal disease 83

peripheral neuropathies 305

peripheral vascular disease 454

peroxisome inhibitors 422

Pfizer Inc. 216, 394

pharmaceutical companies 10, 30, 35, 53, 58, 61, 68–69, 208, 309, 359, 377, 391, 419, 434. *See also* drug companies by name

    political influence by 41–42, 71–72, 95, 112, 191–192, 213–215, 230, 239, 250–251, 326, 382, 399, 406–407, 457, 466

Pharmaceutical Research and Manufacturers of America 393

pharmacies 42–43, 53–54, 56–57, 207–210, 213–214, 229–230, 274, 328–329, 337, 351, 383–384

    "closed-door" 209

    compounding 31–32, 35, 61, 229–230, 337–339, 377–378

    internet 397, 414

Pharmacoepidemiology and Drug Safety 293

pharmacogenetics 291

Pharmacological Basis of Therapeutics, The 293

phenacetin 238–239

phenoxodiol 268–269

phosphatidylserine (PS) 276–277

placebo 75, 129, 132, 139, 172, 200–201, 222, 374, 423, 426, 453

pneumonia 66, 86

Pogliano, Donna 137

polaprezinc 358

policosanol 309

Pomeranz, Bruce H. 406

Pravachol 57, 294, 327, 331

pravastatin 57

Premarin 30–31, 34, 37, 68, 300, 309, 327

Prempro 30–31, 34–35, 37, 300, 327

prescription drugs 40–41, 51, 58–59, 61–62, 70, 80, 85, 95–96, 104, 107, 111–113, 191, 209, 219, 220, 221, 223, 230, 249, 252, 255, 274, 298, 323, 325–329, 332–333, 335, 352, 368, 384

    "black box" warning 143, 305

    counterfeit 207, 212–213, 324, 351, 383, 391

    death from 143–144, 147, 189, 222, 295, 406, 408–409, 415–416, 433–434, 448, 450, 478

    dosage 135, 291–294, 298, 299–301, 304, 307–308, 311–312

    misbranded 15, 384

    pricing of 53, 71, 171, 173, 324, 359, 383, 392

Prevacid 331

Prilosec 57, 298, 327, 331, 333

Prinivil 297–298

Procyte 405

progesterone 30, 35

progestins 30

PROJECT 2000 Research Fund 24–26

PROJECT 2020 Research Fund 26

propanolol 297

Proscar 42, 53, 57

prostaglandin E2 (PGE2) 216

prostatic hypertrophy, benign 286

Provenge 137

Prozac 112, 222, 290, 327, 331

psoriasis 404

Public Citizen 217, 223, 299
    Health Research Group 223, 318, 380

Public Employees for Environmental Responsibility 223

Public Employees for Environmental Responsibility (PEER) 223

puerperal fever 86–87

Pure Encapsulations, Inc. 281, 370

R

Raghavan, Derek 425, 429

ramipril 57

recombinant interferon-alpha 449

Redux 309

Reform FDA Petition 74

Relman, Arnold 309

renal failure 222

restenosis 234

Rezulin 143, 309, 352

ribavirin 357, 445–450

rickets 84

Rinc, Roy 17

Roberts, W. C. 295

Roe versus Wade 465

rosacea 404

Roses, Allen 251

Royal Marsden Hospital 423

RxDepot 273–274

S

Safe Blood: Purifying the Nation's Blood Supply in the Age of AIDS 165

SAMe (S-adenosylmethionine) 96, 454

saw palmetto 286

Schilsky, Richard L. 425, 429

Sectral (acebutolol) 297

Segall, Paul 25

selenium 275–276, 346–347, 453

Seligman, Paul 218

Semmelweis, Ignaz 86

Senate Finance Committee, US 215, 220–221

Senate Investigative Committee, US 66–67

Serevent 222

serotonin 111–113

serotonin reuptake inhibitors (SRIs) 75

Serzone 292

Shalala, Donna 281, 328, 369, 384, 464

Shaman Pharmaceuticals 405

Shapiro, Stephanie 466

shark cartilage 72

Shaw, Sandy 231–232, 234, 281, 282, 370–372, 407, 455

Shaw, Suzanne 223

"Sick Patients Need Cutting-Edge Drugs" 69

Simon, Richard 426

simvastatin 57

Sledge, George W., Jr. 429

Smith, Sheila Weiss 121

Snow, Lurana S. 5, 15, 17–18

Social Security 44, 62, 374

Somers, Suzanne 33–34, 36

SPF (sun protection factor) 182–183

Spiller, Robert 464

spina bifida 374

Sprycel 59

squamous cell carcinoma 126, 182

Squibb. See Bristol-Myers Squibb Company

Standish, Leanna 470

statin drugs 253–257, 331–332

side effects of 255, 305

Strattera 59

stroke 68, 83, 149, 151–153, 173, 188, 192, 216–217, 222, 231, 437, 454

Sullivan, Alan 11

Summers, William 9

sunscreen 181–183

supplements 9, 56, 85–87, 95–96, 112–113, 154–155, 171–174, 189–191, 201–202, 232–234, 241–242, 250, 255–257, 276–277, 280–281, 283–287, 346, 374–375, 402–411, 437–438, 451, 454–456, 457, 469

Supreme Court, US 61, 134, 337, 455–456, 465

Sutent 59

Synthroid 327

T

Tacrine 9, 15, 240, 358

Tambocor 273–274

tamoxifen 421–429

Taxol 268

Taxotere 266

telomerase 264–265, 267

Tenormin (altenolol) 296, 331

testosterone, natural 398

thalidomide 356–357

"The Real FDA Scandal" 105

Thompson, Tommy 133, 271

Thymosin alpha-1 358

thymus gland 24, 358

Tier 1 Initial Approval 129, 133

tobacco 185–186

cigarettes 44–45

topozone oil 469–470

triglycerides 172, 234

Trileptal 57

tryptophan 25, 111–113

Tylenol 122, 237

Type 1b hepatitis C 358

Tysabri 130

U

unapproved therapies 9, 108
Union of Concerned Scientists (UCS) 223–224
United States Pharmacopeia, Drug Information 299
universal healthcare 39
University of Pittsburgh 427
USA Today 380
UV-A light 182
UV-B radiation 182

V

valvular insufficiency 81
Vanderbilt University School of Medicine 217
VanZile, Jon 215
Variability In Drug Therapy: Description, Estimation, And Control. A Sandoz Workshop 293
vascular disease 47, 345, 375, 454
Vasotec 331
verapamil 297
Verelan 297
Viagra 59, 397–399, 415, 434
vinpocetine 241
Vioxx 99, 143, 188–192, 215–225
vitamins
antioxidant 155, 239, 281–282, 371
B1 344
B6 343–344, 375
B12 343–344, 375, 437
C 344, 452
D 47, 81–86
E 280, 444, 452, 458
K 154
von Eschenbach, Edward 104, 270–271
Vumon 265

W

Walford, Roy L. 24
Walker, Steve 127–129, 131, 134
Wall Street Journal 59, 69, 105–106, 147, 308, 360, 384, 393–394
Washington Legal Foundation 127, 130, 261, 419
Washington Post 73
Webster, George C. 25
Weisenberger, Anthony 292
Wellbutrin 292
Wellbutrin SR 57
Wellbutrin XL 71
Wellness Lifestyles, Inc. 233
Wellstone, Paul 383
West Nile virus 168
"When is a Gift Not a Gift?" 406
Whitaker, Julian 253–255, 370
Whitaker vs. Thompson 281–282
Wolfe, Sidney 223
Wolmark, Norman 425
Women's Health Study 30
Wood, Alastair 5, 306
Woodcock, Janet 308
Woosley, Raymond 292, 301, 306

World Health Organization
    392
Wyeth 37, 68

X

Xanax 331

Y

Yale University School of Medi-
    cine 268

Z

zaleplon 57
Zebeta (bisoprolol) 297
Zeneca Pharmaceuticals 421
Zerhouni, Elias A. 271
Zestril (lisinopril) 297–298,
    327, 331
zinc 343, 358
Zithromax 331
Zocor 57, 294–295, 327, 331
Zoloft 112, 222, 292, 327, 331

Why You Should Join the Life Extension Foundation

F OUNDED IN **1980**, THE LIFE EXTENSION FOUNDATION IS A nonprofit organization dedicated to discovering innovative approaches to prevent and treat age-related diseases.

Since its inception, Life Extension has introduced evidence-based therapies that are often decades ahead of conventional medicine. These scientific advances are chronicled in *Life Extension* magazine, read by over 300,000 people each month.

The Life Extension Foundation supports large research programs and utilizes its scientific findings to educate its members about novel methods to help eradicate age-related disease. Unlike today's medical bureaucracy that too often stifles innovation, Life Extension quickly moves discoveries out of the laboratory to patients in need.

Forward-thinking physicians, scientists and lay people join the Life Extension Foundation to obtain the latest information about novel diagnostic procedures and nontoxic treatments that are too often overlooked by the medical mainstream.

Foundation members have free seven-day-a-week phone and email access to knowledgeable health advisors, some with specialized expertise in complimentary approaches to a wide range of age-related ailments including cancer.

Life Extension also maintains an enormous library of hundreds of meticulously referenced protocols that provide unique insight into an array of natural methods to combat the degenerative disease of aging.

It costs $75.00 to join the Life Extension Foundation, and the benefits are too numerous to describe. New members, for instance, receive a 1600-page reference book called *Disease Prevention and Treatment* that provides invaluable health information published by the Foundation over the past three decades. Each month, members are updated about new medical technologies in *Life Extension* magazine. To become a member call 1-800-544-4440 or log on to www.lef.org.